Calcium, Vitamin D and Health

Calcium, Vitamin D and Health

Special Issue Editor

Luis Gracia-Marco

MDPI • Basel • Beijing • Wuhan • Barcelona • Belgrade • Manchester • Tokyo • Cluj • Tianjin

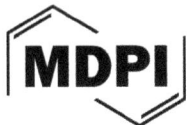

Special Issue Editor
Luis Gracia-Marco
University of Granada
Spain

Editorial Office
MDPI
St. Alban-Anlage 66
4052 Basel, Switzerland

This is a reprint of articles from the Special Issue published online in the open access journal *Nutrients* (ISSN 2072-6643) (available at: https://www.mdpi.com/journal/nutrients/special_issues/calcium_vitaminD_health).

For citation purposes, cite each article independently as indicated on the article page online and as indicated below:

LastName, A.A.; LastName, B.B.; LastName, C.C. Article Title. *Journal Name* **Year**, *Article Number*, Page Range.

ISBN 978-3-03928-564-8 (Hbk)
ISBN 978-3-03928-565-5 (PDF)

© 2020 by the authors. Articles in this book are Open Access and distributed under the Creative Commons Attribution (CC BY) license, which allows users to download, copy and build upon published articles, as long as the author and publisher are properly credited, which ensures maximum dissemination and a wider impact of our publications.

The book as a whole is distributed by MDPI under the terms and conditions of the Creative Commons license CC BY-NC-ND.

Contents

About the Special Issue Editor vii

Luis Gracia-Marco
Calcium, Vitamin D, and Health
Reprinted from: *Nutrients* **2020**, *12*, 416, doi:10.3390/nu12020416 1

Andrea Rabufetti, Gregorio P. Milani, Sebastiano A. G. Lava, Valeria Edefonti, Mario G. Bianchetti, Andreas Stettbacher, Franco Muggli and Giacomo Simonetti
Vitamin D Status Among Male Late Adolescents Living in Southern Switzerland: Role of Body Composition and Lifestyle
Reprinted from: *Nutrients* **2019**, *11*, 2727, doi:10.3390/nu11112727 5

Myriam Abboud, Xiaoying Liu, Flavia Fayet-Moore, Kaye E. Brock, Dimitrios Papandreou, Tara C. Brennan-Speranza and Rebecca S. Mason
Effects of Vitamin D Status and Supplements on Anthropometric and Biochemical Indices in a Clinical Setting: A Retrospective Study
Reprinted from: *Nutrients* **2019**, *11*, 3032, doi:10.3390/nu11123032 17

Alejandro De-la-O, Lucas Jurado-Fasoli, Manuel J. Castillo, Luis Gracia-Marco, Ángel Gutierrez and Francisco J. Amaro-Gahete
Relationship between 1,25-Dihydroxyvitamin D and Body Composition in Middle-Aged Sedentary Adults: The FIT-AGEING Study
Reprinted from: *Nutrients* **2019**, *11*, 2567, doi:10.3390/nu11112567 29

Jose J. Gil-Cosano, Luis Gracia-Marco, Esther Ubago-Guisado, Jairo H. Migueles, Jose Mora-Gonzalez, María V. Escolano-Margarit, José Gómez-Vida, José Maldonado and Francisco B. Ortega
Muscular Fitness Mediates the Association between 25-Hydroxyvitamin D and Areal Bone Mineral Density in Children with Overweight/Obesity
Reprinted from: *Nutrients* **2019**, *11*, 2760, doi:10.3390/nu11112760 39

Marta Rapún-López, Hugo Olmedillas, Alejandro Gonzalez-Agüero, Alba Gomez-Cabello, Francisco Pradas de la Fuente, Luis A. Moreno, José A. Casajús and Germán Vicente-Rodríguez
May Young Elite Cyclists Have Less Efficient Bone Metabolism?
Reprinted from: *Nutrients* **2019**, *11*, 1178, doi:10.3390/nu11051178 49

Patricio Solis-Urra, Carlos Cristi-Montero, Javier Romero-Parra, Juan Pablo Zavala-Crichton, Maria Jose Saez-Lara and Julio Plaza-Diaz
Passive Commuting and Higher Sedentary Time Is Associated with Vitamin D Deficiency in Adult and Older Women: Results from Chilean National Health Survey 2016–2017
Reprinted from: *Nutrients* **2019**, *11*, 300, doi:10.3390/nu11020300 59

Lars Libuda, Björn-Hergen Laabs, Christine Ludwig, Judith Bühlmeier, Jochen Antel, Anke Hinney, Roaa Naaresh, Manuel Föcker, Johannes Hebebrand, Inke R. König and Triinu Peters
Vitamin D and the Risk of Depression: A Causal Relationship? Findings from a Mendelian Randomization Study
Reprinted from: *Nutrients* **2019**, *11*, 1085, doi:10.3390/nu11051085 73

Mariska C Vlot, Laura Boekel, Jolijn Kragt, Joep Killestein, Barbara M. van Amerongen, Robert de Jonge, Martin den Heijer and Annemieke C. Heijboer
Multiple Sclerosis Patients Show Lower Bioavailable 25(OH)D and 1,25(OH)$_2$D, but No Difference in Ratio of 25(OH)D/24,25(OH)$_2$D and FGF23 Concentrations
Reprinted from: *Nutrients* **2019**, *11*, 2774, doi:10.3390/nu11112774 . . . . **85**

Vito Francic, Stan R. Ursem, Niek F. Dirks, Martin H. Keppel, Verena Theiler-Schwetz, Christian Trummer, Marlene Pandis, Valentin Borzan, Martin R. Grübler, Nicolas D. Verheyen, Winfried März, Andreas Tomaschitz, Stefan Pilz, Annemieke C. Heijboer and Barbara Obermayer-Pietsch
The Effect of Vitamin D Supplementation on its Metabolism and the Vitamin D Metabolite Ratio
Reprinted from: *Nutrients* **2019**, *11*, 2539, doi:10.3390/nu11102539 . . . . **101**

Jen-Yin Chen, Yao-Tsung Lin, Li-Kai Wang, Kuo-Chuan Hung, Kuo-Mao Lan, Chung-Han Ho and Chia-Yu Chang
Hypovitaminosis D in Postherpetic Neuralgia—High Prevalence and Inverse Association with Pain: A Retrospective Study
Reprinted from: *Nutrients* **2019**, *11*, 2787, doi:10.3390/nu11112787 . . . . **111**

Rebeca Reyes-Garcia, Antonia Garcia-Martin, Santiago Palacios, Nancy Salas, Nicolas Mendoza, Miguel Quesada-Charneco, Juristo Fonolla, Federico Lara-Villoslada and Manuel Muñoz-Torres
Factors Predicting the Response to a Vitamin D-Fortified Milk in Healthy Postmenopausal Women
Reprinted from: *Nutrients* **2019**, *11*, 2641, doi:10.3390/nu11112641 . . . . **127**

Jaak Jürimäe, Evelin Mäestu, Eva Mengel, Liina Remmel, Priit Purge and Vallo Tillmann
Association between Dietary Calcium Intake and Adiposity in Male Adolescents
Reprinted from: *Nutrients* **2019**, *11*, 1454, doi:10.3390/nu11071454 . . . . **135**

Paula Nascimento Brandão-Lima, Beatriz da Cruz Santos, Concepción Maria Aguilera, Analícia Rocha Santos Freire, Paulo Ricardo Saquete Martins-Filho and Liliane Viana Pires
Vitamin D Food Fortification and Nutritional Status in Children: A Systematic Review of Randomized Controlled Trials
Reprinted from: *Nutrients* **2019**, *11*, 2766, doi:10.3390/nu11112766 . . . . **147**

Rose Marino and Madhusmita Misra
Extra-Skeletal Effects of Vitamin D
Reprinted from: *Nutrients* **2019**, *11*, 1460, doi:10.3390/nu11071460 . . . . **163**

About the Special Issue Editor

Luis Gracia-Marco is Senior Research Fellow in the Faculty of Sport Sciences at the University of Granada (Spain) and former Senior Lecturer at the University of Exeter (U.K.). He was awarded his Ph.D. in 2011 and has published more than 80 peer-reviewed Journal Citation Report (JCR) articles in the fields of body composition, sport sciences, and endocrinology and metabolism. He has supervised a number of B.S., M.S., and Ph.D. students in these areas. He has been involved in studies funded by the European Union and other international and competitive calls as principal investigator and researcher. Dr. Gracia-Marco also leads the bone and exercise research line in the PROFITH (PROmoting FITness and Health through physical activity) Research Group.

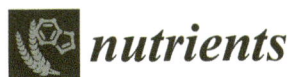

Editorial

Calcium, Vitamin D, and Health

Luis Gracia-Marco

PROFITH "PROmoting FITness and Health through Physical Activity" Research Group, Sport and Health University Research Institute (iMUDS), Department of Physical Education and Sports, Faculty of Sport Sciences, University of Granada, 18071 Granada, Spain; lgracia@ugr.es

Received: 27 January 2020; Accepted: 4 February 2020; Published: 6 February 2020

Calcium is the main mineral in the body. It is involved in a variety of structural and functional roles, but the maintenance of calcium homeostasis is perhaps the most studied function of vitamin D. This Special Issue of *Nutrients*, "Calcium, Vitamin D, and Health" contains 12 original publications and two reviews investigating the contribution of (mainly) vitamin D and calcium on relevant health outcomes in a variety of populations, which reflect the evolving and broad interests of research on this topic.

Three studies were published examining the association between vitamin D and body composition. Rabufetti et al. [1] observed that an increase in body fat percentage was a risk factor for 25-hydroxyvitamin D [25(OH)D] insufficiency in a healthy population of 1045 late adolescent males living in southern Switzerland. Abboud et al. [2], in their study on men and women with overweight/obese and undergoing a weight loss program, found greater weight loss, as well as a larger reduction in body mass index (BMI), and waist circumference in those with higher baseline 25(OH)D levels. Moreover, a similar effect was also observed in those with insufficient baseline 25(OH)D levels but supplemented with vitamin D3 for three months. In a study with middle-aged sedentary adults, De-la-O et al. [3] found negative associations between 1,25-dihydroxyvitamin D (1,25(OH)2D, also known as calcitriol, and BMI, lean mass index, and bone mineral density (BMD). The latter finding backs up the notion that 1,25(OH)2D increases bone resorption via stimulating intestinal calcium absorption after calcium intake.

Two other studies investigated the links between 25(OH)D and bone outcomes in young populations. Gil-Cosano et al. [4] revealed a mediating effect of muscular fitness on the relationship between 25(OH)D levels and BMD in children who were overweight/obese, while Rapun-Lopez et al. [5] showed similar bone remodeling in adolescent male cyclists than age-matched active controls over one year, but lower 25(OH)D. In adult and older women from the Chilean National Health Survey 2016–2017 (total N = 1931), Solis-Urra et al. [6] found a joint association of high sedentary time/passive commuting to be associated with 25(OH)D deficiency, even after controlling for sun exposure. This finding connects with the studies mentioned above [1–3] due to the proposed link between sedentary time and increased adiposity, as well as between adiposity and reduced 25(OH)D levels.

Libuda et al. [7] studied six single nucleotide polymorphisms (SNPs), which were genome-wide significantly associated with 25(OH)D concentrations in more than 79,000 subjects from the SUNLIGHT genome-wide association study (GWAS). However, they did not identify the potential role (from a genetics perspective) of 25(OH)D in the onset of depressive symptoms or broad depression. Multiple sclerosis (MS) has been negatively associated with BMD through various factors, and previous research has suggested that vitamin D could play a role in the pathogenesis of MS by possibly modulating T-lymphocyte subset differentiation. In this regard, Vlot et al. [8] studied the vitamin D-fibroblast-growth-factor-23 (FGF23) and measured multiple vitamin D metabolites and bone turnover markers in a cohort of MS patients and healthy controls. They found lower serum concentrations of total 25(OH)D, free 25(OH)D, free 1.25(OH)2D, and 24,25 dihydroxyvitamin D [24,25(OH)2D] in female MS patients compared with their healthy peers, while serum concentrations of vitamin D binding protein (VDBP) were higher in male MS patients, compared with male controls. This study strengthens the idea that a single measurement of total 25(OH)D may not be enough to fully reflect all changes in vitamin D metabolism in MS patients. In a randomized clinical trial conducted in hypertensive adults, Francic et al. [9] did not support the routine measurement of 24,25 dihydroxycholecalciferol (24,25(OH)2D3) in order to individually optimize the dosage of vitamin D supplementation. Interestingly, the activity of 24-hydroxylase increased after vitamin D supplementation. In patients with postherpetic neuralgia (PHN), Chen et al. [10] showed a higher prevalence of hypovitaminosis D (as reflected by 25(OH)D levels) than in the controls, and those with hypovitaminosis D also had a lower vitamin D supplementation rate and greater pain intensity.

In healthy post-menopausal women, Reyes-Garcia et al. [11] investigated the response of serum 25(OH)D and its predictive factors after a 24-month dietary intervention with milk fortified with vitamin D and calcium. It was found that the improvement in 25(OH)D after the intervention was mainly dependent on the baseline levels of serum 25(OH)D and the percentage of body fat. The study by Jurimae et al. [12] is one of the few studies investigating the association between calcium and adiposity in young populations, and found inverse associations between dietary calcium intake and total body and abdominal adiposity in healthy male adolescents.

Finally, two timely reviews were included in this Special Issue. Brandao-Lima et al. [13] conducted a systematic review of randomized controlled trials aiming to discuss food fortification as a strategy for maintenance or recovery of nutritional status related to vitamin D in children. Marino and Misra [14], in their review, discussed the biological effects of vitamin D beyond the skeleton, using evidence from randomized controlled trials and meta-analyses.

The present Special Issue provides a short summary of the progress on the topic of calcium, vitamin D, and human health in different populations, which will be of interest from a clinical and public health perspective. It also underlines the current limitations and the necessity of more powerful study designs to further advance in the knowledge.

Funding: This research received no external funding.

Acknowledgments: L.G.-M. is supported by "La Caixa" Foundation within the Junior Leader fellowship programme (ID 100010434).

Conflicts of Interest: The author declares no conflict of interest.

References

1. Rabufetti, A.; Milani, G.P.; Lava, S.A.G.; Edefonti, V.; Bianchetti, M.G.; Stettbacher, A.; Muggli, F.; Simonetti, G. Vitamin D Status Among Male Late Adolescents Living in Southern Switzerland: Role of Body Composition and Lifestyle. *Nutrients* **2019**, *11*, 2727. [CrossRef] [PubMed]
2. Abboud, M.; Liu, X.; Fayet-Moore, F.; Brock, K.E.; Papandreou, D.; Brennan-Speranza, T.C.; Mason, R.S. Effects of Vitamin D Status and Supplements on Anthropometric and Biochemical Indices in a Clinical Setting: A Retrospective Study. *Nutrients* **2019**, *11*, 3032. [CrossRef] [PubMed]
3. De-la, O.A.; Jurado-Fasoli, L.; Castillo, M.J.; Gracia-Marco, L.; Gutierrez, A.; Amaro-Gahete, F.J. Relationship between 1,25-Dihydroxyvitamin D and Body Composition in Middle-Aged Sedentary Adults: The FIT-AGEING Study. *Nutrients* **2019**, *11*, 2567. [CrossRef] [PubMed]
4. Gil-Cosano, J.J.; Gracia-Marco, L.; Ubago-Guisado, E.; Migueles, J.H.; Mora-Gonzalez, J.; Escolano-Margarit, M.V.; Gomez-Vida, J.; Maldonado, J.; Ortega, F.B. Muscular Fitness Mediates the Association between 25-Hydroxyvitamin D and Areal Bone Mineral Density in Children with Overweight/Obesity. *Nutrients* **2019**, *11*, 2760. [CrossRef] [PubMed]
5. Rapun-Lopez, M.; Olmedillas, H.; Gonzalez-Aguero, A.; Gomez-Cabello, A.; Pradas de la Fuente, F.; Moreno, L.A.; Casajus, J.A.; Vicente-Rodriguez, G. May Young Elite Cyclists Have Less Efficient Bone Metabolism? *Nutrients* **2019**, *11*, 1178. [CrossRef] [PubMed]
6. Solis-Urra, P.; Cristi-Montero, C.; Romero-Parra, J.; Zavala-Crichton, J.P.; Saez-Lara, M.J.; Plaza-Diaz, J. Passive Commuting and Higher Sedentary Time Is Associated with Vitamin D Deficiency in Adult and Older Women: Results from Chilean National Health Survey 2016(–)2017. *Nutrients* **2019**, *11*, 300. [CrossRef] [PubMed]

7. Libuda, L.; Laabs, B.H.; Ludwig, C.; Buhlmeier, J.; Antel, J.; Hinney, A.; Naaresh, R.; Focker, M.; Hebebrand, J.; Konig, I.R.; et al. Vitamin D and the Risk of Depression: A Causal Relationship? Findings from a Mendelian Randomization Study. *Nutrients* **2019**, *11*, 1085. [CrossRef] [PubMed]
8. Vlot, M.C.; Boekel, L.; Kragt, J.; Killestein, J.; van Amerongen, B.M.; de Jonge, R.; den Heijer, M.; Heijboer, A.C. Multiple Sclerosis Patients Show Lower Bioavailable 25(OH)D and 1,25(OH)2D, but No Difference in Ratio of 25(OH)D/24,25(OH)2D and FGF23 Concentrations. *Nutrients* **2019**, *11*, 2774. [CrossRef] [PubMed]
9. Francic, V.; Ursem, S.R.; Dirks, N.F.; Keppel, M.H.; Theiler-Schwetz, V.; Trummer, C.; Pandis, M.; Borzan, V.; Grubler, M.R.; Verheyen, N.D.; et al. The Effect of Vitamin D Supplementation on its Metabolism and the Vitamin D Metabolite Ratio. *Nutrients* **2019**, *11*, 2539. [CrossRef] [PubMed]
10. Chen, J.Y.; Lin, Y.T.; Wang, L.K.; Hung, K.C.; Lan, K.M.; Ho, C.H.; Chang, C.Y. Hypovitaminosis D in Postherpetic Neuralgia-High Prevalence and Inverse Association with Pain: A Retrospective Study. *Nutrients* **2019**, *11*, 2787. [CrossRef] [PubMed]
11. Reyes-Garcia, R.; Garcia-Martin, A.; Palacios, S.; Salas, N.; Mendoza, N.; Quesada-Charneco, M.; Fonolla, J.; Lara-Villoslada, F.; Munoz-Torres, M. Factors Predicting the Response to a Vitamin D-Fortified Milk in Healthy Postmenopausal Women. *Nutrients* **2019**, *11*, 2641. [CrossRef] [PubMed]
12. Jurimae, J.; Maestu, E.; Mengel, E.; Remmel, L.; Purge, P.; Tillmann, V. Association between Dietary Calcium Intake and Adiposity in Male Adolescents. *Nutrients* **2019**, *11*, 1454. [CrossRef] [PubMed]
13. Brandao-Lima, P.N.; Santos, B.D.C.; Aguilera, C.M.; Freire, A.R.S.; Martins-Filho, P.R.S.; Pires, L.V. Vitamin D Food Fortification and Nutritional Status in Children: A Systematic Review of Randomized Controlled Trials. *Nutrients* **2019**, *11*, 2766. [CrossRef] [PubMed]
14. Marino, R.; Misra, M. Extra-Skeletal Effects of Vitamin D. *Nutrients* **2019**, *11*, 1460. [CrossRef] [PubMed]

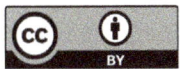

© 2020 by the author. Licensee MDPI, Basel, Switzerland. This article is an open access article distributed under the terms and conditions of the Creative Commons Attribution (CC BY) license (http://creativecommons.org/licenses/by/4.0/).

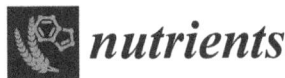

Article

Vitamin D Status Among Male Late Adolescents Living in Southern Switzerland: Role of Body Composition and Lifestyle

Andrea Rabufetti [1,†], Gregorio P. Milani [1,2,3,*,†], Sebastiano A. G. Lava [4], Valeria Edefonti [3], Mario G. Bianchetti [5], Andreas Stettbacher [6], Franco Muggli [6] and Giacomo Simonetti [1,5]

1. Istituto Pediatrico della Svizzera Italiana, 6500 Bellinzona, Switzerland; andrea.rabufetti@eoc.ch (A.R.); Giacomo.Simonetti@eoc.ch (G.S.)
2. Pediatric Unit, Fondazione IRCCS Ca' Granda Ospedale Maggiore Policlinico, 20122 Milan, Italy
3. Department of Clinical Sciences and Community Health, Università degli Studi di Milano, 20122 Milan, Italy; valeria.edefonti@unimi.it
4. Pediatric Cardiology Unit, Department of Pediatrics, Centre Hospitalier Universitaire Vaudois (CHUV), and University of Lausanne, 1011 Lausanne, Switzerland; webmaster@sebastianolava.ch
5. Faculty of Biomedical Sciences, Università della Svizzera Italiana, 6900 Lugano, Switzerland; mario.bianchetti@usi.ch
6. Swiss Federal Department of Defence, 3000 Bern, Switzerland; andreas.stettbacher@vtg.admin.ch (A.S.); fmuggli@bluewin.ch (F.M.)
* Correspondence: milani.gregoriop@gmail.com; Tel.: +39(0)255038727; Fax: +39(0)255032918
† These authors equally contributed to the study.

Received: 27 September 2019; Accepted: 5 November 2019; Published: 11 November 2019

Abstract: Background: Poor vitamin D status is a worldwide health problem. Yet, knowledge about vitamin D status among adolescents in Southern Europe is limited. This study investigated concentrations and modulating factors of vitamin D in a healthy population of male late adolescents living in Southern Switzerland. Methods: All apparently healthy subjects attending for the medical evaluation before the compulsory military service in Southern Switzerland during 2014-2016 were eligible. Dark-skin subjects, subjects on vitamin D supplementation or managed with diseases or drugs involved in vitamin D metabolism were excluded. Anthropometric measurements (body height, weight, fat percentage, mid-upper arm and waist circumference) and blood sampling for total 25-hydroxy-vitamin D, total cholesterol and ferritin concentrations testing, were collected. Participants filled in a structured questionnaire addressing their lifestyle. Characteristics of the subjects with adequate ($\geq$50 nmol/L–$\leq$250 nmol/L) and insufficient (<50 nmol/L) vitamin D values were compared by Kruskal-Wallis test or χ^2 test. Odds ratios for 25-hydroxy-vitamin D insufficiency were calculated by univariate and AIC-selected multiple logistic regression models. Results: A total of 1045 subjects volunteered to participate in the study. Insufficient concentrations of vitamin D were detected in 184 (17%). The season of measurement was the most significant factor associated with vitamin D levels and approximately 40% of subjects presented insufficient vitamin D concentrations in winter. After model selection, body fat percentage, frequency and site of recreational physical activity, and the seasonality were significantly associated with the risk of vitamin D insufficiency. Conclusions: Among healthy male late adolescents in Southern Switzerland, about one every fourth subject presents a poor vitamin D status in non-summer seasons. Body fat percentage, frequent and outdoor recreational physical activity are modulating factors of vitamin D status in this population.

Keywords: macronutrients; sunlight; physical activity; season; body composition

1. Introduction

There are two natural sources of vitamin D: food and especially ultraviolet B radiation on the skin [1]. A limited number of foods naturally contain vitamin D. Fish (mostly fatty fish), egg yolk and liver are good sources of vitamin D_3. On the other hand, vitamin D_2 is contained in various wild mushrooms [1,2]. Among European adolescents, the natural vitamin D intake is low except for countries such as Poland and Norway, which is attributed to high consumption of fish [3].

The amount of cutaneous vitamin D_3 synthesis depends on a number of factors, including time spent outdoors, latitude, season, ethnicity and use of sunscreen [1]. Vitamin D synthesis occurs for about half the year in northern regions above approximately 35° latitude [3,4]. Unsurprisingly, therefore, lower-than desired concentrations of total 25-hydroxy vitamin D have often been detected, especially during the fall and winter months, in countries such Canada, Ireland, the United Kingdom and the northern United States [3,4]. It would be assumed that, in the sunniest areas of the world, this problem would be uncommon. However, in Australia, Brazil, India, Iran, Lebanon and Saudi Arabia many adolescents were found to have lower-than-desired concentrations of vitamin D [3,4].

Limited information is available on vitamin D status in adolescents living in Southern Europe. The objective of the present analysis was to obtain reliable and comparable data on vitamin D status from a large population of late adolescents living in Southern Switzerland, the sunniest region of this country (latitude 46°). The secondary aim was to investigate the role of a broad number of possibly relevant anthropometric, lifestyle and biochemical characteristics on vitamin D status in this population.

2. Methods

This investigation is part of the "CENERI study", a cross sectional study in healthy male adolescents living in Southern Switzerland to investigate risk factors for chronic diseases later in life. In Switzerland, ostensibly male citizens between 18 and 19 years of age have to undertake a medical evaluation before the compulsory military service in the Army [5]. All apparently healthy subjects attending for the medical evaluation before the compulsory military service in Southern Switzerland from January 2014 to December 2016 were eligible for the "CENERI study". Dark-skin subjects (Fitzpatrick skin phototype V or VI), subjects on supplementation with any form of vitamin D and subjects on treatment with anticonvulsant, glucocorticoid, antifungal, and anti-retroviral drugs or with any chronic endocrinologic or metabolic disease potentially affecting vitamin D metabolism, were excluded for the present analysis. Among the 4663 subjects who underwent the medical examination before the compulsory military service, 1045 (22%) Caucasians volunteered to participate in the study.

All measurements and data were collected in the same morning for each subject after an overnight fast. Beyond the routinely collected data on anthropometric measurements (body height and weight), participants were asked to answer a self-administered structured questionnaire addressing their main activity and lifestyle (especially recreational physical activity, smoking behavior and alcohol consumption). Body fat percentage, mid-upper arm and waist circumference were also measured. In addition, blood for total 25-hydroxy-vitamin D, total cholesterol and ferritin concentrations testing, was also collected.

Questions on lifestyle were structured as follows: (i) Frequency of recreational physical activity (never, 1 per week, 2–4 per week, 5–6 per week, every day), (ii) Duration of recreational physical activity session (≤ 1 h, $>1–\leq 2$ h, $>2–\leq 3$ h, >3 h), (iii) Site of recreational physical activity (indoor only, outdoor only, both indoor and outdoor), (iv) Frequency of alcohol consumption (never, 1 per week, 2 per week, 3–4 per week, 5–6 per week, every day), (v) Smoking (never, 1–10 cigarettes per day, 11–20 cigarettes per day, >20 cigarettes per day).

Subjects were weighed (wearing light clothes only) on a calibrated platform scale, with weight being rounded off to the nearest 0.1 kg. Standing height was measured barefooted to the nearest 0.1 cm. These measurements were used to calculate the body mass index. Mid-upper arm circumference was measured to the nearest 0.1 cm midway the acromion and the olecranon in the non-dominant arm. Waist circumference was measured to the nearest 0.5 cm with a non-stretching tape placed around the abdomen at the iliac crest. Body fat percentage was assessed by a validated bioimpedance analysis device (Omron®BF306, Omron Healthcare Europe BV, Hoofddorp, The Netherlands) [6]. After entering demographic and anthropometric data, the subjects were asked to remain in standing position while holding the hand-to-hand bioimpedance device by both hands and straightening both arms forward [7]. All demographics, anthropometric and lifestyle information were prospectively collected by a trained nurse.

An Abbott chemiluminescent microparticle immunoassay, which measures both 25-hydroxy vitamin D_2 and 25-hydroxy vitamin D_3, was applied for the determination of total 25-hydroxy vitamin D concentration in serum [8]. At an average total concentration of 49 nmol/L, 99 nmol/L and 187 nmol/L, the intra-assay coefficient of variation was 3.9%, 4.0%, and 4.0%, respectively. The corresponding inter-assay coefficient was 1.0%, 1.2%, and 2.6% [8]. Accuracy and reliability of the assay are assessed both in the Vitamin D Standardization Program [9] and in the Vitamin D External Quality Assessment Scheme [10]. The circulating levels of total cholesterol (enzyme assay) and ferritin (immunoassay) were measured in serum. All laboratory assessments were performed in the same accredited central laboratory (Viollier, Basel, Switzerland) using an Architect CI8200 (Abbott, Chicago, IL, USA) analyzer. The study was conducted in accordance with the Declaration of Helsinki, and the protocol was approved by the Ethics Committee of Southern Switzerland (RIF CE 2775). Informed written consent was obtained from all subjects to participate in the study.

Data Analysis

Frequency distribution of continuous data were presented as median and interquartile range. Dichotomous data were presented as absolute and relative frequency. Concentrations of total 25-hydroxy-vitamin D were considered adequate if ≥50 nmol/L–≤250 nmol/L, insufficient if <50 nmol/L, deficient if <30 nmol/L or potentially toxic if >250 nmol/L [11]. Anthropometric, lifestyle and further laboratory characteristics of the subjects with adequate (50–250 nmol/L) and insufficient (<50 nmol/L) 25-hydroxy-vitamin D values were compared by Kruskal-Wallis test. χ^2 test was used for comparing frequencies of categorical variables. The Bonferroni test adjustment for multiple comparisons was applied.

Odds ratios (ORs) of 25-hydroxy-vitamin D insufficiency and corresponding 95% confidence intervals (CI) from univariate logistic regression models were calculated for the following variables: age, body height, body weight, body mass index, body fat percentage, frequency/length and site of recreational physical activity, frequency of alcohol consumption, smoking, season (winter from 21 December; spring from 21 March, summer from 21 June and autumn from 21 September), cholesterol and ferritin concentrations. ORs of 25-hydroxy-vitamin D insufficiency and corresponding 95% CI were also derived from the best AIC-selected multiple logistic regression model including the following variables: age, body mass index, body fat percentage, waist circumference frequency/length and site of recreational physical activity, frequency of alcohol consumption, smoking, season, cholesterol and ferritin concentrations. In all analyses, significance was assumed if $p < 0.05$. Statistics was performed using the open source statistical language R, Vienna, version 3.5.3 (11 March, 2019).

3. Results

Body height (178.0 (173.5–182.0) vs. 177.5 (173.0–182.5) cm) and weight (72.2 (65.7–80.0) vs. 72.0 (65.0–80.5) kg) were similar in subjects who volunteered to participate in the study as compared with the remining 3618 subjects. Anthropometric, lifestyle and laboratory findings of the 1045 recruited subjects are given in Table 1. One hundred seventy-nine (17%) subjects presented with concentrations of total 25-hydroxy-vitamin D < 50 nmol/L. Among subjects with a concentration of vitamin D below 50 nmol/L, 24 (13%) had deficient levels of total 25-hydroxy-vitamin D. No subject presented with potentially toxic concentrations of the 25-hydroxy-vitamin D. The concentration of 25-hydroxy-vitamin D_2 was always ≤5 nmol/L. The characteristics of the subjects with adequate or insufficient concentrations of 25-hydroxy-vitamin D are shown in Table 2. A total of 76 (7.2%) out of 1045 had a body mass index ≥ 30 kg/m^2 and 34 (3.3%) ≤ 18.5 kg/m^2.

The season of measurement was the most significant factor associated with insufficient concentrations of 25-hydroxy-vitamin D. The concentrations vitamin D in the four seasons are depicted in Figure 1 (upper panel). Of note, 64 (38%) out of 170 subjects tested for 25-hydroxy-vitamin D level in winter presented insufficient concentrations of this vitamin, 70 (18%) out of 383 in spring, 18 (5.4%) out 331 in summer and 28 (17%) out of 161 in autumn. A total of 13 (7.6%) subjects in winter, 6 (1.6%) in spring and 5 (3.1%) in autumn, presented with deficient concentrations of 25-hydroxy-vitamin D. No subject had a deficient level of 25-hydroxy-vitamin D in summer (Figure 1, lower panel).

Table 1. Baseline characteristics of the enrolled subjects. Data are given as absolute frequency (and percentage) or median (and interquartile range).

N	1045
Main activity	
Student	433 (41)
Worker	612 (59)
Anthropometric characteristics	
Body height, cm	178.0 (173.5–182.0)
Body weight, kg	72.2 (65.7–80.0)
Body mass index, kg/m^2	23.0 (21.0–25.1)
Body fat percentage, %	17.8 (13.7–23.1)
Mid-upper arm circumference, cm	27.0 (25.0–30.0)
Waist circumference, cm	80 (75–87)
Frequency of recreational physical activity	
Never	219 (21)
1 per week	174 (17)
2–4 per week	472 (45)
5–6 per week	88 (8.4)
Every day	92 (8.8)
Length of recreational physical activity session	
≤ 1 h	66 (8.0)
>1–≤ 2 h	602 (73)
>2–≤ 3 h	143 (17)
>3 h	15 (1.8)
Site of recreational physical activity	
Indoor (only)	148 (18)
Outdoor (only)	340 (41)
Both indoor and outdoor	338 (41)
Frequency of alcohol consumption	
Never	201 (19)
1 per week	393 (38)
2 per week	285 (27)
3–4 per week	112 (11)
5–6 per week	42 (4.0)
Every day	12 (1.2)
Smoking	
Never	602 (58)
1–10 cigarettes per day	299 (29)
11–20 cigarettes per day	130 (12)
>20 cigarettes per day	14 (1.3)
Biochemical indices	
Total 25-hydroxy-vitamin D, nmol/L	68 (55–82)
Cholesterol, mmol/L	3.9 (3.5–4.3)
Ferritin, μmol/L	76.0 (52–109)

Table 2. Characteristics of subjects with adequate and insufficient circulating 25-hydroxy-vitamin D. All variables were non-normally distributed. Data are given as absolute frequency (and percentage) or median (and interquartile range). The Kruskal-Wallis test was used for continuous variables. Chi-squared test was used for categorical variables. The Bonferroni test adjustment was applied to account for multiple comparisons.

Subjects Characteristics	25-hydroxy-vitamin D		p-value
	Adequate (≥50 nmol/L)	Insufficient (<50 nmol/L)	
N	866 (83)	179 (17)	
Main activity			
Student	356 (41)	77 (43)	0.7
Worker	510 (59)	102 (67)	
Anthropometric characteristics			
Body height, cm	178.0 (173.0–182.0)	176.0 (171.5–180.0)	0.003 **
Body weight, kg	72.5 (65.9–80.0)	71.3 (64.9–82.0)	0.9
Body mass index, kg/m^2	22.9 (21.0–25.0)	23.0 (20.7–26.3)	0.3
Body fat percentage, %	17.4 (13.4–22.7)	20.1 (14.6–25.2)	<0.0001 ***
Mid-upper arm circumference, cm	27.0 (25.0–29.5)	27.0 (24.0–30.1)	0.4
Waist circumference, cm	80 (75–86)	80 (75–91)	0.1
Frequency of recreational physical activity			
Never	177 (20)	42 (24)	0.03 *
1 per week	134 (16)	40 (22)	
2–4 per week	396 (46)	76 (43)	
5–6 per week	81 (9.4)	7 (3.9)	
Every day	78 (9.0)	14 (7.8)	
Duration of recreational physical activity session			
≤1 h	50 (7.3)	16 (12)	0.3
>1–≤2 h	509 (74)	93 (68)	
>2–≤3 h	118 (17)	25 (18)	
>3 h	12 (1.7)	3 (2.2)	
Site of recreational physical activity			
Indoor (only)	117 (17)	31 (23)	0.1
Outdoor (only)	281 (41)	59 (43)	
Both indoor and outdoor	289 (42)	47 (34)	
Frequency of alcohol consumption			
Never	161 (19)	40 (22)	0.1
1 per week	338 (39)	55 (31)	
2 per week	224 (26)	61 (34)	
3–4 per week	97 (11)	15 (8.4)	
5–6 per week	35 (4.0)	7 (3.9)	
Every day	11 (1.3)	1 (0.6)	
Smoking			
Never	483 (56)	119 (67)	0.018 *
1–10 cigarettes per day	253 (29)	46 (26)	
11–20 cigarettes per day	118 (14)	12 (6.7)	
>20 cigarettes per day	12 (1.4)	2 (1.1)	
Season of measurement			
Winter	106 (12)	64 (36)	<0.0001 ***
Spring	313 (36)	70 (39)	
Summer	313 (36)	18 (10)	
Autumn	134 (16)	27 (15)	
Biochemical indices			
Cholesterol, mmol/L	3.9 (3.5–4.3)	4.0 (3.6–4.4)	0.049 *
Ferritin, µmol/L	76.0 (52.0–109.0)	76.5 (51.0–103.5)	0.9

* $p < 0.05$, ** $p < 0.01$, *** $p < 0.0001$.

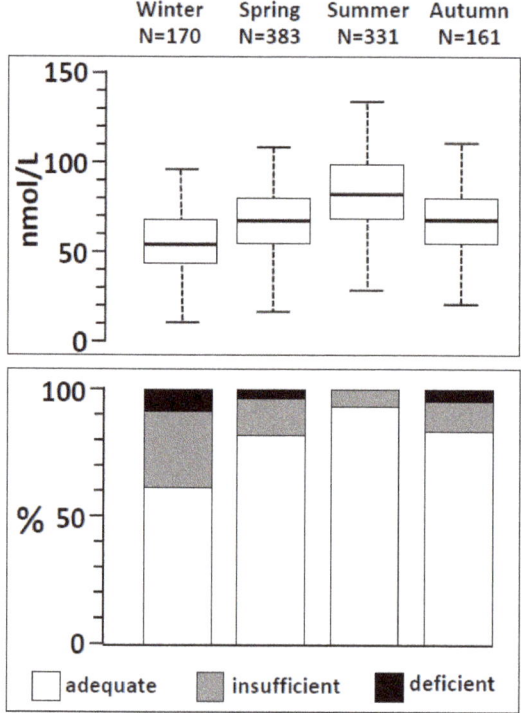

Figure 1. Upper panel. Box-plot of the circulating concentrations of 25-hydroxy-vitamin D across the four seasons. The boxes include values between the 1st and the 3rd quartile (i.e., the interquartile range). The whiskers include values between: 1st quartile − 1.5 times interquartile range and 3rd quartile + 1.5 times interquartile range. **Lower panel.** Frequency of adequate, insufficient or deficient concentrations of 25-hydroxy-vitamin D according to seasonality.

In the univariate logistic regression models (Table 3), body height (ORs 0.96, 95% CI 0.94–0.98), body mass index (OR 1.05, 95% CI 1.00–1.07, body fat percentage (OR 1.04, 95% CI 1.02–1.07), waist circumference (OR 1.02, 95% CI 1.00–1.03), the frequency of recreational physical activity 5–6 per week (OR 0.36, 95% CI 0.16–0.85), cigarettes consumption of 11–20 cigarettes per day (OR 0.41, 95% CI 0.22–0.77), the season (spring, OR 0.37, 95% CI 0.25–0.56, summer, OR 0.09, 95% CI 0.05–0.17, and autumn, OR 0.33, 95% CI 0.20–0.56) and cholesterol (OR 1.29, 95% CI 1.02–1.62) were positively (OR >1) or inversely (OR < 1) associated with the risk of 25-hydroxy-vitamin D insufficiency.

Table 4 shows results from the multiple regression analysis. After model selection based on clinical plausibility and Akaike information criterion, the increase of body fat percentage was a significant risk factor (ORs >1) for 25-hydroxy-vitamin D insufficiency. A frequent (5–6 times per week) and outdoor physical activity and non-winter seasons were significant protective factors (ORs < 1) against 25-hydroxy-vitamin D insufficiency.

Table 3. Odds ratios (ORs) of 25-hydroxy-vitamin D insufficiency and corresponding 95% confidence intervals (CIs) from univariate logistic regression models.

Subject Characteristic	OR	Lower 95%CI	Upper 95%CI	p-Value
Body height, cm	0.96	0.94	0.98	0.004 **
Body weight, kg	1.01	0.99	1.20	0.4
Body mass index, kg/m^2	1.05	1.00	1.07	0.03 *
Body fat percentage, %	1.04	1.02	1.07	<0.0001 ***
Mid-upper arm circumference, cm	0.99	0.95	1.04	0.09
Waist circumference, cm	1.02	1.00	1.03	0.03 *
Frequency of recreational physical activity				
Never	reference			
1 per week	1.26	0.77	2.05	0.4
2–4 per week	0.81	0.53	1.23	0.3
5–6 per week	0.36	0.16	0.85	0.02 *
Every day	0.76	0.39	1.46	0.5
Duration of recreational physical activity session				
≤1 h	reference			
>1–≤2 h	0.57	0.31	1.05	0.06
>2–≤3 h	0.66	0.33	1.35	0.3
>3 h	0.78	0.19	3.12	0.7
Site of recreational physical activity				
Indoor	reference			
Both indoor and outdoor	0.79	0.49	1.29	0.4
Outdoor (only)	0.61	0.37	1.01	0.05
Frequency of alcohol consumption				
Never	reference			
1 per week	0.66	0.42	1.03	0.06
2 per week	1.10	0.70	1.71	0.7
3–4 per week	0.62	0.33	1.19	0.1
5–6 per week	0.80	0.33	1.95	0.6
Every day	0.37	0.05	2.92	0.3
Smoking				
Never	reference			
1–10 cigarettes per day	0.74	0.51	1.07	0.1
11–20 cigarettes per day	0.41	0.22	0.77	0.006 **
>20 cigarettes per day	0.68	0.15	3.06	0.6
Season of measurement				
Winter	reference			
Spring	0.37	0.25	0.56	<0.0001 ***
Summer	0.09	0.05	0.17	<0.0001 ***
Autumn	0.33	0.20	0.56	<0.0001 ***
Biochemical indices				
Cholesterol, mmol/L	1.29	1.02	1.62	0.03 *
Ferritin, µmol/L	1.0	0.99	1.01	0.9

* $p < 0.05$, ** $p < 0.01$, *** $p < 0.0001$.

Table 4. Odds ratios (ORs) of 25-hydroxy-vitamin D insufficiency and corresponding 95% confidence intervals (CIs) as derived from the best Akaike information criterion-selected multiple logistic regression model. The original model included the following variables: body mass index, body fat percentage, mid-upper arm circumference, waist circumference, frequency of recreational physical activity, duration of recreational physical activity session, site of recreational physical activity, season, frequency of alcohol consumption, smoking, cholesterol and ferritin.

Subject Characteristic	OR	Lower 95%CI	Upper 95%CI	p-Value
Body fat percentage, %	1.04	1.01	1.07	0.01 *
Frequency of recreational physical activity				
2–4 per week	0.64	0.40	1.02	0.6
5–6 per week	0.32	0.13	0.78	0.01 *
Every day	0.64	0.31	1.35	0.2
Site of recreational physical activity				
Both indoor and outdoor	0.80	0.47	1.37	0.4
Outdoor (only)	0.56	0.33	0.96	0.04 *
Season of measurement				
Spring	0.31	0.19	0.49	<0.0001 ***
Summer	0.08	0.04	0.17	<0.0001 ***
Autumn	0.24	0.13	0.45	<0.0001 ***
Biochemical indices				
Cholesterol, mmol/L	1.25	0.95	1.66	0.1

* $p < 0.05$, *** $p < 0.0001$.

4. Discussion

This study points out that a large minority (17%) of healthy male late adolescents in Southern Switzerland, a region with a low natural vitamin D intake, has a poor vitamin D status. In this group of subjects, an increase in body fat percentage is a risk factor for vitamin D insufficiency. On the contrary, frequent and outdoor recreational physical activity and, especially, non-winter seasons are protective factors against vitamin D insufficiency. Yet, about one every fifth subject has insufficient concentrations of vitamin D also in spring and autumn.

The prevalence of hypovitaminosis D among adolescents from high-income countries largely varies among studies [12,13]. In the southeastern United States, vitamin D concentrations < 50 nmol/L were observed in about 4% of white male adolescents [14]. In the HELENA study, among 1006 subjects living in ten European countries, about 40% presented vitamin D concentration < 50 nmol/L [15]. Our data point out that insufficient concentrations of vitamin D are frequent among male late adolescents in Southern Switzerland and emphasize that vitamin D concentrations are strongly season dependent. Of note, the frequency of vitamin D insufficiency was very high in winter and still rather important (>15%) in autumn. A previous study suggests that in Ireland (latitude 51–55°) ultraviolet B radiation is effective for some vitamin D synthesis also in October [16]. On the other hand, very low doses were found in November and December. This study did not specifically investigate the ultraviolet B radiation in Southern Switzerland. However, the concentration of 25-hydroxy-vitamin D_2 was always ≤5 nmol/L, confirming that also vitamin D of non-animal origin played a marginal role in vitamin D status in our population.

The peak bone mass is usually reached between 25 and 35 years of age and, in male subjects, is predicted by vitamin D status [17]. Hence, the years preceding the peak bone mass are considered as a critical period to maximize bone strength and maturation [18]. The European Academy of Pediatrics, the American Academy of Pediatrics and Endocrine guidelines currently do not routinely recommend supplying vitamin D in non-dark skinned, non-obese healthy adolescents or young adults [19–21]. The results of this study suggest that longitudinal studies should address the advantages of vitamin D supplementation in Caucasian late adolescents during winter. This finding is even more crucial for the bone metabolism, considering that only vitamins D concentrations >75 nmol/L have a clear-cut antifracture effect [22]. On the other hand, an increasing body of evidence highlights that vitamin D deficiency is associated with chronic and potentially life-threating conditions such as cardiovascular disease later in old adults and elderly [23]. In this study, about one every thirteen subjects had deficient concentrations of vitamin D in winter.

We found an association between vitamin D concentrations, frequent and outdoor physical recreational activity after adjusting for confounders. Although sun-light exposure does not occur exclusively during recreational physical activity, this finding confirms the beneficial role of outdoor activities. Yet, seasonal fluctuations of ultraviolet-B radiations might decrease the effects of sun-light exposure during non-summer seasons and especially in winter [22,23]. Differently from previous observations [24,25], this study did not identify any association between vitamin D and a marker of inflammation such as ferritin. This might be due to the fact that the population of this study exclusively included healthy late adolescents without any chronic disease. Also, we did not find any association with cholesterol or alcohol consumption. A possible explanation is that most prior studies have included subjects with a much broader range of age and the mentioned factors could become determinant when persisting for long-term periods [26]. Previous studies found body mass index to be inversely associated with vitamin D concentrations. However, residual confounding such as physical activity or body composition assessment have not always been considered [27]. Furthermore, body mass index cannot distinguish lean from fat mass, especially in youth [28]. One of the advantages of this study is that many anthropometric characteristics were explored disclosing an association between body fat percentage and vitamin D concentrations levels after adjusting for confounders. A tendency to accumulate vitamin D (a liposoluble compound) in fat depots or an impaired vitamin D intestinal absorption or hydroxylation in adipose tissue are likely to underly this association [29]. Of note, some studies have also hypothesized that vitamin D insufficiency itself could reduce weight loss or favoring weight gain [29].

This study has many strengths and limitations. The main strengths are the large number of apparently healthy subjects enrolled with a narrow range of age and the concomitant determination of many potential modulators of vitamin D including the body fat percentage. Furthermore, Southern Switzerland is considered the sunniest region of Switzerland: therefore, it is possible that the number of late adolescents with vitamin D insufficiency might be even higher in the other parts of Switzerland. The main limitation of this study is the exclusion of females. Second, results are partly based on self-reports, which might not always correspond to the actual behavior of the responders. Third, its cross-sectional nature prevents to longitudinally evaluate vitamin D concentrations throughout the seasons. Fourth, we did not analyze some common inflammatory indices, such as C-reactive protein. Finally, the use of sunscreen, which is usually not very common among male adolescents and young adults in Switzerland [30], was not investigated.

5. Conclusions

This study showed that about one every fourth healthy male late adolescent in Southern Switzerland presents insufficient concentrations of vitamin D during non-summer seasons. Low body fat and both frequent and outdoor recreational physical activity are associated with adequate vitamin D level this population.

Author Contributions: Conceptualization, F.M., M.G.B., A.S. and G.S.; Methodology, F.M., A.R., S.A.G.L., V.E. and G.P.M.; Formal Analysis, V.E. and G.P.M.; Investigation, F.M., A.S., S.A.G.L. and M.G.B; Data Curation, A.R., G.P.M. and G.S. Writing—Original Draft Preparation, G.S., M.G.B., F.M. G.P.M.; Writing—Review & Editing, A.R., S.A.G.L., V.E., A.S.; Supervision, G.S.; Project Administration, F.M.; Funding Acquisition, F.M.

Funding: The study was supported by the Swiss Society of Hypertension.

Acknowledgments: Authors thank Silvia Muggli for data check.

Conflicts of Interest: The authors declare no conflicts of interest.

References

1. Santi, F.; Tamone, C.; D'Amelio, P. Vitamin D: Nutrient, hormone, and immunomodulator. *Nutrients* **2018**, *10*, 1656. [CrossRef]
2. Lamberg-Allardt, C. Vitamin D in foods and as supplements. *Prog. Biophys. Mol. Biol.* **2006**, *92*, 33–38. [CrossRef] [PubMed]
3. Smith, T.J. Lanham-New SA, Hart KH. Vitamin D in adolescents: Are current recommendations enough? *J. Steroid Biochem. Mol. Biol.* **2017**, *173*, 265–272. [CrossRef] [PubMed]
4. Stoffman, N.; Gordon, C.M. Vitamin D and adolescents: What do we know? *Curr. Opin. Pediatr.* **2009**, *21*, 465–471. [CrossRef] [PubMed]
5. Santi, M.; Lava, S.A.; Simonetti, G.D.; Stettbacher, A.; Bianchetti, M.G.; Muggli, F. Clustering of cardiovascular disease risk factors among male youths in Southern Switzerland: Preliminary study. *Swiss Med. Wkly.* **2016**, *146*, w14338. [CrossRef] [PubMed]
6. Lintsi, M.; Kaarma, H.; Kull, I. Comparison of hand-to-hand bioimpedance and anthropometry equations versus dual-energy X-ray absorptiometry for the assessment of body fat percentage in 17-18-year-old conscripts. *Clin. Physiol. Funct. Imaging* **2004**, *24*, 85–90. [CrossRef] [PubMed]
7. Deurenberg, P.; Andreoli, A.; Borg, P.; Kukkonen-Harjula, K.; de Lorenzo, A.; van Marken Lichtenbelt, W.D.; Testolin, G.; Vigano, R.; Vollaard, N. The validity of predicted body fat percentage from body mass index and from impedance in samples of five European populations. *Eur. J. Clin. Nutr.* **2001**, *55*, 973–979. [CrossRef] [PubMed]
8. Annema, W.; Nowak, A.; von Eckardstein, A.; Saleh, L. Evaluation of the new restandardized Abbott Architect 25-OH Vitamin D assay in vitamin D-insufficient and vitamin D-supplemented individuals. *J. Clin. Lab. Anal.* **2018**, *32*, e22328. [CrossRef] [PubMed]
9. Durazo-Arvizu, R.A.; Tian, L.; Brooks, S.P.J.; Sarafin, K.; Cashman, K.D.; Kiely, M.; Merkel, J.; Myers, G.L.; Coates, P.M.; Sempos, C.T. The Vitamin D Standardization Program (VDSP) Manual for Retrospective Laboratory Standardization of Serum 25-Hydroxyvitamin D Data. *J. AOAC Int.* **2017**, *100*, 1234–1243. [CrossRef] [PubMed]
10. Burdette, C.Q.; Camara, J.E.; Nalin, F.; Pritchett, J.; Sander, L.C.; Carter, G.D.; Jones, J.; Betz, J.M.; Sempos, C.T.; Wise, S.A. Establishing an Accuracy Basis for the Vitamin D External Quality Assessment Scheme (DEQAS). *J. AOAC Int.* **2017**, *100*, 1277–1287. [CrossRef] [PubMed]
11. Lava, S.A.; Simonetti, G.D.; Bianchetti, A.A.; Ferrarini, A.; Bianchetti, M.G. Prevention of vitamin D insufficiency in Switzerland: A never-ending story. *Int. J. Pharm.* **2013**, *457*, 353–356. [CrossRef] [PubMed]
12. Cashman, K.D.; Dowling, K.G.; Škrabáková, Z.; Gonzalez-Gross, M.; Valtueña, J.; De Henauw, S.; Moreno, L.; Damsgaard, C.T.; Michaelsen, K.F.; Mølgaard, C.; et al. Vitamin D deficiency in Europe: Pandemic? *Am. J. Clin. Nutr.* **2016**, *103*, 1033–1044. [CrossRef] [PubMed]
13. Schleicher, R.L.; Sternberg, M.R.; Looker, A.C.; Yetley, E.A.; Lacher, D.A.; Sempos, C.T.; Taylor, C.L.; Durazo-Arvizu, R.A.; Maw, K.L.; Chaudhary-Webb, M.; et al. National Estimates of Serum Total 25-Hydroxyvitamin D and Metabolite Concentrations Measured by Liquid Chromatography-Tandem Mass Spectrometry in the US Population during 2007–2010. *J. Nutr.* **2016**, *146*, 1051–1061. [CrossRef] [PubMed]
14. Dong, Y.; Pollock, N.; Stallmann-Jorgensen, I.S.; Gutin, B.; Lan, L.; Chen, T.C.; Keeton, D.; Petty, K.; Holick, M.F.; Zhu, H. Low 25-hydroxyvitamin D levels in adolescents: Race, season, adiposity, physical activity, and fitness. *Pediatrics* **2010**, *125*, 1104–1111. [CrossRef] [PubMed]
15. González-Gross, M.; Valtueña, J.; Breidenassel, C.; Moreno, L.A.; Ferrari, M.; Kersting, M.; De Henauw, S.; Gottrand, F.; Azzini, E.; Widhalm, K.; et al. Vitamin D status among adolescents in Europe: The Healthy Lifestyle in Europe by Nutrition in Adolescence study. *Br. J. Nutr.* **2012**, *107*, 755–764. [CrossRef] [PubMed]
16. Cashman, K.D.; van den Heuvel, E.G.; Schoemaker, R.J.; Préveraud, D.P.; Macdonald, H.M.; Arcot, J. 25-Hydroxyvitamin D as a Biomarker of Vitamin D Status and Its Modeling to Inform Strategies for Prevention of Vitamin D Deficiency within the Population. *Adv. Nutr.* **2017**, *8*, 947–957. [CrossRef] [PubMed]
17. Högström, M.; Nordström, A.; Nordström, P. Relationship between vitamin D metabolites and bone mineral density in young males: A cross-sectional and longitudinal study. *Calcif. Tissue Int.* **2006**, *79*, 95–101. [CrossRef] [PubMed]

18. Levine, M.A. Assessing bone health in children and adolescents. *Indian J. Endocrinol. Metab.* **2012**, *16*, S205–S212. [CrossRef] [PubMed]
19. Golden, N.H.; Abrams, S.A.; Committee on Nutrition. Optimizing bone health in children and adolescents. *Pediatrics* **2014**, *134*, 2014–2173. [CrossRef] [PubMed]
20. Grossman, Z.; Hadjipanayis, A.; Stiris, T.; Del Torso, S.; Mercier, J.C.; Valiulis, A.; Shamir, R. Vitamin D in European children-statement from the European Academy of Paediatrics (EAP). *Eur. J. Pediatr.* **2017**, *176*, 829–831. [CrossRef] [PubMed]
21. Holick, M.F.; Binkley, N.C.; Bischoff-Ferrari, H.A.; Gordon, C.M.; Hanley, D.A.; Heaney, R.P.; Murad, M.H.; Weaver, C.M.; Endocrine Society. Evaluation, treatment, and prevention of vitamin D deficiency: An Endocrine Society clinical practice guideline. *J. Clin. Endocrinol. Metab.* **2011**, *96*, 1911–1930. [CrossRef] [PubMed]
22. Rusińska, A.; Płudowski, P.; Walczak, M.; Borszewska-Kornacka, M.K.; Bossowski, A.; Chlebna-Sokół, D.; Czech-Kowalska, J.; Dobrzańska, A.; Franek, E.; Helwich, E.; et al. Vitamin D Supplementation Guidelines for General Population and Groups at Risk of Vitamin D Deficiency in Poland-Recommendations of the Polish Society of Pediatric Endocrinology and Diabetes and the Expert Panel With Participation of National Specialist Consultants and Representatives of Scientific Societies-2018 Update. *Front. Endocrinol. (Lausanne)* **2018**, *9*, 246. [CrossRef] [PubMed]
23. Holick, M.F. Ultraviolet B Radiation: The Vitamin D Connection. *Adv. Exp. Med. Biol.* **2017**, *996*, 137–154. [CrossRef] [PubMed]
24. Munasinghe, L.L.; Ekwaru, J.P.; Mastroeni, M.F.; Mastroeni, S.S.B.S.; Veugelers, P.J. The association of serum 25-hydroxyvitamin D concentrations with elevated serum ferritin levels in normal weight, overweight and obese Canadians. *PLoS ONE* **2019**, *14*, e0213260. [CrossRef] [PubMed]
25. Tønnesen, R.; Hovind, P.H.; Jensen, L.T.; Schwarz, P. Determinants of vitamin D status in young adults: Influence of lifestyle, sociodemographic and anthropometric factors. *BMC Public Health* **2016**, *16*, 385. [CrossRef] [PubMed]
26. Sanada, F.; Taniyama, Y.; Muratsu, J.; Otsu, R.; Shimizu, H.; Rakugi, H.; Morishita, R. Source of Chronic Inflammation in Aging. *Front. Cardiovasc. Med.* **2018**, *5*, 12. [CrossRef] [PubMed]
27. Cheng, S.; Massaro, J.M.; Fox, C.S.; Larson, M.G.; Keyes, M.J.; McCabe, E.L.; Robins, S.J.; O'Donnell, C.J.; Hoffmann, U.; Jacques, P.F.; et al. Adiposity, cardiometabolic risk, and vitamin D status: The Framingham Heart Study. *Diabetes* **2010**, *59*, 242–248. [CrossRef] [PubMed]
28. Witt, K.A.; Bush, E.A. College athletes with an elevated body mass index often have a high upper arm muscle area, but not elevated triceps and subscapular skinfolds. *J. Am. Diet. Assoc.* **2005**, *105*, 599–602. [CrossRef] [PubMed]
29. Migliaccio, S.; Di Nisio, A.; Mele, C.; Scappaticcio, L.; Savastano, S.; Colao, A. Obesity Programs of nutrition, Education, Research and Assessment (OPERA) Group. Obesity and hypovitaminosis D: Causality or casualty? *Int. J. Obes. Suppl.* **2019**, *9*, 20–31. [CrossRef] [PubMed]
30. Berret, J.; Liardet, S.; Scaletta, C.; Panizzon, R.; Hohlfeld, P.; Applegate, L.A. Use of sunscreens in families living in Switzerland. *Dermatology* **2002**, *204*, 202–208. [CrossRef] [PubMed]

© 2019 by the authors. Licensee MDPI, Basel, Switzerland. This article is an open access article distributed under the terms and conditions of the Creative Commons Attribution (CC BY) license (http://creativecommons.org/licenses/by/4.0/).

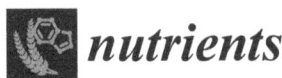

Article

Effects of Vitamin D Status and Supplements on Anthropometric and Biochemical Indices in a Clinical Setting: A Retrospective Study

Myriam Abboud [1,2], Xiaoying Liu [1], Flavia Fayet-Moore [3], Kaye E. Brock [1], Dimitrios Papandreou [2], Tara C. Brennan-Speranza [1] and Rebecca S. Mason [1,*]

1. Department of Physiology & Bosch Institute, School of Medical Sciences, Faculty of Medicine and Health, University of Sydney, Sydney NSW 2006, Australia; Myriam.abboud@zu.ac.ae (M.A.); xliu0534@uni.sydney.edu.au (X.L.); kaye.brock@sydney.edu.au (K.E.B.); tara.speranza@sydney.edu.au (T.C.B.-S.)
2. Department of Health Sciences, Zayed University, P.O. Box 144534 Dubai, UAE; Dimitrios.Papandreou@zu.ac.ae
3. School of Molecular Bioscience, University of Sydney NSW 2006, Australia & Nutrition Research Australia, Sydney, NSW 2000, Australia; flavia@nraus.com
* Correspondence: rebecca.mason@sydney.edu.au; Tel.: +61-(2)-9351-2561; Fax: +61-(2)-9351-2510

Received: 18 November 2019; Accepted: 10 December 2019; Published: 12 December 2019

Abstract: Context: Obesity and low vitamin D status are linked. It is not clear that weight loss through lifestyle intervention is influenced by vitamin D status. Objective: The aim of this study was to investigate the effect of baseline vitamin D status and vitamin D supplementation on weight loss and associated parameters for participants on a weight loss program in a primary care setting. Design: A retrospective analysis of clinical records of patients who underwent an individually tailored weight loss program at a single dietetic clinic in Sydney, Australia. Setting: Primary care centers. Patients: 205 overweight and obese men and women aged from 18 to 50 years. Interventions: Patients were referred to a dietetic clinic for a weight loss program. Patients with low serum 25-hydroxyvitamin D (25(OH)D) concentrations at baseline were advised to increase sun exposure and take multivitamins supplemented with 2000 IU or 4000 IU per day of vitamin D3, according to the preference of their primary care physician. Main outcome measures: Clinical parameters of weight, height, waist circumference, and serum 25(OH)D, as well as blood pressure and fasting lipid profile were collected from both baseline and three-month follow-up consultations. Results: Subjects with sufficient baseline 25(OH)D levels ($\geq$50 nmol/L) experienced significantly greater weight loss (-7.7 ± 5.9 kg vs. -4.2 ± 3.3 kg) and reductions in BMI (-2.6 ± 1.8 kg/m^2 vs. -1.5 ± 1.1 kg/m^2) and waist circumference (-5.2 ± 3.5 cm vs. -3.1 ± 3.1 cm) as compared with those who were vitamin D insufficient at baseline ($p < 0.001$ for all). Vitamin D insufficient patients who were supplemented with daily 2000 IU or 4000 IU vitamin D experienced significantly greater decreases in weight (-5.3 ± 3.6 kg vs. -2.3 ± 1.6 kg), BMI (-1.9 ± 1.2 kg/m^2 vs. -0.8 ± 0.6 kg/m^2) and waist circumference (-4.2 ± 3.4 cm vs. -1.2 ± 1.3 cm) as compared with those not supplemented ($p < 0.001$ for all). We also observed a greater decrease in low-density lipoprotein (LDL) cholesterol (-0.4 ± 0.5 mmol/L vs. -0.2 ± 0.5 mmol/L) in subjects insufficient at baseline and supplemented as compared with those insufficient at baseline and not supplemented ($p < 0.01$). Conclusion: In a weight loss setting in a dietetic clinic, adequate vitamin D status at baseline, or achieved at three months through supplementation, was associated with significantly greater improvement of anthropometric measures. The study has implications for the management of vitamin D status in obese or overweight patients undergoing weight loss programs.

Keywords: vitamin D deficiency; 25-hydroxyvitamin D; vitamin D supplements; weight loss; low-density lipoprotein (LDL) cholesterol; high-density lipoprotein (HDL) cholesterol; triglycerides (TG); blood pressure

1. Introduction

Vitamin D has multiple pleiotropic functions beyond its traditional role in calcium homeostasis, as well as bone and muscle function [1]. Actions of the vitamin D hormone, calcitriol, have been demonstrated in many tissues, including adipocytes [2] and the cardiovascular system [3]. The first evidence of a relationship between vitamin D and body fat was described in 1972 by Mawer et al. [4]. Inadequate vitamin D status, obesity, and chronic noncommunicable disease often cluster [1,3,5–7]. They are important public health issues that contribute significantly to modern healthcare costs, morbidity, and mortality [8,9]. Many studies support the proposal that obesity could be driving low serum 25(OH)D concentrations mainly due to decreased bioavailability of vitamin D through sequestration in body fat compartments [4,10–13]. There is limited human research which indicates that vitamin D could potentiate weight loss and improvements in metabolic markers [14,15]. A recent randomized controlled trial in postmenopausal women reported that while supplementation with vitamin D did not alter weight loss or associated parameters overall as compared with a placebo group, women in the supplemented group who reached 25(OH)D concentrations of ≥32 ng/mL (≥80 nmol/L), had greater improvement in several measured weight loss parameters as compared with those women whose final 25(OH)D concentrations were below 80 nmol/L [16].

In this study, we hypothesized that overweight and obese patients presenting adequate 25(OH)D levels will have a greater reduction in body weight, body mass index (BMI), and waist circumference as compared with those with inadequate vitamin D levels while undergoing a three-month clinic-specific individually tailored weight loss management program. Furthermore, we expect that vitamin D repletion of those who were insufficient at baseline, through short-term daily vitamin D supplementation would enhance weight loss, decrease waist circumference, and improve biochemical markers. This was investigated using clinic records of a population of overweight and obese men and premenopausal women who participated in an individually tailored three month weight loss program.

2. Study Design and Population

This study is a retrospective analysis of a clinical databank that was recorded in a health giver-receiver setting. The Human Ethics Committee at the University of Sydney approved the research protocol (Protocol 2013/206). Between September 2011 and March 2013, a total of 935 patients who attended three medical centers in Sydney, Australia, were referred to a dietetic clinic (established by author MA) to assist with a program for weight loss, under the Chronic Disease Management Plan of Medicare Australia [17]. This care plan entitled each patient to five consultations with a dietician or another allied health professional. Under an agreed protocol, patients had blood taken for 25(OH)D and blood lipid measurements at the initial visit with the primary care physician. These patients were seen by the dietician fortnightly for the first month and then monthly after that. Thus, the initial visit was the first visit, then, after two weeks (second visit), then, another two weeks (third visit), then, after one month (fourth visit), then, after one month (fifth visit). This fifth visit coincided with the three-month follow-up, when the follow-up blood for testing was taken. The referring doctors differed in their approach to management of patients who had 25(OH)D concentrations less than 50 nmol/L at baseline. Some referring doctors advised their patients to take supplements of vitamin D3 at 2000 IU per day, and some at 4000 IU per day. The remaining patients with low baseline 25OHD were advised to increase their sun exposure and take multivitamins (with only small amounts, 40 IU of vitamin D). The dietician performed anthropometric measures at each visit. Weight was measured using the same scales, which were calibrated monthly. Height and waist circumference were measured at the initial and final visits. Waist circumference was measured with the patient standing, at a level midway between the iliac tubercle and lower lateral rib margin, and hip circumference was measured at the level of the iliac tubercle.

For the individually tailored weight loss protocol, at the initial consultation with the dietician, each patient's daily estimated energy requirement (EER) was calculated using the Harris-Benedict equation [18] and physical activity factors (see more detailed information in the supplementary Tables S1–S3). Overweight and obese individual caloric goals were calculated to be 300 and 500 Kcal/day, respectively, less than their EER. Once the EER was calculated, a meal plan was designed by the dietitian and given to the participant at the initial consultation, and adherence was checked via a 24-h recall method during each of the follow-up visits. The reported intake was relatively compliant with the prescribed energy intake. The participants were not seen by any exercise physiologist and did not undertake any major changes in physical activity that could have altered their energy needs.

As part of continuing care, a report was sent to the referring primary care physician requesting a follow-up on 25(OH)D and other biochemical markers at three months from the initial consultation, which coincided with the final dietary consultation. This blood test was performed on the same day as the final dietary consultation.

All 935 records of patients who were referred to this program between September 2011 and March 2013 were examined. Of these, 676 records were excluded based on the following predetermined exclusion criteria: a history of diabetes mellitus, polycystic ovary syndrome, parathyroid disorder, kidney or liver disease, osteopenia or osteoporosis, or current pregnancy, or taking any medication known to affect body weight (such as steroids) or supplements such as calcium or vitamin D (>400 IU of vitamin D2 or vitamin D3, not prescribed as part of this intervention). A further 47 patients were excluded as they did not complete the follow-up blood test at three months. There were seven subjects in the group which had sufficient 25(OH)D concentrations (≥50 nmol/L) at baseline, who received vitamin D supplements. These were also excluded from the analysis.

Records of 205 healthy men and premenopausal women between the ages of 18 and 50 were coded for analysis. Clinical parameters including blood pressure; fasting lipid profile, i.e., total cholesterol (TC), low-density lipoprotein (LDL) cholesterol, high-density lipoprotein (HDL) cholesterol, and triglycerides (TG), and serum 25 hydroxyvitamin D (25(OH)D; as well as anthropometric measurements (weight, height, and waist circumference) were collected from both baseline and three-month follow-up consultations. Patients reported sun exposure frequency at baseline and exercise levels.

Overweight and obesity were classified according to BMI (overweight 25 to 29.9 kg/m^2 and obesity ≥30 kg/m^2) and waist circumference (overweight men 94.0 to 101.9 cm, women 80.0 to 87.9 cm, obesity men ≥102.0 cm, and women ≥88.0 cm).

Biochemistry

Plasma levels of cholesterols and triglycerides were determined by standard laboratory methods and were all performed by Laverty Laboratory, North Ryde, Sydney, Australia. They were measured using an enzyme-based Siemens platform, where LDL was calculated in accordance with the Friedewald equation (18). Normal ranges for lipid profile were provided by the commercial laboratory: TC (3.5–5.4 mmol/L), LDL (2.1–4 mmo/L), HDL (>=1 mmol/L), TG (0.1–2 mmol/L). Plasma 25(OH)D concentrations were all determined at the Laverty Laboratory using the Diasorin Siemens chemiluminescent assay and vitamin D insufficiency was defined as 25(OH)D level <50 nmol/L [19]. The assay characteristics are described in [20].

3. Statistical Analysis

All analyses were performed using SPSS for Windows (version 17.0 SPSS, Inc., Chicago, IL, USA). Analyzed data were collected from a clinical setting with intention-to-treat approach. Differences in anthropometric and blood parameters between patients who had sufficient baseline 25(OH)D, and insufficient baseline 25(OH)D with or without prescription of vitamin D supplementation, were assessed by one-way ANOVA followed by Tukey's post-test. Comparisons for the within-group changes in Table 1 were made using paired Student t-tests. Correlations were assessed by calculating Pearson correlation coefficients. LOESS plots [21] were calculated by the SPSS program. Multivariate analysis of changes in weight, BMI, and waist circumference were regressed against 25(OH)D concentrations at follow-up using stepwise linear regression models using the following independent variables: 25(OH)D values at follow-up, adjusting for age, sex, season of baseline appointment, sun exposure, and exercise and were split by prescription of vitamin D supplements. In the initial analyses, the subjects who were vitamin D insufficient at baseline (25(OH)D <50 nmol/L) and supplemented with 2000 IU vitamin D3 per day, were analyzed separately from those who were supplemented with 4000 IU/day. There were no differences between these groups in terms of baseline parameters, except for baseline 25(OH)D which was significantly lower at 31 ± 13 nmol/L in the subjects who were prescribed 4000 IU per day, as compared with 39 ± 16 nmol/L in those prescribed 2000 IU per day ($p < 0.02$). For ease of data presentation and statistical power, these supplemented groups have been combined.

Table 1. Baseline and follow-up characteristics for all subjects.

Parameters	Baseline N = 205 Mean ± SD	Follow Up N = 205 Mean ± SD	p value
Weight, kg	88.5 ± 18.3	82.9 ± 17.6	<0.001
BMI, kg/m^2	31 ± 5.3	29.1 ± 5.2	<0.001
Waist circumference, cm	97.7 ± 14.1	93.7 ± 13.8	<0.001
25(OH)D, mmol/L	45.2 ± 18.7	54.0 ± 16.8	<0.001
BP systolic, mm Hg	126.1 ± 14.3	122.9 ± 11.4	<0.001
BP diastolic, mm Hg	77.8 ± 10.4	78.0 ± 8.5	NS
Total cholesterol, mmol/L	5.7 ± 3.7	5.1 ± 0.9	0.02
LDL, mmol/L	3.2 ± 0.9	2.9 ± 0.8	<0.001
HDL, mmol/L	1.5 ± 0.4	1.4 ± 0.3	NS
Triglycerides, mmol/L	1.6 ± 1.1	1.4 ± 0.8	<0.001

25(OH)D indicates serum 25-hydroxyvitamin D; HDL, high-density lipoprotein; LDL, low-density lipoprotein; and BP, blood pressure. Data are shown as mean values ± SD data from 205 subjects, except for total cholesterol and triglycerides (204), LDL (194), and HDL (197). p values show differences between baseline and follow-up values, NS, non-significant $p > 0.05$.

4. Results

4.1. Subject Characteristics

As shown in Table 1, there was a significant overall reduction in weight, BMI, waist circumference, systolic blood pressure, LDL, and triglycerides after the three-month weight loss program.

There were 70 men and 135 women whose records were included in the study. Although the men were significantly older (mean 39 years vs. 37 years, $p = 0.007$) and had significantly higher weight, waist circumference, blood pressure, LDL, and triglyceride values, and lower HDL, at baseline, they were not significantly different from the women in terms of baseline BMI, 25(OH)D, or the proportion who were vitamin D sufficient (see Supplementary Table S1). At three months, there were again no significant differences between males and females in terms of BMI, 25(OH)D concentrations, or the proportion who were vitamin D sufficient, but differences in the other parameters persisted (Supplementary Table S2). Sex had no significant effect on changes in weight, BMI, waist circumference, 25(OH)D concentration, or total cholesterol over the three-month period of analysis (p values of >0.05 for all). For this reason, in Table 1 and subsequent tables, data for male and female subjects have been combined.

Consistent with the high prevalence of vitamin D insufficiency with obesity, the mean baseline serum 25(OH)D concentration was insufficient (45 ± 19 nmol/L) and the mean baseline BMI classified subjects as obese overall. At baseline, 3% of the baseline subjects were in the normal weight range, 50% were overweight, and 47% were obese. After three months on a weight loss program and supplementation with vitamin D for some individuals, the mean serum 25(OH)D level was significantly higher than that of the baseline at 54 ± 17 nmol/L ($p < 0.001$) with a three month median and interquartile range of 55 and 23 nmol/L, respectively, while the mean BMI and waist circumference were significantly lower than that of the baseline (Table 1). After three months on the program, 22% of subjects were normal weight, 45% were overweight, and 33% were obese.

4.2. Effect of Vitamin D Status and Supplementation on Anthropomorphic Measures and Other Parameters

Baseline serum 25(OH)D was significantly higher in the sufficient group as compared with the deficient group (64 ± 11 vs. 33 ± 10 nmol/L, $p < 0.001$, Table 2). After three months on the program, 25(OH)D concentrations were similar to baseline values in both vitamin D sufficient and vitamin D insufficient individuals not given supplemental vitamin D, despite advice to increase sun exposure and take multivitamins (Table 2).

Table 2. Baseline values for anthropomorphic measures, lipids, and blood pressure, and baseline and follow-up values for 25(OH)D with or without the three month supplementation with vitamin D. Values are presented as means ± SDs.

Parameters	Sufficient at Baseline	Insufficient at Baseline			ANOVA p-Value [#]
	Suf	Total	Non-Supplemented (Insuf-NonSup)	Supplemented (Insuf-Sup)	
N	82	123	48	75	
Age (years)	37 ± 8.2	38 ± 7.5	37 ± 7.4	38 ± 7.6	0.485
% Female	60%	70%	67%	73%	
Weight, kg	89 ± 17	88 ± 19	88 ± 17	87 ± 21	0.764
BMI, kg/m^2	31 ± 5	31 ± 5	31 ± 4	31 ± 6	0.534
Waist, cm	97 ± 14	98 ± 14	98 ± 13	98 ± 15	0.922
Baseline 25(OH)D nmol/L	64 ± 11 [a,b]	33 ± 10	34 ± 10	32 ± 10	**<0.001**
Follow-up 25(OH)D nmol/L	62 ± 11 [a,b]	49 ± 18	35 ± 11	57 ± 16 [c]	**<0.001**
BP-systolic, mmHg	126 ± 14	126 ± 15	127 ± 13	125 ± 16	0.793
BP-diastolic mmHg	77 ± 10	78 ± 11	78 ± 10	78 ± 11	0.908
Total cholesterol mmol/L	5.9 ± 5.8	5.5 ± 1.1	5.5 ± 1.2	5.5 ± 1.0	0.704
LDL mmol/L	3.2 ± 0.8	3.2 ± 1.0	3.1 ± 1.1	3.3 ± 0.9	0.647
HDL mmol/L	1.5 ± 0.4	1.5 ± 0.4	1.5 ± 0.5	1.5 ± 0.4	0.950
triglyceride mmol/L	1.4 ± 0.9	1.7 ± 1.2	1.8 ± 1.4	1.6 ± 1.1	0.203

[#] For differences between sufficient at baseline, Insuf-NonSup and Insuf-Sup. The total column is presented for information. [a] $p < 0.05$ Suf vs. Insuf-NonSup (Tukey's post hoc test); [b] $p < 0.05$ Suf vs. Insuf-Sup (Tukey's post hoc test); [c] $p < 0.05$ Insuf-NonSup vs. Insuf-Sup (Tukey's post hoc test). Significant p values are shown in bold.

At three months, the subjects who were vitamin D sufficient at baseline experienced significantly greater body weight loss, BMI decrease, and waist circumference reduction than those with baseline vitamin D deficiency ($p < 0.001$ for all, Table 3). The season of baseline appointment did not affect the weight changes at three months.

Table 3. Changes in 25(OH)D, weight, BMI, waist circumference, lipids, and blood pressure with or without the three month supplementation with vitamin D. Values are presented as means ± SDs.

Change (Δ) in Parameters	Sufficient at Baseline Suf	Total	Insufficient at Baseline Non-Supplemented (Insuf-NonSup)	Supplemented (Insuf-Sup)	ANOVA p-Value [#]
N	82	123	48	75	
Δ25(OH)D, mmol/L	−1.7 ± 7 [b]	16 ± 17	1.0 ± 4.8	25 ± 16 [c]	<0.001
Δweight, kg	−7.7 ± 5.9 [a,b]	−4.2 ± 3.3	−2.3 ± 1.6	−5.3 ± 3.6 [c]	<0.001
ΔBMI, kg/m^2	−2.6 ± 1.8 [a,b]	−1.5 ± 1.1	−0.8 ± 0.6	−1.9 ± 1.2 [c]	<0.001
Δwaist circum-ference, cm	−5.2 ± 3.5 [a]	−3.1 ± 3.1	−1.3 ± 1.3	−4.2 ± 3.4 [c]	<0.001
Δsystolic BP, mmHg	−4.8 ± 9.2	−2.2 ± 11	−3.1 ± 8.4	−1.6 ± 12	0.165
Δdiastolic BP, mmHg	−0.2 ± 8.6	0.4 ± 9.1	1.4 ± 8.2	−0.2 ± 9.6	0.553
ΔTotal Cholesterol mmol/L	−1.0 ± 5.6	−0.3 ± 0.5	−0.2 ± 0.4	−0.4 ± 0.5	0.378
ΔLDL mmol/L	−0.4 ± 0.4 [a]	−0.26 ± 0.5	−0.1 ± 0.4	−0.4 ± 0.5 [c]	**0.002**
ΔHDL mmol/L	−0.1 ± 0.2	−0.1 ± 0.2	−0.1 ± 0.2	−0.1 ± 0.2	0.380
Δtriglycerides mmol/L	−0.2 ± 0.4	−0.2 ± 0.7	−0.2 ± 0.9	−0.2 ± 0.5	0.920

[#] For differences between sufficient at baseline, Insuf-NonSup and Insuf-Sup. The total column is presented for information. [a] $p < 0.05$ Suf vs. Insuf-NonSup (Tukey's post hoc test); [b] $p < 0.05$ Suf vs. Insuf-Sup (Tukey's post hoc test); [c] $p < 0.05$ Insuf-NonSup vs. Insuf-Sup (Tukey's post hoc test). Significant p values are shown in bold.

Of the subjects with baseline vitamin D insufficiency, 60% received vitamin D supplements, which raised 25(OH)D concentrations significantly ($p < 0.001$, Tables 2 and 3). The initially low vitamin D status subjects who received supplemental vitamin D also experienced significantly greater body weight loss, as well as a greater reduction in BMI and waist circumference than those who were not supplemented ($p < 0.001$ for all parameters, Table 3). Vitamin D supplementation resulted in a significant decrease in LDL-cholesterol levels in this group as compared with the non-supplemented subjects ($p < 0.01$, Table 3). However, there were no significant differences in the changes in total cholesterol, HDL-cholesterol, TG, diastolic, or systolic BP between the subjects who received supplements and those who did not. Even with supplementation, the reductions in weight, BMI, and waist circumference in the initially vitamin D deficient group were significantly lower than those of the initially vitamin D sufficient group ($p < 0.001$).

The increase in 25(OH)D concentrations in those subjects who were initially vitamin D deficient and prescribed 2000 IU/day ($n = 40$) was 15 ± 7 nmol/L, significantly lower than the 37 ± 15 nmol/L increase in 25(OH)D concentrations in those subjects prescribed 4000 IU/day of vitamin D ($n = 30$) ($p < 0.02$ as compared with the lower dose group). Those subjects who were vitamin D deficient at baseline and who were prescribed 4000 IU of vitamin D3 daily, lost significantly more weight (−6.9 vs. −4.4 kg; $p < 0.001$), significantly reduced their BMI to a greater extent (−2.5 vs. −1.5 kg/m^2; $p = 0.001$), and reduced their waist circumference more effectively (−5.3 vs. −3.3 cm; $p < 0.001$) than those who were told to take 2000 IU daily. The dose of supplemental vitamin D did not significantly affect changes in LDL, HDL, and total cholesterol.

The relationship between changes in weight, BMI, and waist circumference, and concentrations of 25(OH)D at three months, for all patients are shown in Figure 1a–c. In general, the largest decreases in each of these measurements were in patients whose follow-up 25(OH)D was above 50 nmol/L. After adjusting for age, sex, season, sun exposure, and exercise, a stepwise multivariate regression model for changes in weight, BMI, and waist circumference showed that body weight loss, and decreases in BMI and waist circumference reduction were all significantly associated with 25(OH)D concentrations as the independent variable at three months (Table 4).

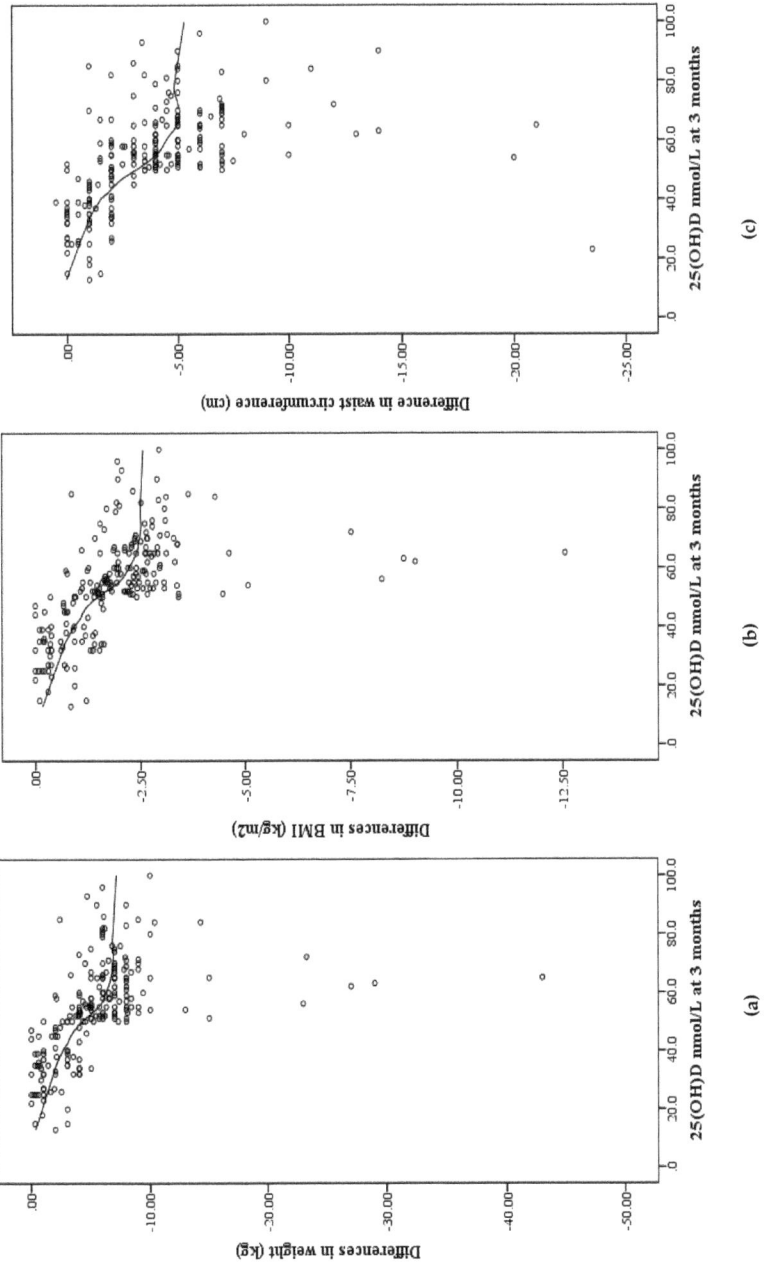

Figure 1. Shows changes in weight (**a**), BMI (**b**), and waist circumference (**c**) between baseline and 3 months plotted against serum 25(OH)D concentrations at 3 months for all 205 participants.

Table 4. Multivariate regression model [#] for the association between changes in weight, BMI, and waist circumference with concentrations of 25(OH)D at 3 months.

	Insufficient at Baseline N = 123		All Subjects N = 205	
Change (Δ) in Parameters over 3 Months	Non-Supplemented (Insuf-NonSup)	Supplemented (Insuf-Sup)	Non-Supplemented	Supplemented
N	48	75	130	75
Δweight, kg	−0.45 ***	−0.61 ***	−0.47 ***	−0.60 ***
ΔBMI, kg/m^2	−0.45 ***	−0.63 ***	−0.46 ***	−0.63 ***
Δwaist circumference, cm	−0.75 ***	−0.29 ***	−0.55 ***	−0.29 ***

Data expressed as adjusted beta coefficients [#] Adjusted for age, sex, season, sun exposure, and exercise. Difference = (follow-up − baseline) values, *** $p < 0.001$.

5. Discussion

The results presented here, derived from clinical dietetic practice, showed that higher baseline vitamin D status was associated with significantly greater weight loss and larger reductions in BMI and in waist circumference during a weight loss program. The analysis also showed that, on this individually tailored weight loss program, vitamin D supplementation for those participants who were vitamin D insufficient at baseline, enhanced weight loss, BMI reductions, and reductions in waist circumference.

Although there have been a number of studies on the effects of vitamin D status and vitamin D supplementation on weight loss and related parameters over time (reviewed in [22–24]), most of these studies did not include subjecting participants to an individually tailored weight loss regimen. Overall, the results of meta-analyses of studies which did not include a specific weight loss regimen, showed that while better vitamin D status before or during a randomized controlled trial of vitamin D supplementation predicted greater weight or fat loss over time in a few studies, overall there was no effect of vitamin D supplementation on body mass index or fat mass, even in larger studies of longer duration, such as that of Sneve et al. [25]. A recent publication reported a significant reduction in waist circumference in subjects in a randomized controlled trial of 16 weeks of high dose vitamin D supplements vs. placebo [26]. The subjects were of Asian ethnicity living in Melbourne, Australia and this was a secondary analysis of the trial, which did not include instructions on weight loss. Vitamin D status has been reported to affect weight loss and related parameters in some trials involving weight loss regimens [27,28], but not in the majority of such studies, although body weight or composition were secondary outcomes in most of these studies [22,23]. A recent review by Bassatne et al. (2019) found no clear evidence for a beneficial effect of vitamin D supplementation on cardiometabolic parameters in obese individuals and the authors concluded that Vitamin D supplementation had no effect on weight loss [24], although data on biochemical parameters and weight loss are very scarce. In a study of children with variants in the fat mass and obesity-associated gene (FTO), which affect adiposity in an age-dependent manner, it was reported that FTO genotype re9939609 was associated with a significant weight gain in children who were vitamin D insufficient, defined as <75 nmol/L, but no significant genetic effects were observed in vitamin D sufficient children [29].

There have been very few randomized controlled trials which were designed to examine the effect of vitamin D supplementation on weight loss and body composition during a weight loss program. Zittermann et al. [14] randomized 200 healthy overweight men and women, with mean 25(OH)D of 30 nmol/L, who were on an individually tailored weight loss program, to either vitamin D3 supplementation (83 ug = 3332 IU/day) or a placebo. At the end of 12 months, 25(OH)D concentrations were 55 nmol/L higher in the supplemented group, but there was no significant difference in weight loss over this time between the two groups. Mason et al. [16] enrolled 218 overweight or obese women over 50 years, with baseline 25(OH)D between 25 and 80 nmol/L (mean 53 nmol/L) and randomized them to a weight loss program with 2000 IU/d of vitamin D3 or to weight loss with a placebo. Although changes in weight, BMI, and waist circumference were similar between the groups overall at 12 months, those women whose 25(OH)D rose to above 80 nmol/L (≥32 ng/mL) lost significantly more weight and reduced their waist circumference and percent body fat to a significantly greater extent than women who achieved a 25(OH)D of <80 nmol/L [16].

In our study there was no effect of vitamin D status at baseline or of vitamin D supplementation on changes in systolic or diastolic blood pressure, or changes in total cholesterol, HDL, or triglycerides. The decrease in LDL, however, was significantly greater in the baseline sufficient subjects as compared with the deficient group as a whole, and in the latter group, was significantly greater in those supplemented with vitamin D (Table 3). Mason et al. [16] did not report lipid data but did show a significant decrease in C-reactive protein in the vitamin D supplemented group amongst those with complete pill counts (97%) as compared with a placebo. Although Zitterman et al. [14] showed no effect of vitamin D supplementation on weight loss in their 12-month randomized controlled trial, vitamin D supplementation resulted in significant decreases in triglyceride and TNF-α concentrations, but a significant increase in LDL cholesterol. There have been inconsistent results reported in several studies, overall showing no effect on cardiovascular or inflammatory markers with vitamin D supplementation, although these were not carried out in conjunction with an individually tailored weight loss program [30].

The current analysis examined data was neither randomized nor blinded, and therefore the potential effects of conscious or unconscious bias cannot be discounted. Another limitation is the use of 24 h recall to assess adherence to the dietary plan, which is known to be biased by misreporting [31,32], specifically underreporting. Due to this limitation, which is difficult to overcome, it is not possible to properly assess the role that different energy intakes affected weight loss. The initial data included all records of those who attended the clinic for the standardized chronic disease management plan in the period September 2011 to March 2013. The criteria for exclusion were decided in advance of the data collection and, as expected, excluded a very large number of subjects. Nevertheless, the cohort of patients whose data were analyzed were all part of a standardized chronic disease management plan established through a clinical partnership between three medical centers and a dietetics clinic. The main variable was the referring primary care physician's preference for improvement of vitamin D status in the patients (either advice to increase sun exposure + multivitamins (in Australia, multivitamins have negligible vitamin D), or supplementation with either 2000 IU/d or 4000 IU/d of vitamin D3). Based on the data in Table 2, the groups were well matched. As patients were not randomized, there is a possibility that the effects of vitamin D supplementation were chance findings. The patient numbers in each of these groups were limited, so it is difficult to make definitive interpretations, although the apparently greater weight loss in the group supplemented with 4000 IU/day, who achieved higher 25(OH)D concentrations than those supplemented with 2000 IU/day, is intriguing and may at least provide preliminary data for future studies. Critical for vitamin D studies that are interpretable [33], the mean baseline 25(OH)D concentrations in the deficient group in this study were both well below 50 nmol/L, nearly 60% of subjects were deficient at baseline, and, although tablet counts were not performed, those who were supplemented increased their 25(OH)D concentrations by an average of 25 nmol/L (baseline deficient group).

A strength of this analysis is that the female and male subjects in the clinical cohort were relatively young, with a mean age <40 y. BMI and 25(OH)D concentrations did not differ between men and women at baseline or at three months (Supplementary Tables S1 and S2). Sex had no significant effect on changes in BMI, waist circumference, or 25(OH)D, and therefore males and females were combined for further analysis to increase statistical power. Nevertheless, there were effects of sex on other parameters tested. A further limitation of the analysis is that the data in Tables 2 and 3 were not adjusted for sex or other factors, unlike Table 4, which may have influenced the outcomes reported.

As indicated by the multivariate analysis (Table 4), the effect of the achieved 25(OH)D concentration on changes in weight, BMI, and waist circumference was present even after adjustment for age, sex, season, and physical activity, indicating that these factors did not explain the effect of vitamin D supplementation. The mechanisms which might explain an effect of vitamin D status on weight loss are poorly understood. It is generally agreed that high body fat is likely to cause low vitamin D status, due to sequestration of vitamin D in adipose tissue [11]. A Mendelian randomization approach has also reported that a higher BMI leads to low vitamin D status and not the other way around [13]. Possible explanations about how vitamin D status could influence adiposity are still speculative. Since low vitamin D results in increased parathyroid hormone, this increased parathyroid hormone could increase calcium influx into adipocytes, which in turn, could inhibit lipolysis and stimulate lipogenesis [34]. Adipocytes express 1α-hydroxylase [35] and actively accumulate 25(OH)D [36]. As reviewed by Ding et al. [2] the vitamin D receptor (VDR) is expressed in adipocytes and preadipocytes and its expression has been shown to be dynamically upregulated during adipogenesis. Paradoxically, VDR knockdown in adipocytes inhibited adipogenesis and VDR knockout mice showed less body fat and were resistant to diet-induced obesity [37]. Effects of vitamin D status on central control of appetite are also plausible, considering the wide expression of the VDR in the central nervous system, including the hypothalamus [38].

Decreases in anthropomorphic parameters in our study were generally greater in those subjects who were initially vitamin D sufficient, regardless of later supplementation. In those who were vitamin D deficient at baseline, supplementation with vitamin D improved the weight loss parameters measured. After initiation of a supplementation regimen, it takes approximately three months for 25(OH)D to reach a plateau [39,40], and therefore the initially deficient patients would have remained relatively deficient for part of the study period.

On the basis of these findings, we cannot discard the hypothesis that sufficient serum 25(OH)D concentrations could be a determinant of the success of a weight loss program. Since vitamin D is synthesized endogenously, it would not be possible to show an effect of supplementation in subjects who are already "sufficient" by whatever criteria this is determined. Indeed, in this study, a large proportion (60%) of the clinic population were vitamin D deficient at baseline. The results of the study support the proposal that correction of low levels of 25(OH)D could benefit weight loss and the lipid profile of some overweight or obese patients, leading to the conclusion that, in clinical practice, it is important to individualize vitamin D therapy and educate the patient on the need for supplementation only when necessary.

Supplementary Materials: The following are available online at http://www.mdpi.com/2072-6643/11/12/3032/s1, Table S1: Baseline characteristics of men and women; Table S2: 3-month follow up characteristics of men and women; Table S3. The Harris–Benedict equations.

Author Contributions: Conceptualization, M.A. and R.S.M.; methodology, M.A. and R.S.M.; software, X.L., T.C.B.-S. and K.E.B.; validation R.S.M.; formal analysis, X.L., F.F.-M. and K.E.B.; investigation M.A.; resources, D.P.; data curation, M.A., X.L., F.F.-M., K.E.B., and R.S.M.; writing—original draft preparation, M.A. and R.S.M.; writing—review and editing, X.L., D.P., T.C.B.-S. and R.S.M.; visualization, X.L., F.F.-M., K.E.B. and T.C.B.-S.; supervision, R.S.M.; project administration, M.A.

Funding: M.A., F.F.-M., K.E.B. have nothing to declare. R.S.M. has received lecture fees from Amgen Australia and Australian Doctor Group supported by an educational grant from Sanofi Pty Ltd.

Acknowledgments: The authors declare that apart from speaker fees from Amgen and the Australian Doctor Group (R.S.M.), they have no conflict of interest and they thank the managers of the medical centers who agreed to take part in this investigation by providing access to patients' medical records, and the nurses who made sure to remind the patients for follow-up appointments with the dietician.

Conflicts of Interest: The authors declare no conflict of interest.

References

1. Bouillon, R.; Marcocci, C.; Carmeliet, G.; Bikle, D.; White, J.; Dawson-Hughes, B.; Lips, P. Skeletal and extra-skeletal actions of vitamin D: Current evidence and outstanding questions. *Endocr. Rev.* **2019**, *40*. [CrossRef] [PubMed]
2. Ding, C.; Gao, D.; Wilding, J.; Trayhurn, P.; Bing, C. Vitamin D signalling in adipose tissue. *Br. J. Nutr.* **2012**, *108*, 1915–1923. [CrossRef] [PubMed]

3. Gouni-Berthold, I.; Krone, W.; Berthold, H.K. Vitamin D and cardiovascular disease. *Curr. Vasc. Pharmacol.* **2009**, *7*, 414–422. [CrossRef] [PubMed]
4. Mawer, E.B.; Backhouse, J.; Lumb, G.A.; Stanbury, S.W. Evidence for formation of 1,25-dihydroxycholecalciferol during metabolism of vitamin D in man. *Nat. New Biol.* **1971**, *232*, 188–189. [CrossRef] [PubMed]
5. Hewison, M. Vitamin D and the immune system: New perspectives on an old theme. *Endocrinol. Metab. Clin. N. Am.* **2010**, *39*, 365–379. [CrossRef] [PubMed]
6. Renehan, A.G.; Roberts, D.L.; Dive, C. Obesity and cancer: Pathophysiological and biological mechanisms. *Arch. Physiol. Biochem.* **2008**, *114*, 71–83. [CrossRef] [PubMed]
7. Johnson, A.R.; Milner, J.J.; Makowski, L. The inflammation highway: Metabolism accelerates inflammatory traffic in obesity. *Immunol. Rev.* **2012**, *249*, 218–238. [CrossRef]
8. Arredondo, A.; Azar, A.; Recamán, A.L. Diabetes, a global public health challenge with a high epidemiological and economic burden on health systems in Latin America. *Glob. Public Health* **2018**, *13*, 780–787. [CrossRef]
9. Wang, Y.; Beydoun, M.A.; Liang, L.; Caballero, B.; Kumanyika, S.K. Will all Americans become overweight or obese? estimating the progression and cost of the US obesity epidemic. *Obesity (Silver Spring)* **2008**, *16*, 2323–2330. [CrossRef]
10. Vaes, A.M.M.; Tieland, M.; de Regt, M.F.; Wittwer, J.; van Loon, L.J.C.; de Groot, L.C.P.G.M. Dose-response effects of supplementation with calcifediol on serum 25-hydroxyvitamin D status and its metabolites: A randomized controlled trial in older adults. *Clin. Nutr.* **2018**, *37*, 808–814. [CrossRef]
11. Wortsman, J.; Matsuoka, L.Y.; Chen, T.C.; Lu, Z.; Holick, M.F. Decreased bioavailability of vitamin D in obesity. *Am. J. Clin. Nutr.* **2000**, *72*, 690–693. [CrossRef]
12. Ortega, R.M.; Lopez-Sobaler, A.M.; Aparicio, A.; Bermejo, L.M.; Rodriguez-Rodriguez, E.; Perea, J.M.; Andres, P. Vitamin D status modification by two slightly hypocaloric diets in young overweight/obese women. *Int. J. Vitam. Nutr. Res.* **2009**, *79*, 71–78. [CrossRef]
13. Vimaleswaran, K.S.; Berry, D.J.; Lu, C.; Tikkanen, E.; Pilz, S.; Hiraki, L.T.; Cooper, J.D.; Dastani, Z.; Li, R.; Houston, D.K.; et al. Causal relationship between obesity and vitamin D status: Bi-directional Mendelian randomization analysis of multiple cohorts. *PLoS Med.* **2013**, *10*, e1001383. [CrossRef]
14. Zittermann, A.; Frisch, S.; Berthold, H.K.; Gotting, C.; Kuhn, J.; Kleesiek, K.; Stehle, P.; Koertke, H.; Koerfer, R. Vitamin D supplementation enhances the beneficial effects of weight loss on cardiovascular disease risk markers. *Am. J. Clin. Nutr.* **2009**, *89*, 1321–1327. [CrossRef]
15. Nagpal, J.; Pande, J.N.; Bhartia, A. A double-blind, randomized, placebo-controlled trial of the short-term effect of vitamin D3 supplementation on insulin sensitivity in apparently healthy, middle-aged, centrally obese men. *Diabet. Med.* **2009**, *26*, 19–27. [CrossRef]
16. Mason, C.; Xiao, L.; Imayama, I.; Duggan, C.; Wang, C.Y.; Korde, L.; McTiernan, A. Vitamin D3 supplementation during weight loss: A double-blind randomized controlled trial. *Am. J. Clin. Nutr.* **2014**, *99*, 1015–1025. [CrossRef]
17. Health AGDo. Chronic Disease Management (formerly Enhanced Primary Care or EPC)—GP services. 2014. Available online: http://www.health.gov.au/internet/main/publishing.nsf/content/mbsprimarycare-chronicdiseasemanagement (accessed on 10 March 2014).
18. Japur, C.C.; Penaforte, F.R.; Chiarello, P.G.; Monteiro, J.P.; Vieira, M.N.; Basile-Filho, A. Harris-Benedict equation for critically ill patients: Are there differences with indirect calorimetry? *J. Crit. Care* **2009**, *24*, 628.e621–628.e625. [CrossRef]
19. Nowson, C.A.; McGrath, J.; Ebeling, P.R.; Haikerwal, A.; Daly, R.M.; Sanders, K.; Seibel, M.J.; Mason, R.S. Vitamin D and Health in Adults in Australia and New Zealand: A position statement. *Med. J. Aust.* **2012**, *196*, 686–687. [CrossRef]
20. Farrell, C.J.; Martin, S.; McWhinney, B.; Straub, I.; Williams, P.; Herrmann, M. State-of-the-art vitamin D assays: A comparison of automated immunoassays with liquid chromatography-tandem mass spectrometry methods. *Clin. Chem.* **2012**, *58*, 531–542. [CrossRef]
21. Cleveland, W.S.; Devlin, S.J. Locally Weighted Regression—An Approach to Regression-Analysis by Local Fitting. *J. Am. Stat. Assoc.* **1988**, *83*, 596–610. [CrossRef]
22. Soares, M.J.; Chan She Ping-Delfos, W.; Ghanbari, M.H. Calcium and vitamin D for obesity: A review of randomized controlled trials. *Eur. J. Clin. Nutr.* **2011**, *65*, 994–1004. [CrossRef]

23. Soares, M.J.; Pathak, K. Vitamin D Supplementation for Obesity: Potential Mechanisms of Action and an Update of Randomized Controlled Trials. *Curr. Nutr. Food Sci.* **2014**, *10*, 29–35. [CrossRef]
24. Bassatne, A.; Chakhtoura, M.; Saad, R.; Fuleihan, G.E. Vitamin D supplementation in obesity and during weight loss: A review of randomized controlled trials. *Metabolism* **2019**. [CrossRef]
25. Sneve, M.; Figenschau, Y.; Jorde, R. Supplementation with cholecalciferol does not result in weight reduction in overweight and obese subjects. *Eur. J. Endocrinol.* **2008**, *159*, 675–684. [CrossRef]
26. Scott, D.; Mousa, A.; Naderpoor, N.; De Courten, M.; De Courten, B. Vitamin D supplementation improves waist-to-hip ratio and fasting blood glucose in vitamin D deficient, overweight or obese Asians: A pilot secondary analysis of a randomised controlled trial. *J. Steroid Biochem. Mol. Biol.* **2019**, *186*, 136–141. [CrossRef]
27. Shahar, D.R.; Schwarzfuchs, D.; Fraser, D.; Vardi, H.; Thiery, J.; Fiedler, G.M.; Bluher, M.; Stumvoll, M.; Stampfer, M.J.; Shai, I.; et al. Dairy calcium intake, serum vitamin D, and successful weight loss. *Am. J. Clin. Nutr.* **2010**, *92*, 1017–1022.
28. Ortega, R.M.; Aparicio, A.; Rodriguez-Rodriguez, E.; Bermejo, L.M.; Perea, J.M.; Lopez-Sobaler, A.M.; Ruiz-Roso, B.; Andres, P. Preliminary data about the influence of vitamin D status on the loss of body fat in young overweight/obese women following two types of hypocaloric diet. *Br. J. Nutr.* **2008**, *100*, 269–272. [CrossRef]
29. Lourenco, B.H.; Qi, L.; Willett, W.C.; Cardoso, M.A.; Team, A.S. FTO genotype, vitamin D status, and weight gain during childhood. *Diabetes* **2014**, *63*, 808–814. [CrossRef]
30. Autier, P.; Boniol, M.; Pizot, C.; Mullie, P. Vitamin D status and ill health: A systematic review. *Lancet Diabetes Endocrinol.* **2014**, *2*, 76–89. [CrossRef]
31. Lopes, T.S.; Luiz, R.R.; Hoffman, D.J.; Ferriolli, E.; Pfrimer, K.; Moura, A.S.; Sichieri, R.; Pereira, R.A. Misreport of energy intake assessed with food records and 24-h recalls compared with total energy expenditure estimated with DLW. *Eur. J. Clin. Nutr.* **2016**, *70*, 1259–1264. [CrossRef]
32. Tam, K.W.; Veerman, J.L. Prevalence and characteristics of energy intake under-reporting among Australian adults in 1995 and 2011 to 2012. *Nutr. Diet.* **2019**, *76*, 546–559. [CrossRef]
33. Lappe, J.M.; Heaney, R.P. Why randomized controlled trials of calcium and vitamin D sometimes fail. *Derm.-Endocrinol.* **2012**, *4*, 95–100. [CrossRef]
34. Zemel, M.B.; Shi, H.; Greer, B.; Dirienzo, D.; Zemel, P.C. Regulation of adiposity by dietary calcium. *FASEB J.* **2000**, *14*, 1132–1138. [CrossRef]
35. Friedewald, W.T.; Levy, R.I.; Fredrickson, D.S. Estimation of the concentration of low-density lipoprotein cholesterol in plasma, without use of the preparative ultracentrifuge. *Clin. Chem.* **1972**, *18*, 499–502.
36. Abboud, M.; Gordon-Thomson, C.; Hoy, A.J.; Balaban, S.; Rybchyn, M.S.; Cole, L.; Su, Y.; Brennan-Speranza, T.C.; Fraser, D.R.; Mason, R.S. Uptake of 25-hydroxyvitamin D by muscle and fat cells. *J. Steroid Biochem. Mol. Biol.* **2013**, *144*, 232–236. [CrossRef]
37. Wong, K.E.; Szeto, F.L.; Zhang, W.; Ye, H.; Kong, J.; Zhang, Z.; Sun, X.J.; Li, Y.C. Involvement of the vitamin D receptor in energy metabolism: Regulation of uncoupling proteins. *Am. J. Physiol. Endocrinol. Metab.* **2009**, *296*, E820–E828. [CrossRef]
38. Eyles, D.W.; Smith, S.; Kinobe, R.; Hewison, M.; McGrath, J.J. Distribution of the vitamin D receptor and 1 alpha-hydroxylase in human brain. *J. Chem. Neuroanat.* **2005**, *29*, 21–30. [CrossRef]
39. Camozzi, V.; Frigo, A.C.; Zaninotto, M.; Sanguin, F.; Plebani, M.; Boscaro, M.; Schiavon, L.; Luisetto, G. 25-Hydroxycholecalciferol response to single oral cholecalciferol loading in the normal weight, overweight, and obese. *Osteoporos. Int.* **2016**, *27*, 2593–2602. [CrossRef]
40. Ish-Shalom, S.; Segal, E.; Salganik, T.; Raz, B.; Bromberg, I.L.; Vieth, R. Comparison of daily, weekly, and monthly vitamin D3 in ethanol dosing protocols for two months in elderly hip fracture patients. *J. Clin. Endocrinol. Metab.* **2008**, *93*, 3430–3435. [CrossRef]

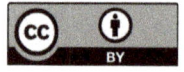

© 2019 by the authors. Licensee MDPI, Basel, Switzerland. This article is an open access article distributed under the terms and conditions of the Creative Commons Attribution (CC BY) license (http://creativecommons.org/licenses/by/4.0/).

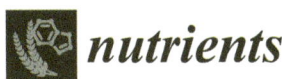

Article

Relationship between 1,25-Dihydroxyvitamin D and Body Composition in Middle-Aged Sedentary Adults: The FIT-AGEING Study

Alejandro De-la-O [1,*], Lucas Jurado-Fasoli [1], Manuel J. Castillo [1], Luis Gracia-Marco [2], Ángel Gutierrez [1,†] and Francisco J. Amaro-Gahete [1,2,*,†]

1. EFFECTS 262 Research Group, Department of Physiology, Faculty of Medicine, University of Granada, 18071 Granada, Spain; juradofasoli@ugr.es (L.J.-F.); gutierre@ugr.es (Á.G.); mcgarzon@ugr.es (M.J.C.)
2. PROFITH "PROmoting FITness and Health Through Physical Activity" Research Group, Sport and Health University Research Institute (iMUDS), Department of Physical Education and Sports, Faculty of Sport Sciences, University of Granada, 18071 Granada, Spain; lgracia@ugr.es
* Correspondence: delao@ugr.es (A.D.-l.-O.); amarof@ugr.es (F.J.A.-G.); Tel.: +34-958-243-540 (A.D.-l.-O. & F.J.A.-G.)
† These authors contributed equally to this work.

Received: 29 September 2019; Accepted: 21 October 2019; Published: 24 October 2019

Abstract: Vitamin D deficiency is a worldwide health problem that, in addition to its well-known negative effects on musculoskeletal health, has been related to a wide range of acute and chronic age-related diseases. However, little is known about the association of body composition with the active, hormonal form of vitamin D, 1,25-dihydroxyvitamin D plasma levels (1,25(OH)$_2$D). Therefore, the aim of this study was to investigate the association of 1,25(OH)$_2$D with body composition including lean and fat body mass as well as bone mineral density (BMD) in middle-aged sedentary adults. A total of 73 (39 women) middle-aged sedentary adults (53.7 ± 5.1 years old) participated in the current study. We measured weight and height, and we used dual energy X-ray absorptiometry to measure lean body mass, fat body mass and BMD. Body mass index (BMI), lean mass index (LMI), and fat mass index (FMI) were calculated. 1,25(OH)$_2$D was measured using a DiaSorin Liaison®immunochemiluminometric analyzer. The results showed a negative association of 1,25(OH)$_2$D with BMI, LMI and BMD ($\beta = -0.274$, $R^2 = 0.075$, $p = 0.019$; $\beta = -0.268$, $R^2 = 0.072$, $p = 0.022$; and $\beta = -0.325$, $R^2 = 0.105$, $p = 0.005$, respectively), which persisted after controlling for age and sex. No significant differences in 1,25(OH)$_2$D across body weight status were observed after controlling for the same covariates. In summary, our results suggest that 1,25(OH)$_2$D could be negatively associated with BMI, LMI and BMD whereas no association was found with FMI in middle-aged sedentary adults.

Keywords: vitamin D; calcitriol; body mass index; lean mass; fat mass; bone mineral density

1. Introduction

As the world´s population ages, the prevalence of chronic diseases increases, particularly over the last decades, becoming one of the great challenges that society faces [1,2]. Abnormalities in body composition such as a decrease of lean body mass and/or bone mineral density (BMD) or an increment in fat body mass are powerful predictors of morbidity and mortality risk as well as overall quality of life [3]. Epidemiologic studies indicate that these body composition changes are closely related to obesity, sarcopenia and/or osteoporosis in the elderly population [3,4]. However, these chronic diseases are progressive and initiate at a younger age [5,6]. Their high prevalence and concomitant health risk make them a particularly relevant worldwide public health problem and a social and economic burden [7–9].

Vitamin D is a fat-soluble vitamin essential for normal homeostasis of calcium and phosphorus, as well as for bone health [10] and preventing falls [11] and fractures [12]. Globally, vitamin D deficiency has been considered as a major public health problem affecting not only musculoskeletal health but also a wide range of several age-related chronic diseases [13]. 25-hydroxyvitamin D (25(OH)D) is the most commonly used biomarker when evaluating the relationship of vitamin D status with health-related outcomes [14–17]. However, 25(OH)D is thought to be largely inactive since it requires to be metabolized in the kidney by the enzyme 25-hydroxyvitamin D-1α-hydroxylase to be active. Therefore, 1,25-dihydroxyvitamin D (1,25(OH)$_2$D), also known as calcitriol, is responsible for most, if not all, of its biological effects [18,19]. The association between 1,25(OH)$_2$D and body composition parameters has been hard to establish for several reasons: (i) previously there was not a reliable and sensitive assay for calcitriol [20,21] and (ii) 25(OH)D has a higher concentration and longer half-life than 1,25(OH)$_2$D, thus requiring less sample volume for reliable measurements [22].

Consequently, epidemiological data are scarce, and a review of the scientific literature found no large studies examining the relationship between 1,25(OH)$_2$D and body composition outcomes. There is some evidence of the existence of an inverse association of 1,25(OH)$_2$D with body mass index (BMI) and fat body mass [23,24], however these data are conflicting with other studies [25–28]. In contrast, data are scarce on the potential relationship between 1,25(OH)$_2$D and lean body mass. Two recent studies found a significant association between low 1,25(OH)$_2$D and low lean body mass [29,30], which is highly dependent on the individual's age [29]. Similarly, controversial findings have been discovered regarding the role of 1,25(OH)$_2$D in bone health. Previous cross-sectional studies have reported an inverse association between 1,25(OH)$_2$D and BMD [31–33], whereas other studies found that 1,25(OH)$_2$D was unrelated to bone mineral content [34], bone loss [33,35] or hip fracture risk [36,37].

There are limited data on the study of body composition parameters in relation to 1,25(OH)$_2$D status in middle-aged adults. Thus, understanding whether 1,25(OH)$_2$D is associated with body composition parameters in this population is of clinical interest since, as previously established, the interventions to delay or reverse body composition related diseases are preferable when individuals are still relatively young and healthy [38,39].

Therefore, the aim of this study was to investigate the association of 1,25(OH)$_2$D with body composition including lean and fat body mass as well as BMD in middle-aged sedentary adults.

2. Materials and Methods

2.1. Study Design and Participants

The present cross-sectional study was conducted under the framework of the FIT-AGEING study (clinicaltrial.gov: ID: NCT03334357) [40]. The Ethics Committee on Human Research of the Regional Government of Andalucía approved the rationale, design, and methodology of the study [0838-N-2017] and all participants signed written informed consent in accordance with the Declaration of Helsinki (last revision guidelines, 2013).

Seventy-three middle-aged sedentary adults were recruited via electronic media, social networks and leaflets. The inclusion criteria were as follows: (i) to be sedentary (i.e., less than 20 min of physical activity on less than 3 days/week), (ii) not to have had greater body weight changes than 3 kg in the past 3 months, (iii) to be aged between 45 and 65 years old, (iv) not to be a smoker, (v) to be taking no long-term medication, (vi) not to be pregnant and (vii) not to suffer from any chronic cardiometabolic disease.

All tests were performed during September–October 2016/17 at the Sport and Health University Research Institute (iMUDS, Granada, Spain) and at the "Campus de la Salud" Hospital (Granada, Spain).

2.2. Anthropometric Parameters and Body Composition Assessment

A pre-validated Seca model 799 scale and stadiometer (Seca, Hamburg, Germany) was used to measure body weight and height with light clothing and without shoes. BMI was subsequently calculated as weight (kg)/height (m^2). Body composition outcomes were determined by a dual-energy X-ray absorptiometry scanner (Discovery Wi, Hologic, Inc., Bedford, MA, USA) obtaining lean body mass in kg, fat body mass in kg, and BMD in g/cm^2. A spine phantom quality check scan was conducted on each study day. A whole-body scan was performed considering all manufacturer's guidelines (i.e., the positioning of participants, the analysis of results and the quality controls among others). The APEX 4.0.2. software was used to draw an automatic delineation of anatomic regions. The lean mass index (LMI) was calculated as lean body mass (kg)/body height (m^2). Similarly, we calculated the fat mass index (FMI) as fat body mass (kg)/body height (m^2). Fat mass was also expressed as a percentage of the total body mass. The participants were categorized into three groups on the basis of BMI levels: (i) normal weight (BMI ≥ 18.5 and <25 kg/m^2), (ii) overweight (BMI ≥ 25 and <30 kg/m^2), and (iii) obese (BMI ≥ 30 kg/m^2).

2.3. Dietary Intake Assessment

We performed a total of three 24-hour dietary recalls collected on non-consecutive days (one weekend day included). This validated method is able to determine the energy intake to within 8–10% of the current energy intake [41]. The interviews were meal sequence-based, in which a detailed description of the food consumed by the participants was recorded. The 24-hour dietary recalls were collected by an experimented and qualified research dietitian (L.J.-F.), using a photograph guide to improve the quality of the information provided on portion sizes of food and assisting participants in the estimation of the consumed food quantity [42]. The software EvalFINUT® updated with data from USDA (U.S. Department of Agriculture) and BEDCA ("Base de Datos Española de Composición de Alimentos") was used to calculate energy and micronutrient (i.e., vitamin D, calcium and phosphorus) intake derived from the 24-hour recalls.

2.4. Physical Activity Assessment

Physical activity levels were objectively assessed with a wrist-worn accelerometer (ActiGraph GT3X+, Pensacola, FL, United States) for 7 consecutive days (24 hours/day) [40]. The sampling frequency was previously set at 100 Hz to store raw accelerations [43]. The ActiLife v.6.13.3 software (ActiGraph, Pensacola, FL, United States) and the GGIR package (v.1.5-12^2) in R (v.3.1.2^3) were used to process these files [44,45]. The participants came to the laboratory and specific information about how to wear the accelerometer was given. They were also reminded to remove it only during water-based activities such as swimming or bathing. Only the participants who wore the accelerometer for ≥16 hours/day for 4 days (including 1 weekend day) were included in the analysis.

2.5. Blood Samples Assessment

A 10 mL peripheral blood sample was taken from the antecubital vein after overnight fasting. It was collected using the Vacutainer SST system (Becton Dickinson, Plymouth, UK) in ethylenediamine tetra-acetic acid-containing tubes. Blood samples were centrifuged at four thousand revolution per minute for seven minutes at 4 °C and stored at −80 °C. Plasma levels of 1,25(OH)$_2$D were measured using a DiaSorin Liaison®immunochemiluminometric analyzer (DiaSorin Ltd, Wokingham, Berkshire, UK) and expressed in pg/mL.

2.6. Statistical Analysis

Data were checked for normality with the use of distribution plots (i.e., visual check of histograms, and Q-Q plots) and the Shapiro-Wilk test. The descriptive parameters were reported as mean and standard deviation.

Differences between sexes were examined using an independent samples T test. Given that no interaction for sex was observed ($p > 0.05$), data are presented for men and women together. Simple linear regression models were built to test the association of 1,25(OH)$_2$D and body composition outcomes (i.e., BMI, LMI, FMI, and BMD). We also performed multiple linear regression models to analyze these associations controlling for age (Model 1), sex (Model 2), and age and sex (Model 3). Additionally, we also adjusted these models for total energy, vitamin D, calcium, phosphorus intake and/or physical activity levels (i.e., light, moderate-vigorous and total physical activity). To test whether 1,25(OH)$_2$D was different across body weight status (i.e., normal-weight, overweight and obese individuals), an analysis of variance (ANOVA) was conducted. Moreover, we performed an analysis of covariance to test the differences of 1,25(OH)$_2$D across weight status adjusting for age and sex.

Data were analyzed with the use of the Statistical Package for Social Sciences (SPSS, v. 22.0, IBM SPSS Statistics, IBM Corporation, Armonk, NY, USA). Graphical plots were built using the GraphPad Prism 5 (GraphPad Software, San Diego, CA, USA). The level of significance was fixed at <0.05.

3. Results

Table 1 shows the descriptive parameters of our study participants by sex. No significant differences in 1,25(OH)$_2$D were observed between men and women ($p = 0.576$).

Table 1. Descriptive characteristics of participants.

	N	All		N	Men		N	Women	
Age (years)	73	53.7	(5.1)	34	54.6	(5.2)	39	53	(5.0)
Body composition parameters									
Body mass index (kg/m^2)	73	26.7	(3.8)	34	28.3	(3.6)	39	25.3	(3.3) *
Lean mass (kg)	73	43.2	(11.7)	34	53.9	(6.5)	39	34.1	(5.8) *
Lean mass index (kg/m^2)	73	15.2	(2.9)	34	17.5	(2.0)	39	13.2	(1.8) *
Fat mass (%)	73	40.1	(8.9)	34	34.7	(8.0)	39	44.5	(7.4) *
Fat mass (kg)	73	30.1	(8.5)	34	30.9	(9.8)	39	29.2	(7.1)
Fat mass index (kg/m^2)	73	10.8	(3.1)	34	10.0	(3.2)	39	11.4	(2.9)
Bone mineral density (g/cm^2)	73	1.1	(0.1)	34	1.2	(0.1)	39	1.0	(0.1) *
Dietary intake									
Total Energy intake (kcal/day)	72	2071.7	(455.4)	34	2312.1	(402.9)	38	1854.6	(390.3) *
Vitamin D intake (µg/day)	72	5.0	(6.0)	34	3.8	(3.3)	38	6.1	(7.6)
Calcium intake (mg/day)	72	763.4	(340.5)	34	867.3	(396.9)	38	670.5	(251.4) *
Phosphorus intake (mg/day)	72	1324.7	(558.9)	34	1507.6	(689.6)	38	1161.0	(342.2) *
Physical activity parameters									
LPA (min/day)	70	173.7	(45.4)	33	169.9	(52.7)	37	178.0	(40.7)
MVPA (min/day)	70	95.8	(35.6)	33	96.4	(37.1)	37	96.6	(35.7)
Total PA (min/day)	70	269.5	(75.1)	33	265.2	(79.3)	37	273.3	(72.0)
Blood parameters									
1,25 Dihydroxyvitamin D (pg/ml)	73	40.3	(14.1)	34	38.3	(13.4)	39	42.0	(14.6)

Data are presented as means (standard deviation). Abbreviations: LPA, light physical activity; MVPA, moderate-vigorous physical activity; PA, physical activity. * Significance differences between sexes ($p < 0.05$) obtained by the independent sample T test.

Figure 1 shows the associations between 1,25(OH)$_2$D and body composition related parameters. There was a significant negative association of 1,25(OH)$_2$D with BMI ($\beta = -0.274$, $R^2 = 0.075$, $p = 0.019$, Figure 1A), LMI ($\beta = -0.268$, $R^2 = 0.072$, $p = 0.022$, Figure 1B) and BMD ($\beta = -0.325$, $R^2 = 0.105$, $p = 0.005$, Figure 1D), which persisted after including age, sex, and age and sex in the model (all $p \leq 0.042$, Table 2). 1,25(OH)$_2$D was not significantly associated with FMI ($\beta = -0.080$, $R^2 = 0.006$, $p = 0.502$; Figure 1C), which did not change adjusting for age, sex, and age and sex (all $p \geq 0.35$, Table 2). The results remained unchanged after further adjusting for total energy, vitamin D, calcium, phosphorus intake and/or physical activity levels (i.e., light, moderate-vigorous and total physical activity) (data not shown, all $p > 0.1$).

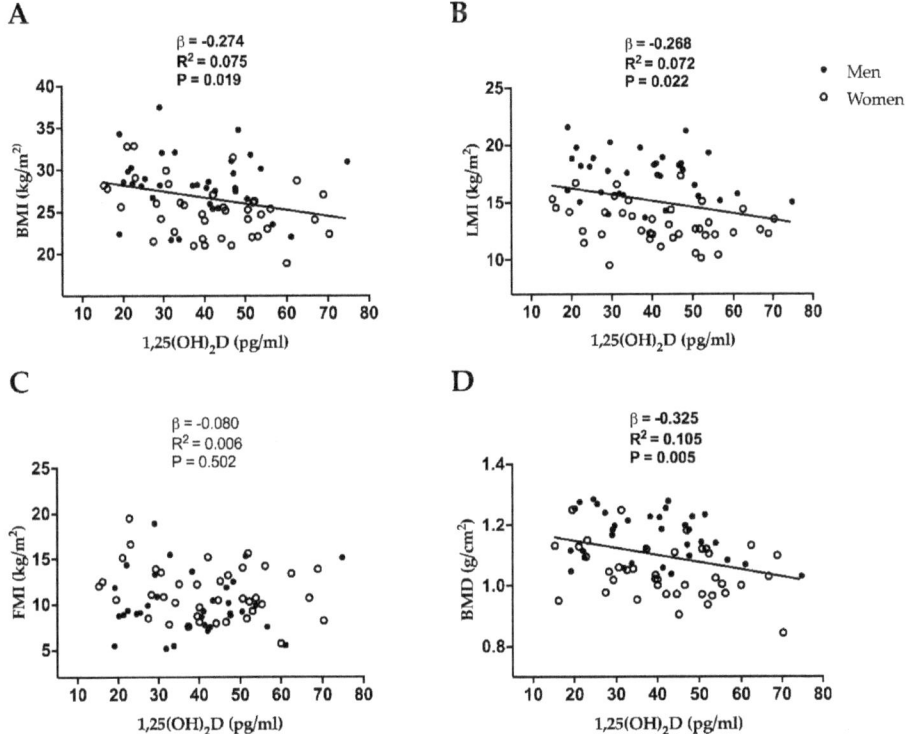

Figure 1. Simple linear regression graphs between 1,25-Dihydroxyvitamin D (1,25(OH)$_2$D) and body mass index (BMI) (**A**), lean mass index (LMI) (**B**), fat mass index (FMI) (**C**), and bone mineral density (BMD) (**D**) in middle-aged sedentary adults. β (standardized regression coefficient), R^2, and P from a simple linear regression analysis.

Table 2. Association of 1,25-Dihydroxyvitamin D with body mass index, lean mass index, fat mass index and bone mineral density.

	1,25-Dihydroxyvitamin D					
	Model 1		Model 2		Model 3	
	p value	β	p value	β	p value	β
Body mass index (kg/m^2)	**0.020**	−0.274	**0.040**	−0.263	**0.042**	−0.262
Lean mass index (kg/m^2)	**0.023**	−0.269	**0.030**	−0.383	**0.032**	−0.383
Fat mass index (kg/m^2)	0.505	−0.080	0.354	−0.112	0.356	−0.113
Bone mineral density (g/cm^2)	**0.005**	−0.325	**0.009**	−0.370	**0.009**	−0.377

Model 1 was adjusted for age; Model 2 was adjusted for sex; and Model 3 was adjusted for age and sex. p value of multiple-regression analysis. β (standardized regression coefficient). Values in bold indicate significance differences ($p < 0.05$).

ANOVA revealed no significant differences in 1,25(OH)$_2$D across body weight status (45.3 ± 13.3 pg/mL in normal-weight, 37.8 ± 13.1 pg/mL in overweight and 38.4 ± 16.7 pg/mL in obese individuals; Figure 2), which persisted after including age and sex as a covariate (44.8 ± 13.1 pg/mL in normal-weight; 37.9 ± 12.3 pg/mL in overweight and 38.9 ± 14.0 in obese individuals; $p = 0.2$).

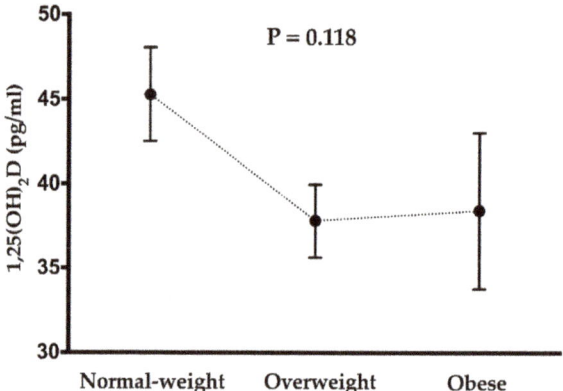

Figure 2. 1,25-Dihydroxyvitamin D (1,25(OH)$_2$D) by body weight status categories in middle-aged adults. Values are presented as means and standard error. p value obtained from the analysis of the variance to compare 1,25(OH)$_2$D across weight status (normal-weight, over-weight, and obese).

4. Discussion

The main results of the present study suggest that 1,25(OH)$_2$D is negatively associated with BMI, LMI and BMD independently of age and sex, whereas no association was found between 1,25(OH)$_2$D and FMI in middle-aged sedentary adults.

There is a controversy in the scientific literature regarding the 1,25(OH)$_2$D status of obese individuals. It has been described in classical studies that there are greater levels of 1,25(OH)$_2$D (~20 to 30%) in both obese men and women [25–28,46]. However, although we did not find any significant differences between BMI groups, we observed that overweight and obese individuals have ~16.6% and ~15.3% lower 1,25(OH)$_2$ than normal-weight individuals, which agrees with a previous large cohort that reported a ~18% lower 1,25(OH)$_2$D in the obese group compared with their lean counterparts [23,24]. These discrepancies between studies cannot be attributed to the individual's age, sex and/or BMI, since the participants had similar biological characteristics. A seasonal effect might explain these controversial results as the 1,25(OH)$_2$D assessment was conducted in winter months [46] or spring months [27] in some studies, while others did not control the season in which the blood samples were taken [24]. Given that the effects of ultraviolet ray exposure on 25(OH)D could be different for obese and lean individuals, the time of the year when the study was conducted may be of importance. However, previous studies have suggested that the season of the year does not present the same influence on 1,25(OH)$_2$D as it has on 25(OH)D [47]. The different 1,25(OH)$_2$D assay methods used across the studies could be one important factor to consider. While older studies applied radioreceptor assays [25–28,46] in which lipid interferences have been described when samples are not pure enough [48], more recent studies including our own study used modern immuno assays for the assessment of 1,25(OH)$_2$D [30,32]. Taken all together, it is likely that obese subjects present low 1,25(OH)$_2$D. This fact could be explained because obesity is associated with poor levels of 25(OH)D, and it has been demonstrated that 1,25(OH)$_2$D depends on substrate availability [23,49]. A higher fat body mass offers a greater distribution space for both fat-soluble compounds. Additionally, obese individuals are usually exposed to negative lifestyle factors (i.e., unhealthy dietary habits and sedentary behaviour, among others), [50] and to lower sunlight exposure [51]. These lifestyle factors have been shown to have a negative influence on vitamin D status [52,53].

The use of 25(OH)D as a key marker of vitamin D status has logical advantages summarized as greater serum stability and a longer half-life than other markers (e.g., 1,25(OH)$_2$D) [22]. However, it is important to consider that it is biologically inactive and therefore could not be the best vitamin D function indicator [54]. The shorter half-life of 1,25(OH)$_2$D could be one of the reasons why the relationship of 1,25(OH)$_2$D and lean body mass has not been deeply studied. Hassan-Smith et al. reported a positive association between 1,25(OH)$_2$D and lean body mass [29]. These findings differ from those observed in our study in which we obtained higher 1,25(OH)$_2$D in individuals with lower lean body mass. These discrepancies could be explained by the different biological characteristics of the subjects of the study (i.e., our cohort was older than the Hassan-Smith et al. study [29]) and by the different assay methods used to determine 1,25(OH)$_2$D. New studies measuring 1,25(OH)$_2$D are necessary to clarify this issue.

We also found a negative association between 1,25(OH)$_2$D and BMD in our study cohort which concurs with a previous study that reported a positive association of 1,25(OH)$_2$D and the bone resorption marker β-cTX [32]. These results are consistent with the notion that 1,25(OH)$_2$D increases bone resorption via stimulating intestinal calcium absorption after calcium intake [32]. Moreover, recent animal and in vitro studies have proposed that 1,25(OH)$_2$D has a direct effect on osteoclasts inducing bone resorption by its interaction with the receptor activator of nuclear factor-κβ/receptor activator of nuclear factor-κβ ligand signaling pathway [55,56]. Taking this into consideration, an inverse association would be expected between 1,25(OH)$_2$D and bone mineral density. In addition, it seems plausible that 1,25(OH)$_2$D is produced when BMD is low and once BMD is recovered 25 (OH)D is transformed into the inactive 24,25(OH)$_2$D. Although this argument could explain our findings, further intervention studies are needed to understand this issue.

Our study has some limitations. The cross-sectional design does not allow ascribing causality to the observed relationships. Further, our study population was limited to sedentary healthy middle-aged adults (45–65 years old) and hence these results may not be generalizable to younger, older, and/or physically active individuals. This study, like most clinical studies, was based on a single assay of 1,25(OH)$_2$D. We did not assess the 24-hydroxyvitamin D$_2$ plasma levels. In addition, a whole-body DXA scan was conducted, so future studies are necessary to investigate whether spine and hip bone mineral density have the same association pattern. Finally, due to the relatively small sample size of the current study, the data should be interpreted with caution. One of the strengths of this study is that body composition was measured using a gold-standard technology, such as dual-energy X-ray absorptiometry. In addition, the measurement of objective physical activity data and dietary intake to be used as covariates represent further strengths.

5. Conclusions

In conclusion, our results suggest that 1,25(OH)$_2$D could be negatively associated with BMI, LMI and BMD independently of age and sex, while no significant relationship was obtained between 1,25(OH)$_2$D and FMI in middle-aged sedentary adults. Intervention studies are needed to understand whether changes in body composition status are associated with changes in 1,25(OH)$_2$D in this age-population.

Author Contributions: Conceptualization, A.D.-l.-O., L.J.-F., M.J.C., L.G.-M., Á.G. and F.J.A.-G.; methodology, A.D.-l.-O., L.J.-F. and F.J.A.-G.; formal analysis, A.D.-l.-O. and F.J.A.-G.; writing—Original draft, A.D.-l.-O. and F.J.A.-G.; writing—review and editing, A.D.-l.-O., L.J.-F., L.G.-M., Á.G., M.J.C. and F.J.A.-G.

Funding: A.D.-l.-O. is funded by the Spanish Ministry of Education (FPU15/03960). L.G.-M. is supported by a fellowship from "la Caixa" Foundation (ID 100010434) and the fellowship code is LCF/BQ/PR19/11700007. F.J.A.-G. is funded by the Spanish Ministry of Education (FPU14/04172), the University of Granada *Plan Propio de Investigación 2016*-Excellence actions: Unit of Excellence on Exercise and Health (UCEES)-and *Plan Propio de Investigación 2018-Programa Contratos-Puente*.

Acknowledgments: The authors would like to thank all the participants that took part in the study for their time and effort. We are grateful to Ana Yara Postigo Fuentes for her assistance with the English language. This study is part of a PhD Thesis conducted in the Official Doctoral Program in Biomedicine of the University of Granada, Spain.

Conflicts of Interest: The authors declare no conflict of interest.

References

1. Jin, K.; Simpkins, J.W.; Ji, X.; Leis, M.; Stambler, I. The Critical Need to Promote Research of Aging and Aging-related Diseases to Improve Health and Longevity of the Elderly Population. *Aging Dis.* **2015**, *6*, 1–5. [CrossRef] [PubMed]
2. Fulop, T.; Larbi, A.; Witkowski, J.M.; McElhaney, J.; Loeb, M.; Mitnitski, A.; Pawelec, G. Aging, frailty and age-related diseases. *Biogerontology* **2010**, *11*, 547–563. [CrossRef] [PubMed]
3. Hamer, M.; O'Donovan, G. Sarcopenic obesity, weight loss, and mortality: The English Longitudinal Study of Ageing. *Am. J. Clin. Nutr.* **2017**, *106*, 125–129. [CrossRef] [PubMed]
4. Kohara, K. Sarcopenic obesity in aging population: Current status and future directions for research. *Endocrine* **2014**, *45*, 15–25. [CrossRef] [PubMed]
5. Hirschfeld, H.P.; Kinsella, R.; Duque, G. Osteosarcopenia: Where bone, muscle, and fat collide. *Osteoporos. Int.* **2017**, *28*, 2781–2790. [CrossRef]
6. Prado, C.M.; Purcell, S.A.; Alish, C.; Pereira, S.L.; Deutz, N.E.; Heyland, D.K.; Goodpaster, B.H.; Tappenden, K.A.; Heymsfield, S.B. Implications of low muscle mass across the continuum of care: A narrative review. *Ann. Med.* **2018**, *50*, 675–693. [CrossRef]
7. Harvey, N.; Dennison, E.; Cooper, C. Osteoporosis: Impact on health and economics. *Nat. Rev. Rheumatol.* **2010**, *6*, 99. [CrossRef]
8. Withrow, D.; Alter, D.A. The economic burden of obesity worldwide: A systematic review of the direct costs of obesity. *Obes. Rev.* **2011**, *12*, 131–141. [CrossRef]
9. Bruyère, O.; Beaudart, C.; Ethgen, O.; Reginster, J.-Y.; Locquet, M. The health economics burden of sarcopenia: A systematic review. *Maturitas* **2018**, *119*, 61–69. [CrossRef]
10. Holick, M.F.; Chen, T.C. Vitamin D deficiency: A worldwide problem with health consequences. *Am. J. Clin. Nutr.* **2008**, *87*, 1080S–1086S. [CrossRef]
11. Bischoff-Ferrari, H.A.; Dawson-Hughes, B.; Staehelin, H.B.; Orav, J.E.; Stuck, A.E.; Theiler, R.; Wong, J.B.; Egli, A.; Kiel, D.P.; Henschkowski, J. Fall prevention with supplemental and active forms of vitamin D: A meta-analysis of randomised controlled trials. *BMJ* **2009**, *339*, b3692. [CrossRef] [PubMed]
12. Looker, A.C. Serum 25-hydroxyvitamin D and risk of major osteoporotic fractures in older U.S. adults. *J. Bone Miner. Res.* **2013**, *28*, 997–1006. [CrossRef] [PubMed]
13. Zittermann, A.; Gummert, J.F. Nonclassical vitamin D action. *Nutrients* **2010**, *2*, 408–425. [CrossRef] [PubMed]
14. Autier, P.; Boniol, M.; Pizot, C.; Mullie, P. Vitamin D status and ill health: A systematic review. *Lancet Diabetes Endocrinol.* **2014**, *2*, 76–89. [CrossRef]
15. Cranney, A.; Horsley, T.; O'Donnell, S.; Weiler, H.; Puil, L.; Ooi, D.; Atkinson, S.; Ward, L.; Moher, D.; Hanley, D.; et al. Effectiveness and safety of vitamin D in relation to bone health. *Evid. Rep. Technol. Assess. (Full. Rep.)* **2007**, 1–235.
16. Visser, M.; Deeg, D.J.H.; Lips, P. Low vitamin D and high parathyroid hormone levels as determinants of loss of muscle strength and muscle mass (sarcopenia): The Longitudinal Aging Study Amsterdam. *J. Clin. Endocrinol. Metab.* **2003**, *88*, 5766–5772. [CrossRef]
17. Afzal, S.; Brondum-Jacobsen, P.; Bojesen, S.E.; Nordestgaard, B.G. Vitamin D concentration, obesity, and risk of diabetes: A mendelian randomisation study. *lancet. Diabetes Endocrinol.* **2014**, *2*, 298–306. [CrossRef]
18. Holick, M.F. Vitamin D deficiency. *N. Engl. J. Med.* **2007**, *357*, 266–281. [CrossRef]
19. Norman, A.W. From vitamin D to hormone D: Fundamentals of the vitamin D endocrine system essential for good health. *Am. J. Clin. Nutr.* **2008**, *88*, 491S–499S. [CrossRef]
20. Jenkinson, C.; Taylor, A.E.; Hassan-Smith, Z.K.; Adams, J.S.; Stewart, P.M.; Hewison, M.; Keevil, B.G. High throughput LC-MS/MS method for the simultaneous analysis of multiple vitamin D analytes in serum. *J. Chromatogr. B Anal. Technol. Biomed. Life Sci.* **2016**, *1014*, 56–63. [CrossRef]
21. Casetta, B.; Jans, I.; Billen, J.; Vanderschueren, D.; Bouillon, R. Development of a method for the quantification of 1alpha,25(OH)2-vitamin D3 in serum by liquid chromatography tandem mass spectrometry without derivatization. *Eur. J. Mass Spectrom. (Chichester Eng.)* **2010**, *16*, 81–89. [CrossRef] [PubMed]
22. Lips, P. Relative value of 25(OH)D and 1,25(OH)2D measurements. *J. Bone Miner. Res.* **2007**, *22*, 1668–1671. [CrossRef] [PubMed]
23. Konradsen, S.; Ag, H.; Lindberg, F.; Hexeberg, S.; Jorde, R. Serum 1,25-dihydroxy vitamin D is inversely associated with body mass index. *Eur. J. Nutr.* **2008**, *47*, 87–91. [CrossRef] [PubMed]

24. Parikh, S.J.; Edelman, M.; Uwaifo, G.I.; Freedman, R.J.; Semega-Janneh, M.; Reynolds, J.; Yanovski, J.A. The relationship between obesity and serum 1,25-dihydroxy vitamin D concentrations in healthy adults. *J. Clin. Endocrinol. Metab.* **2004**, *89*, 1196–1199. [CrossRef]
25. Bell, N.H.; Epstein, S.; Greene, A.; Shary, J.; Oexmann, M.J.; Shaw, S. Evidence for alteration of the vitamin D-endocrine system in obese subjects. *J. Clin. Investig.* **1985**, *76*, 370–373. [CrossRef]
26. Hey, H.; Stokholm, K.H.; Lund, B.; Lund, B.; Sorensen, O.H. Vitamin D deficiency in obese patients and changes in circulating vitamin D metabolites following jejunoileal bypass. *Int. J. Obes.* **1982**, *6*, 473–479.
27. Liel, Y.; Ulmer, E.; Shary, J.; Hollis, B.W.; Bell, N.H. Low circulating vitamin D in obesity. *Calcif. Tissue Int.* **1988**, *43*, 199–201. [CrossRef]
28. Kerstetter, J.; Caballero, B.; O'Brien, K.; Wurtman, R.; Allen, L. Mineral homeostasis in obesity: Effects of euglycemic hyperinsulinemia. *Metabolism* **1991**, *40*, 707–713. [CrossRef]
29. Hassan-Smith, Z.K.; Jenkinson, C.; Smith, D.J.; Hernandez, I.; Morgan, S.A.; Crabtree, N.J.; Gittoes, N.J.; Keevil, B.G.; Stewart, P.M.; Hewison, M. 25-hydroxyvitamin D3 and 1,25-dihydroxyvitamin D3 exert distinct effects on human skeletal muscle function and gene expression. *PLoS ONE* **2017**, *12*, e0170665. [CrossRef]
30. Marantes, I.; Achenbach, S.J.; Atkinson, E.J.; Khosla, S.; Melton III, L.J.; Amin, S. Is vitamin D a determinant of muscle mass and strength? *J. Bone Miner. Res.* **2011**, *26*, 2860–2871. [CrossRef]
31. Fujiyoshi, A.; Polgreen, L.E.; Hurley, D.L.; Gross, M.D.; Sidney, S.; Jacobs, D.R.J. A cross-sectional association between bone mineral density and parathyroid hormone and other biomarkers in community-dwelling young adults: The CARDIA study. *J. Clin. Endocrinol. Metab.* **2013**, *98*, 4038–4046. [CrossRef] [PubMed]
32. Vanderschueren, D.; Pye, S.R.; O'Neill, T.W.; Lee, D.M.; Jans, I.; Billen, J.; Gielen, E.; Laurent, M.; Claessens, F.; Adams, J.E.; et al. Active vitamin D (1,25-dihydroxyvitamin D) and bone health in middle-aged and elderly men: The European Male Aging Study (EMAS). *J. Clin. Endocrinol. Metab.* **2013**, *98*, 995–1005. [CrossRef] [PubMed]
33. Swanson, C.M.; Srikanth, P.; Lee, C.G.; Cummings, S.R.; Jans, I.; Cauley, J.A.; Bouillon, R.; Vanderschueren, D.; Orwoll, E.S.; Nielson, C.M. Associations of 25-Hydroxyvitamin D and 1,25-Dihydroxyvitamin D with Bone Mineral Density, Bone Mineral Density Change, and Incident Nonvertebral Fracture. *J. Bone Miner. Res.* **2015**, *30*, 1403–1413. [CrossRef] [PubMed]
34. Orwoll, E.; Kane-Johnson, N.; Cook, J.; Roberts, L.; Strasik, L.; McClung, M. Acute parathyroid hormone secretory dynamics: Hormone secretion from normal primate and adenomatous human tissue in response to changes in extracellular calcium concentration. *J. Clin. Endocrinol. Metab.* **1986**, *62*, 950–955. [CrossRef] [PubMed]
35. Stone, K.; Bauer, D.C.; Black, D.M.; Sklarin, P.; Ensrud, K.E.; Cummings, S.R. Hormonal predictors of bone loss in elderly women: A prospective study. The Study of Osteoporotic Fractures Research Group. *J. Bone Miner. Res.* **1998**, *13*, 1167–1174. [CrossRef]
36. Cummings, S.R.; Browner, W.S.; Bauer, D.; Stone, K.; Ensrud, K.; Jamal, S.; Ettinger, B. Endogenous hormones and the risk of hip and vertebral fractures among older women. Study of Osteoporotic Fractures Research Group. *N. Engl. J. Med.* **1998**, *339*, 733–738. [CrossRef]
37. Lips, P.; Netelenbos, J.C.; Jongen, M.J.; van Ginkel, F.C.; Althuis, A.L.; van Schaik, C.L.; van der Vijgh, W.J.; Vermeiden, J.P.; van der Meer, C. Histomorphometric profile and vitamin D status in patients with femoral neck fracture. *Metab. Bone Dis. Relat. Res.* **1982**, *4*, 85–93. [CrossRef]
38. Fontana, L.; Kennedy, B.K.; Longo, V.D.; Seals, D.; Melov, S. Medical research: Treat ageing. *Nature* **2014**, *511*, 405–407. [CrossRef]
39. Belsky, D.W.; Caspi, A.; Houts, R.; Cohen, H.J.; Corcoran, D.L.; Danese, A.; Harrington, H.; Israel, S.; Levine, M.E.; Schaefer, J.D.; et al. Quantification of biological aging in young adults. *Proc. Natl. Acad. Sci. USA* **2015**, *112*, E4104–E4110. [CrossRef]
40. Amaro-Gahete, F.J.; De-la-O, A.; Jurado-Fasoli, L.; Espuch-Oliver, A.; Robles-Gonzalez, L.; Navarro-Lomas, G.; de Haro, T.; Femia, P.; Castillo, M.J.; Gutierrez, A. Exercise training as S-Klotho protein stimulator in sedentary healthy adults: Rationale, design, and methodology. *Contemp. Clin. Trials Commun.* **2018**, *11*, 10–19. [CrossRef]
41. Halliday, T.M.; Davy, B.M.; Clark, A.G.; Baugh, M.E.; Hedrick, V.E.; Marinik, E.L.; Flack, K.D.; Savla, J.; Winett, S.; Winett, R.A. Dietary intake modification in response to a participation in a resistance training program for sedentary older adults with prediabetes: Findings from the Resist Diabetes study. *Eat. Behav.* **2014**, *15*, 379–382. [CrossRef] [PubMed]

42. López, M.D.R.; Martín-Lagos, R.A.; Martin-Lagos, R.A. *Guía para Estudios Dietéticos: Álbum Fotográfico de Alimentos*; Editorial Universidad de Granada: Granada, Spain, 2010; ISBN 9788433851673.
43. Migueles, J.H.; Cadenas-Sanchez, C.; Ekelund, U.; Delisle Nystrom, C.; Mora-Gonzalez, J.; Lof, M.; Labayen, I.; Ruiz, J.R.; Ortega, F.B. Accelerometer Data Collection and Processing Criteria to Assess Physical Activity and Other Outcomes: A Systematic Review and Practical Considerations. *Sports Med.* **2017**, *47*, 1821–1845. [CrossRef] [PubMed]
44. Hildebrand, M.; Hansen, B.H.; van Hees, V.T.; Ekelund, U. Evaluation of raw acceleration sedentary thresholds in children and adults. *Scand. J. Med. Sci. Sports* **2017**, *27*, 1814–1823. [CrossRef] [PubMed]
45. Hildebrand, M.; VAN Hees, V.T.; Hansen, B.H.; Ekelund, U. Age group comparability of raw accelerometer output from wrist- and hip-worn monitors. *Med. Sci. Sports Exerc.* **2014**, *46*, 1816–1824. [CrossRef]
46. Zamboni, G.; Soffiati, M.; Giavarina, D.; Tato, L. Mineral metabolism in obese children. *Acta Paediatr. Scand.* **1988**, *77*, 741–746. [CrossRef]
47. Zittermann, A. Vitamin D in preventive medicine: Are we ignoring the evidence? *Br. J. Nutr.* **2003**, *89*, 552–572. [CrossRef]
48. Clarke, A.D.; Rowbury, C.S. Removal of lipids before liquid chromatography of vitamin D in serum. *Clin. Chem.* **1985**, *31*, 657–658.
49. Zittermann, A. Vitamin D and disease prevention with special reference to cardiovascular disease. *Prog. Biophys. Mol. Biol.* **2006**, *92*, 39–48. [CrossRef]
50. Mozaffarian, D. Foods, obesity, and diabetes-are all calories created equal? *Nutr. Rev.* **2017**, *75*, 19–31. [CrossRef]
51. Vimaleswaran, K.S.; Berry, D.J.; Lu, C.; Tikkanen, E.; Pilz, S.; Hiraki, L.T.; Cooper, J.D.; Dastani, Z.; Li, R.; Houston, D.K.; et al. Causal relationship between obesity and vitamin D status: Bi-directional Mendelian randomization analysis of multiple cohorts. *PLoS Med.* **2013**, *10*, e1001383. [CrossRef]
52. Skaaby, T.; Husemoen, L.L.N.; Thuesen, B.H.; Pisinger, C.; Hannemann, A.; Jorgensen, T.; Linneberg, A. Longitudinal associations between lifestyle and vitamin D: A general population study with repeated vitamin D measurements. *Endocrine* **2016**, *51*, 342–350. [CrossRef] [PubMed]
53. Need, A.G.; Morris, H.A.; Horowitz, M.; Nordin, C. Effects of skin thickness, age, body fat, and sunlight on serum 25-hydroxyvitamin D. *Am. J. Clin. Nutr.* **1993**, *58*, 882–885. [CrossRef] [PubMed]
54. Ryan, Z.C.; Craig, T.A.; Folmes, C.D.; Wang, X.; Lanza, I.R.; Schaible, N.S.; Salisbury, J.L.; Nair, K.S.; Terzic, A.; Sieck, G.C. 1α, 25-dihydroxyvitamin D3 regulates mitochondrial oxygen consumption and dynamics in human skeletal muscle cells. *J. Biol. Chem.* **2016**, *291*, 1514–1528. [CrossRef] [PubMed]
55. Lieben, L.; Carmeliet, G.; Masuyama, R. Calcemic actions of vitamin D: Effects on the intestine, kidney and bone. *Best Pract. Res. Clin. Endocrinol. Metab.* **2011**, *25*, 561–572. [CrossRef]
56. Lips, P. Vitamin D physiology. *Prog. Biophys. Mol. Biol.* **2006**, *92*, 4–8. [CrossRef]

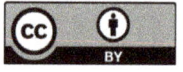

© 2019 by the authors. Licensee MDPI, Basel, Switzerland. This article is an open access article distributed under the terms and conditions of the Creative Commons Attribution (CC BY) license (http://creativecommons.org/licenses/by/4.0/).

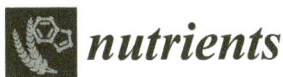

Article

Muscular Fitness Mediates the Association between 25-Hydroxyvitamin D and Areal Bone Mineral Density in Children with Overweight/Obesity

Jose J. Gil-Cosano [1,*], Luis Gracia-Marco [1,2,*], Esther Ubago-Guisado [1,3], Jairo H. Migueles [1], Jose Mora-Gonzalez [1], María V. Escolano-Margarit [4], José Gómez-Vida [4], José Maldonado [5,6] and Francisco B. Ortega [1]

[1] PROFITH "PROmoting FITness and Health through Physical Activity" Research Group, Sport and Health University Research Institute (iMUDS), Department of Physical Education and Sports, Faculty of Sport Sciences, University of Granada, 18071 Granada, Spain; esther.ubago@gmail.com (E.U.-G.); jairohm@ugr.es (J.H.M.); jmorag@ugr.es (J.M.-G.); ortegaf@ugr.es (F.B.O.)
[2] Growth, Exercise, Nutrition and Development Research Group, University of Zaragoza, 50009 Zaragoza, Spain
[3] Universidad de Castilla-La Mancha, Health and Social Research Center, 16002 Cuenca, Spain
[4] Department of Pediatrics, San Cecilio Hospital, 18012 Granada, Spain; mv.escolano@hotmail.com (M.V.E.-M.); gomezvida@gmail.com (J.G.-V.)
[5] Department of Pediatrics, School of Medicine, University of Granada, 18016 Granada, Spain; jmaldon@ugr.es
[6] The Institute of Biomedicine Research (Instituto de Investigación Biosanitaria (IBS), 18014 Granada, Spain
* Correspondence: josejuangil@ugr.es (J.J.G.-C.); lgracia@ugr.es (L.G.-M.); Tel.: +34-958-244-352 (J.J.G.-C.)

Received: 30 September 2019; Accepted: 11 November 2019; Published: 14 November 2019

Abstract: The association between vitamin D [25(OH)D] and bone health has been widely studied in children. Given that 25(OH)D and bone health are associated with muscular fitness, this could be the cornerstone to understand this relationship. Hence, the purpose of this work was to examine if the relation between 25(OH)D and areal bone mineral density (aBMD) was mediated by muscular fitness in children with overweight/obesity. Eighty-one children (8–11 years, 53 boys) with overweight/obesity were included. Body composition was measured with dual energy X-ray Absorptiometry (DXA), 25(OH)D was measured in plasma samples and muscular fitness was assessed by handgrip and standing long jump tests (averaged z-scores were used to represent overall muscular fitness). Simple mediation analyses controlling for sex, years from peak height velocity, lean mass and season were carried out. Our results showed that muscular fitness z-score, handgrip strength and standing long jump acted as mediators in the relationship between 25(OH)D and aBMD outcomes (percentages of mediation ranged from 49.6% to 68.3%). In conclusion, muscular fitness mediates the association of 25(OH)D with aBMD in children with overweight/obesity. Therefore, 25(OH)D benefits to bone health could be dependent on muscular fitness in young ages.

Keywords: Vitamin D; strength; bone health; mediation; childhood; obesity

1. Introduction

The World Health Organization defines osteoporosis as a systemic skeletal disease characterized by low bone density and microarchitectural deterioration of bone tissue [1]. Acquiring an optimal bone mineral accrual during childhood (i.e., late childhood and peripubertal years) is considered an important factor for reducing the risk of osteoporosis later in life [2]. In general, children with overweight/obesity usually have a greater areal bone mineral density (aBMD) than normal-weight children as they mature earlier, tend to be taller and have greater lean mass [2]. Notwithstanding,

Rokoff et al. [3] recently showed central adiposity to be inversely associated with aBMD Z-score at the total body less head (TBLH) in children with high levels of abdominal fat.

Childhood obesity is associated with a deficient 25(OH)D status in Spain [4]. Vitamin D status is reflected by 25-hydroxyvitamin D (25(OH)D) levels and its concentration in children with obesity is influenced by vitamin D intake, season, ethnicity/race, decreased exposure to sunlight as a consequence of the sedentary lifestyle, or by 25(OH)D sequestration through adipose tissue [5]. This prohormone is essential for bone development and remodeling processes, as well as for normal calcium and phosphorus homeostasis [6]. Some studies evidenced that 25(OH)D-deficient children had lower aBMD Z-score at the lumbar spine (LS) and the total body, probably influenced by the consequent increase in parathormone levels [7,8].

Moderate-to-high muscular fitness at a young age is a powerful determinant of health [9]. In this regard, Torres-Costoso et al. [10] found that children with good performance in handgrip and standing long jump had better and worse bone health, respectively. The latter associations were fully mediated by lean mass, whose function seems to be influenced by 25(OH)D levels [11]. When calcitriol (1,25(OH)$_2$D, an active metabolite of vitamin D) activates the nuclear vitamin D receptor (VDR), several slow pathways are activated leading to cytoskeletal protein synthesis important for muscle function (i.e., calmodulin, calbindin D-9K or insulin-like growth factor binding protein-3) [12–14]. Moreover, the activation of the nuclear VDR also increases phosphate metabolism via increases in the uptake and accumulation of phosphate and ATP, resulting in positive effects on muscle contraction [15]. In addition, the 1,25(OH)$_2$D activation of the membranous VDR stimulates rapid actions that affect Ca^{2+} handling and muscle cell proliferation and differentiation [16].

Although the relationship between 25(OH)D and muscular fitness has been described in youth, no study has jointly examined the association of these predictors with aBMD outcomes. Most published studies have been conducted using statistical multivariate procedures in order to control for potential confounders, but these statistical procedures are unable to distinguish between confounding and mediating variables. Mediation analysis allows us to clarify the process underlying the relationship between two variables and the extent to which this relationship can be modified or confounded by a third variable [17]. Therefore, the aim of this study was to examine whether the relationship between 25(OH)D and aBMD outcomes is mediated by muscular fitness in children with overweight/obesity.

2. Materials and Methods

2.1. Design

A cross-sectional analysis was conducted of the baseline measurements of the ActiveBrains project (registered at Clinicaltrials.gov, number NCT02295072). A detailed description of the study has been published elsewhere [18]. The ActiveBrains project measured 110 children with overweight/obesity aged 8–11 years from Granada (south of Spain) according to the following inclusion criteria: (1) to be overweight or obese based on the World Obesity Federation (formerly named International Obesity Task Force) cut-off points (2) to be 8 to 11 years old, (3) not to have any physical disabilities or neurological disorder that affects their physical performance, and (4) in the case of girls, not to have started the menstruation at the moment of the assessments.

A total of 81 children with overweight/obesity (10.0 ± 1.2 years old, 65% boys) with valid data on 25(OH)D, muscular fitness variables, body composition (i.e., bone, fat and lean mass) and sexual maturation were included in this report. Participants were recruited from the Pediatric Unit of the "San Cecilio" and "Virgen de las Nieves" University Hospitals in the province of Granada, Spain. Furthermore, we contacted several schools of Granada and we advertised the study in the local media, inviting any child meeting the inclusion criteria. The study protocol was approved by the Ethics Committee on Human Research (CEIH) of the University of Granada (Reference: 848, February 2014). Written consent was obtained from parents for the participation of their children.

2.2. Measures

2.2.1. Anthropometrics and Sexual Maturation

Participants were weighed using an electronic scale (SECA 861, Hamburg, Germany) with an accuracy of 100 g. A precision stadiometer was used to assess height (cm) and sitting height (SECA 225, Hamburg, Germany) to the nearest 0.1 cm. BMI was calculated as body mass (kg)/height (m^2) and the participants were classified as overweight or obese according to sex- and age-specific BMI cut-offs defined by Cole et al. [19].

Somatic maturity offset was assessed as years from peak height velocity (PHV) from age, height and sitting height using validated algorithms for children [20]. In boys: −8.128741 + (0.0070346 × (age × sitting height)), where R^2 = 0.906 and the standard error of the estimate = 0.514. In girls: −7.709133 + (0.0042232 × (age × height)), where R^2 = 0.898 and the standard error of the estimate = 0.528. PHV is the period of time of maximum growth in stature and therefore, years from PHV are considered in terms of time before and time after the PHV.

2.2.2. Vitamin D

Venous blood samples were obtained between 8:00 a.m. and 9:00 a.m. by venipuncture after an overnight fast (at least 12 h) from September 2015 to February 2016 (Autumn and Winter). Blood samples in tubes containing EDTA were spun immediately at 30,000 g for 10 min. Plasma was isolated and stored at −80 °C until assayed. Plasma 25(OH)D was analyzed by immunoturbidimetry (Alinity i 25-OH Vitamin D Reagent Kit ref. 08P4522, Abbot, IL, USA) with a sensitivity of 3.5 ng/mL and an intra-assay coefficient of variation of 2.5%.

2.2.3. Muscular Fitness

Upper-body muscular fitness was assessed using the handgrip strength test through a dynamometer with an adjustable grip (TKK 5101 Grip D, Takey, Tokyo Japan). Participants were instructed to squeeze continuously for ≥2 s with the elbow in full extension position. The test was repeated twice (right and left hands alternately). The best score of the 2 attempts for each hand was chosen and averaged [21]. Finally, relative upper-body muscular fitness was expressed per kg of body mass (Handgrip strength (kg/kg)). Lower-body muscular fitness was assessed by the standing long jump test. Participants were instructed to push off vigorously and jump as far forward as possible, trying to land on both feet. The distance reached was taken in centimeters from the take-off line and the heel of the nearest foot at landing. The longest attempt from 3 was recorded (cm). The scientific rationale for the selection of these tests, as well as their validity and reliability, has previously been demonstrated in children and adolescents [21].

A muscular fitness score (muscular fitness z-score) was computed by combining the standardized values of handgrip strength (kg/kg) and standing long jump (cm). Each of these variables was standardized as follows: z-score = (ith value − mean)/SD. The muscular fitness z-score was calculated as the mean of the 2 standardized scores (handgrip strength and standing long jump).

2.2.4. Body Composition

Children were scanned with dual-energy X-ray Absorptiometry (DXA) using the Hologic Discovery Wi (Hologic Series Discovery QDR, Bedford, MA, USA). The DXA equipment was calibrated at the start of each testing day by using a lumbar spine phantom as recommended by the manufacturer. All DXA scans and analyses were performed using the GE encore software (version 4.0.2) following the same protocol by the same researcher. The positioning of the participants and the analyses of the results were undertaken following recommendations from the International Society of Clinical Densitometry [22]. The total body scan was used to obtain fat mass, lean mass, and aBMD at the TBLH, arms, and legs.

2.3. Statistical Analysis

Descriptive characteristics of the participants are presented as mean ± standard deviation (SD) or percentages. All variables were checked for normality using visual check of histograms, Q-Q and box plots. Interaction analyses were performed for sex and since no significant interactions were found ($p \leq 0.28$), analyses were performed for boys and girls together.

A partial correlation analysis controlling for sex and years from PHV was performed to examine the relationship between 25(OH)D, muscular fitness variables, TBLH lean mass, and TBLH fat mass.

We carried out a mediation analysis controlling for sex, years from PHV, TBLH lean mass and season to test whether the association between 25(OH)D and aBMD outcomes was mediated by muscular fitness. These covariates were selected because of their well-known association with aBMD [23,24]. The PROCESS macro version 3.1, model 4, with 10,000 bias-corrected bootstrap samples and 95% confidence intervals was used for these analyses. In a nutshell, the mediation analysis is composed of ordinary least squared regression-based equations (paths) that allow us to answer the question of how a predictor transmits its effect (total effect) on an outcome being partitioned into direct (c′ path) and indirect effect (a × b path). Most contemporary analysts focus on the indirect effect by stating 2 steps in establishing mediation [25]: (1) show that the causal variable is correlated with the mediator (path a); (2) show that the mediator affects the outcome variable controlling for the predictor (path b). Thus, mediation is assessed by the indirect effect of the 25(OH)D (predictor) on aBMD (outcome) through muscular fitness (mediator). The total (c path), direct (c′ path), and indirect effects (a × b paths) are presented (Figure 1). Indirect effects with confidence intervals not including zero were interpreted as statistically significant [25] regardless of the significance of the total effect (the effect of 25(OH)D on aBMD outcomes) and the direct effect (the effect on aBMD outcomes when both 25(OH)D and muscular fitness are included as independent variables). The percentage of mediation (P_M) was calculated as "(indirect effect/total effect) × 100" to know how much of the total effect was explained by the mediation when the following assumptions were achieved: the total effect is larger than the indirect effect and of the same sign. All the analyses were performed using the IBM SPSS Statistics for Windows version 20.0 (IBM Corp: Armonk, NY, USA), and the level of significance was set to $p < 0.05$.

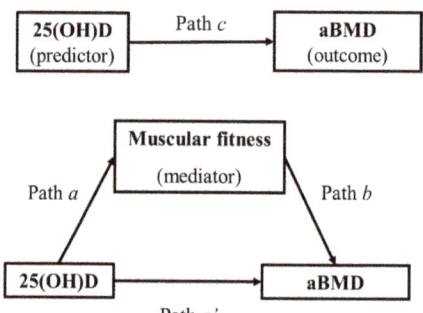

Figure 1. Causal diagram reflecting the simple mediation analyses. Path c shows the association between the predictor and the outcome. Arrows a × b show the natural indirect effect pathway, and c′ shows the natural direct effect pathway. *aBMD*: areal bone mineral density.

3. Results

Table 1 shows the raw descriptive characteristics of the participants at baseline (mean ± SD). Briefly, the mean age of the participants was 10.0 ± 1.2 years and they were 2.4 ± 0.9 years below PHV, overweight and obesity was evident in 28.4% and 71.6% of them, respectively; the mean 25(OH)D concentration was 31.5 nmol/L and only 6.2% of the children measured fell above the suggested cut-off of 50 nmol/L [26].

Table 1. Characteristics of the study sample by sex.

Variables	All (n = 81)	Boys (n = 53)	Girls (n = 28)
Age (years)	10.0 ± 1.2	10.2 ± 1.2	9.7 ± 1.2
Years from PHV (years)	−2.4 ± 0.9	−2.6 ± 0.9	−1.8 ± 1.1
Height (cm)	143.9 ± 8.7	144.5 ± 8.1	142.7 ± 9.8
Body mass (kg)	54.8 ± 10.7	55.8 ± 10.7	53.1 ± 10.8
TBLH fat mass (kg) [a]	21.9 ± 5.8	22.1 ± 5.9	21.5 ± 5.8
TBLH lean mass (kg) [a]	26.6 ± 5.2	27.3 ± 4.9	25.5 ± 5.3
BMI (kg·m^{-2})	26.3 ± 3.4	26.5 ± 3.4	25.9 ± 3.3
Overweight (%)	28.4	26.4	32.1
Obesity (%)	71.6	73.6	67.9
Autumn (%)	91.4	90.6	92.9
Winter (%)	8.6	9.4	7.1
25(OH)D (nmol/L) [a,*]	31.5 ± 9.5	32.7 ± 9.6	29.2 ± 8.9
Deficiency (%)	46.9	43.4	53.6
Insufficiency (%)	46.9	49.1	42.9
Sufficiency (%)	6.2	7.5	3.6
Muscular fitness z-score [b]	0.000 ± 1.000	0.032 ± 0.098	−0.061 ± 1.037
Handgrip strength (kg)/body mass (kg) [a]	0.307 ± 0.059	0.309 ± 0.058	0.303 ± 0.059
Standing long jump (cm) [a]	106.2 ± 17.8	106.5 ± 17.9	105.7 ± 17.9
TBLH (g·m^{-2}) [a]	0.772 ± 0.059	0.775 ± 0.059	0.766 ± 0.058
Arms (g·m^{-2}) [a]	0.607 ± 0.041	0.613 ± 0.041	0.596 ± 0.040
Legs (g·m^{-2}) [a]	0.913 ± 0.079	0.917 ± 0.082	0.906 ± 0.074

PHV peak height velocity; TBLH total body less head; BMI body mass index; 25(OH)D 25-hydroxyvitamin D; aBMD areal bone mineral density; [a] Values were Blom-transformed before analysis, but non-transformed values are presented; [b] Z-score mean computed from handgrip strength (kg/kg) and standing long jump (cm) tests; * Vitamin D status was defined as follows [26]: Sufficiency, > 50 nmol·L^{-1}; Insufficiency, 30–50 nmol·L^{-1}; Deficiency, <30 nmol/L^{-1}.

Partial correlations between 25(OH)D, muscular fitness variables, TBLH fat mass and TBLH lean mass after adjustment for sex and years from PHV are presented in Table 2. 25(OH)D was positively correlated with muscular fitness z-score and handgrip strength ($r = 0.28$ and $r = 0.29$, respectively). Muscular fitness z-score was positively correlated with TBLH aBMD and arms aBMD ($r = 0.24$ and $r = 0.35$, respectively), whilst handgrip strength was positively correlated with arms aBMD ($r = 0.32$). Finally, standing long jump was positively correlated with aBMD at TBLH, arms and legs ($r = 0.27$, $r = 0.29$ and $r = 0.23$, respectively).

Table 2. Partial coefficients of the independent variable with muscular fitness variables and aBMD outcomes adjusted for sex and years from PHV.

	Muscular Fitness z-Score [b]	Handgrip Strength/Body Mass	Standing Long Jump	TBLH aBMD	Arms aBMD	Legs aBMD
25(OH)D	0.275 *	0.285 *	0.186	0.039	0.043	−0.011
Muscular fitness z-score [b]	-	0.881 **	0.869 **	0.244 *	0.352 *	0.182
Handgrip strength/body mass		-	0.540 **	0.165	0.320 *	0.089
Standing long jump			-	0.266 *	0.295 *	0.233 *
TBLH aBMD				-	0.764 **	0.894 **
Arms aBMD					-	0.577 **

PHV peak height velocity; 25(OH)D 25-hydroxyvitamin D; TBLH total body less head: aBMD areal bone mineral density; [b] Z-score mean computed from handgrip strength (kg/kg) and standing long jump (cm) tests; Boldface indicates statistical significance: * $p < 0.050$, ** $p < 0.001$.

Mediation Analysis

Mediation analysis models are depicted in Figure 2. 25(OH)D was not significantly associated with any of the aBMD outcomes (c, total effect). Regarding path a, 25(OH)D was positively associated with muscular fitness z-score (Figure 2A, β = 0.277, p = 0.023) and handgrip strength (Figure 2B, β = 0.252, p = 0.038). In the path b, in all mediation models, muscular fitness was positively associated with TBLH aBMD (Figure 2A, β = 0.210, p = 0.004), arms aBMD (Figure 2B, β = 0.319, p < 0.001) and legs aBMD (Figure 2C, β = 0.204, p = 0.007). Finally, when 25(OH)D and muscular fitness were simultaneously included as independent variables (c', direct effect), aBMD outcomes were not predicted. There was a significant mediating effect of muscular fitness on the relationship of 25(OH)D with TBLH aBMD, arms aBMD and legs aBMD (P_M ranged from 49.6 to 68.3%).

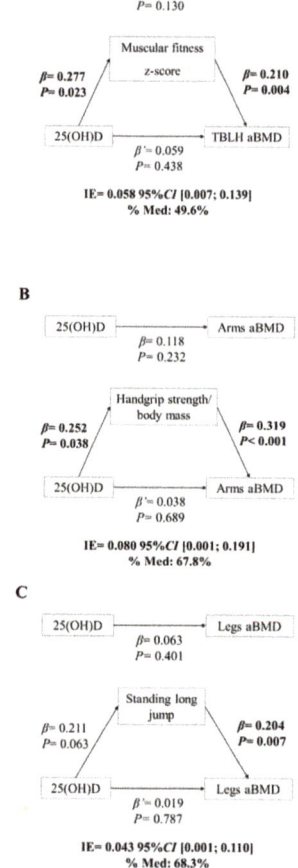

Figure 2. Simple mediation models of the relationship between 25(OH)D and aBMD outcomes using muscular fitness as a mediator, controlling for sex, years from PHV, TBLH lean mass and season. Muscular fitness z-score was used as a mediator in panel (**A**), handgrip strength/body mass was used as mediator in panel (**B**) and standing long jump was used as a mediator in panel (**C**). Z-score mean computed from handgrip strength (kg/kg) and standing long jump (cm) tests; *PHV* peak height velocity; *TBLH* total body less head; *25(OH)D* 25-hydroxyvitamin D; *aBMD* areal bone mineral density

4. Discussion

In the present study, we revealed a mediating effect of muscular fitness on the relationship between 25(OH)D levels and aBMD at the TBLH, arms, and legs after controlling for sex, years from PHV, TBLH lean mass and season. To the best of our knowledge, this is the first study in children with overweight/obesity analyzing whether muscular fitness acts as mediator in the association between 25(OH)D and aBMD outcomes.

Our results show no significant association between 25(OH)D and aBMD outcomes after adjusting for sex, years from PHV, TBLH lean mass and season (path c, total effect). This finding agrees with Hauksson et al. [27] who found no significant association between 25(OH)D levels and bone mineral accrual in Icelandic children at ages 7 and 9. On the contrary, Pekkinen et al. [7] reported that 25(OH)D status was a key determinant of aBMD in children and adolescents. In this regard, 25(OH)D status has been highlighted as a significant predictor of peak bone mass in males but not in females during childhood [28]. Likewise, non-significant associations between 25(OH)D and bone outcomes have been reported in American prepubertal girls after adjusting for potential cofounders [29] and in Finnish prepubertal girls after adjustment for maturation and BMI [8]. This could be explained by the differences in sex hormone effects on bone since estrogens may counteract the effects of lower 25(OH)D levels in females, whereas in males this compensatory effect is absent [28]. Nevertheless, we did not find sex interaction between 25(OH)D and aBMD outcomes, suggesting that these sex differences in hormonal effects on bone might not occur in prepubertal children with overweight/obesity since estradiol levels may be high in both boys and girls [30,31].

A few studies have assessed the effect of 25(OH)D in relation to muscular fitness in children [32–34]. In addition, the present study does so, taking into account different ways of measuring muscular fitness in the upper and lower limbs. The results of the present investigation confirm a relationship between 25(OH)D levels and muscular fitness z-score, handgrip strength and standing long jump (path a). These results agree with Foo et al. [32] who observed that adolescent girls with sufficient 25(OH)D status performed significantly better in handgrip strength compared with those with deficient or severely deficient status. Moreover, our results partly concur with Ward et al. [33] who found a positive association between 25(OH)D levels and the performance in countermovement jump in British adolescent girls. Otherwise, a study carried out with children did not find any relationship between handgrip strength and 25(OH)D status [34].

In this study, muscular fitness z-score, handgrip strength, and standing long jump were positively associated with TBLH aBMD, arms aBMD and legs aBMD, respectively (path b). Torres-Costoso et al. [10] reported a positive association between handgrip strength and aBMD outcomes in children aged 8–11 years, although a negative association between standing long jump and aBMD outcomes was found. The latter inverse association contrasts with our results. A possible explanation for these differences could be the different weight status of the participants included in both studies (BMI, 18.8 ± 3.8 vs. 26.3 ± 3.4). In addition, the fact that our results were adjusted for TBLH lean mass (but not in Torres-Costoso's study) could modify the direction of the association. Our findings agree with the literature and support the fact that bones adapt their resistance to the mechanical stimuli (i.e., body mass and muscle contractions) placed on them [35]. Moreover, it should be noted that the performance in the standing long jump test may be affected by the coordination skills [9], which might not be fully developed in 8–11-year-old children.

Our results show that the total effect of 25(OH)D on aBMD outcomes was mediated by muscular fitness z-score, handgrip strength and standing long jump (P_M ranged from 49.6 to 68.3%). Since the mediation analysis assumes that the predictor variable causes the mediator [17], muscular fitness may be an intermediate step in the causal pathway of 25(OH)D with aBMD. There is consistent evidence regarding the bivariate association of muscular fitness with both 25(OH)D [36] and aBMD outcomes [37,38]. Otherwise, the relationship between 25(OH)D and bone in children remains controversial [27,32]. In addition, a recent study has reported that the association between muscular fitness and aBMD is fully mediated by lean mass, whose function appears to be affected by 25(OH)D levels [11]. Together with our results, this evidence indicates that increasing 25(OH)D levels may increase muscular fitness and, ultimately, the aBMD. As an optimal bone mineral accrual is critical during childhood in order to prevent osteoporosis later in life [2], public health policies should start at an early age. Therefore, school-based interventions aiming at improving outdoor physical activity levels are justified among children to synthesize 25(OH)D and, ultimately, improve muscular fitness.

Strengths and Limitations

The current study has several limitations that should be acknowledged. First, our cross-sectional design rules out the possibility of identifying cause-effect relationships. Thus, the reported findings need to be confirmed prospectively. Second, the number of participants with complete data in all studied variables is relatively small. Third, although we did not find interaction by sex, our results need to be confirmed by studying boys and girls separately. Finally, calcium intake was not available and therefore, we did not include it in the model as a cofounder (i.e., vitamin D interacts with calcium affecting bone health [6]).

The present study has also several strengths, such as the use of relevant sets of cofounders (i.e., sex, years from PHV, TBLH lean mass and season) that are crucial to analyze the association of 25(OH)D with bone outcomes in children. Furthermore, valid and reliable tests for assessing muscular fitness were chosen from the ALPHA-Fitness battery [21]. Finally, we used DXA for assessing aBMD bone outcomes which are the gold standard for measuring bone outcomes and have been used worldwide in the pediatric population [22].

5. Conclusions

Muscular fitness plays a key role in the relationship between 25(OH)D levels and aBMD at the TBLH and arms. Increasing 25(OH)D levels may improve muscular fitness and, ultimately, aBMD in children with overweight/obesity. Future longitudinal studies must be conducted in order to confirm these findings.

Author Contributions: J.J.G.-C. was involved in the data collection and conceived the hypothesis, analyzing and drafting the manuscript. J.H.M., J.M.-G., M.V.E.-M., J.G.-V., J.M., and F.B.O. were involved in the study design, data collection, and critical revision. L.G.-M., E.U.-G. and F.B.O. participated in the interpretation of the results and critical revision. All authors have read and approved the final version of the submitted manuscript.

Funding: This study was supported by the Spanish Ministry of Economy and Competitiveness (Reference DEP2013-47540). This study takes place thanks to the additional funding from the University of Granada, UGR Research and Knowledge Transfer Fund (PPIT) 2016, Excellence actions: Units of Scientific Excellence; Scientific Unit of Excellence on Exercise and Health (UCEES) and the European Regional Development Funds (ERDF, ref. SOMM17/6107/UGR). In addition, this study was further supported by the SAMID III network, RETICS, funded by the PN I+D+I 2017-2021 (Spain), ISCIII-Sub-Directorate General for Research Assessment and Promotion and the European Regional Development Fund (ERDF) (Ref. RD16/0022). L.G-M is supported by a fellowship from "la Caixa" Foundation (ID 100010434) and the fellowship code is LCF/BQ/PR19/11700007. J.H.M. and J.M.-G. are supported by the Spanish Ministry of Education, Culture and Sport (FPU15/02645 and FPU14/06837, respectively).

Acknowledgments: The author gratefully acknowledge the children, parents, coaches, hospitals and schools who helped and participated in this study. We are grateful to Ana Yara Postigo Fuentes for her assistance with the English language.

Conflicts of Interest: The authors declare that they have no conflict of interest.

References

1. World Health Organization. Who Scientific Group on the Assessment of Osteoporosis At Primary Health. *World Health* **2007**. Available online: https://www.who.int/chp/topics/Osteoporosis.pdf (accessed on 3 April 2019).
2. Kelley, J.C.; Crabtree, N.; Zemel, B.S. Bone Density in the Obese Child: Clinical Considerations and Diagnostic Challenges. *Calcif. Tissue Int.* **2017**, *100*, 514–527. [CrossRef] [PubMed]
3. Rokoff, L.B.; Rifas-Shiman, S.L.; Switkowski, K.M.; Young, J.G.; Rosen, C.J.; Oken, E.; Fleisch, A.F. Body composition and bone mineral density in childhood. *Bone* **2019**, *121*, 9–15. [CrossRef]

4. Durá-Travé, T.; Gallinas-Victoriano, F.; Chueca-Guindulain, M.J.; Berrade-Zubiri, S. Prevalence of hypovitaminosis D and associated factors in obese Spanish children. *Nutr. Diabetes* **2017**, *7*, e248.
5. Alemzadeh, R.; Kichler, J.; Babar, G.; Calhoun, M. Hypovitaminosis D in obese children and adolescents: Relationship with adiposity, insulin sensitivity, ethnicity, and season. *Metabolism* **2008**, *57*, 183–191. [CrossRef] [PubMed]
6. Gil, Á.; Plaza-Diaz, J.; Mesa, M.D. Vitamin D: Classic and Novel Actions. *Ann. Nutr. Metab.* **2018**, *72*, 87–95. [CrossRef]
7. Pekkinen, M.; Viljakainen, H.; Saarnio, E.; Lamberg-Allardt, C.; Mäkitie, O. Vitamin D is a major determinant of bone mineral density at school age. *PLoS ONE* **2012**, *7*, e40090. [CrossRef]
8. Cheng, S.; Tylavsky, F.; Kröger, H.; Kärkkäinen, M.; Lyytikainen, A.; Koistinen, A.; Mahonen, A.; Alen, M.; Halleen, J.; Väänänen, K.; et al. Association of low 25-hydroxyvitamin D concentrations with elevated parathyroid hormone concentrations and low cortical bone density in early pubertal and prepubertal Finnish girls. *Am. J. Clin. Nutr.* **2003**, *78*, 485–492. [CrossRef]
9. Ortega, F.B.; Ruiz, J.R.; Castillo, M.J.; Sjöström, M. Physical fitness in childhood and adolescence: A powerful marker of health. *Int. J. Obes.* **2008**, *32*, 1–11. [CrossRef]
10. Torres-Costoso, A.; Gracia-Marco, L.; Sánchez-López, M.; García-Prieto, J.C.; García-Hermoso, A.; Díez-Fernández, A.; Martínez-Vizcaíno, V. Lean mass as a total mediator of the influence of muscular fitness on bone health in schoolchildren: A mediation analysis. *J. Sports Sci.* **2015**, *33*, 817–830. [CrossRef]
11. Hazell, T.J.; Deguire, J.R.; Weiler, H.A. Vitamin D: An overview of its role in skeletal muscle physiology in children and adolescents. *Nutr. Rev.* **2012**, *70*, 520–533. [CrossRef] [PubMed]
12. Brunner, A.; de Boland, A.R. 1,25-Dihydroxyvitamin D3 Affects the Synthesis, Phosphorylation and in vitro Calmodulin Binding of Myoblast Cytoskeletal Proteins. *Zeitschrift für Naturforschung C* **2018**, *45*, 1156–1160. [CrossRef] [PubMed]
13. Zanello, S.B.; Boland, R.L.; Norman, A.W. cDNA sequence identity of a vitamin D-dependent calcium-binding protein in the chick to calbindin D-9K. *Endocrinology* **1995**, *136*, 2784–2787. [CrossRef] [PubMed]
14. Barton-Davis, E.R.; Shoturma, D.I.; Musaro, A.; Rosenthal, N.; Sweeney, H.L. Viral mediated expression of insulin-like growth factor I blocks the aging-related loss of skeletal muscle function. *Proc. Natl. Acad. Sci. USA* **1998**, *95*, 15603–15607. [CrossRef] [PubMed]
15. Boland, R.; de Boland, A.R.; Marinissen, M.J.; Santillan, G.; Vazquez, G.; Zanello, S. Avian muscle cells as targets for the secosteroid hormone 1,25-dihydroxy-vitamin D3. *Mol. Cell. Endocrinol.* **1995**, *114*, 1–8. [CrossRef]
16. De Boland, A.R.; Nemere, I. Rapid actions of vitamin D compounds. *J. Cell. Biochem.* **1992**, *49*, 32–36. [CrossRef]
17. Baron, R.M.; Kenny, D.A. The moderator-mediator variable distinction in social psychological research: Conceptual, strategic, and statistical considerations. *J. Pers. Soc. Psychol.* **1986**, *51*, 1173–1182. [CrossRef]
18. Cadenas-Sánchez, C.; Mora-González, J.; Migueles, J.H.; Martín-Matillas, M.; Gómez-Vida, J.; Escolano-Margarit, M.V.; Maldonado, J.; Enriquez, G.M.; Pastor-Villaescusa, B.; de Teresa, C.; et al. An exercise-based randomized controlled trial on brain, cognition, physical health and mental health in overweight/obese children (ActiveBrains project): Rationale, design and methods. *Contemp. Clin. Trials* **2016**, *47*, 315–324. [CrossRef]
19. Cole, T.J.; Lobstein, T. Extended international (IOTF) body mass index cut-offs for thinness, overweight and obesity. *Pediatr. Obes.* **2012**, *7*, 284–294. [CrossRef]
20. Moore, S.A.; McKay, H.A.; Macdonald, H.; Nettlefold, L.; Baxter-Jones, A.D.G.; Cameron, N.; Brasher, P.M.A. Enhancing a somatic maturity prediction model. *Med. Sci. Sports Exerc.* **2015**, *47*, 1755–1764. [CrossRef]
21. Ruiz, J.R.; Castro-piñero, J.; España-romero, V.; Artero, E.G.; Ortega, F.B.; Cuenca, M.M.; Jimenez-pavón, D.; Chillón, P.; Girela-rejón, M.J.; Mora, J.; et al. Field-based fitness assessment in young people: The ALPHA health-related fitness test battery for children and adolescents. *Br. J. Sports Med.* **2011**, *45*, 518–524. [CrossRef] [PubMed]
22. Crabtree, N.J.; Arabi, A.; Bachrach, L.K.; Fewtrell, M.; El-Hajj Fuleihan, G.; Kecskemethy, H.H.; Jaworski, M.; Gordon, C.M. Dual-energy x-ray absorptiometry interpretation and reporting in children and adolescents: The revised 2013 ISCD pediatric official positions. *J. Clin. Densitom.* **2014**, *17*, 225–242. [CrossRef] [PubMed]

23. Ubago-Guisado, E.; Vlachopoulos, D.; Fatouros, I.G.; Deli, C.K.; Leontsini, D.; Moreno, L.A.; Courteix, D.; Gracia-Marco, L. Longitudinal determinants of 12-month changes on bone health in adolescent male athletes. *Arch. Osteoporos.* **2018**, *13*, 106. [CrossRef] [PubMed]
24. Vlachopoulos, D.; Ubago-Guisado, E.; Barker, A.R.; Metcalf, B.S.; Fatouros, I.G.; Avloniti, A.; Knapp, K.M.; Moreno, L.A.; Williams, C.A.; Gracia-Marco, L. Determinants of Bone Outcomes in Adolescent Athletes at Baseline: The PRO-BONE Study. *Med. Sci. Sports Exerc.* **2017**, *49*, 1389–1396. [CrossRef] [PubMed]
25. Hayes, A.F. Beyond Baron and Kenny: Statistical Mediation Analysis in the New Millennium. *Commun. Monogr.* **2009**, *76*, 408–420. [CrossRef]
26. Munns, C.F.; Shaw, N.; Kiely, M.; Specker, B.L.; Thacher, T.D.; Ozono, K.; Michigami, T.; Tiosano, D.; Mughal, M.Z.; Mäkitie, O.; et al. Global Consensus Recommendations on Prevention and Management of Nutritional Rickets. *J. Clin. Endocrinol. Metab.* **2016**, *101*, 394–415. [CrossRef]
27. Hauksson, H.H.; Hrafnkelsson, H.; Magnusson, K.T.; Johannsson, E.; Sigurdsson, E.L. Vitamin D status of Icelandic children and its influence on bone accrual. *J. Bone Miner. Metab.* **2016**, *34*, 580–586. [CrossRef]
28. Zhu, K.; Oddy, W.H.; Holt, P.; Ping-Delfos, W.C.S.; Mountain, J.; Lye, S.; Pennell, C.; Hart, P.H.; Walsh, J.P. Tracking of Vitamin D status from childhood to early adulthood and its association with peak bone mass. *Am. J. Clin. Nutr.* **2017**, *106*, 276–283. [CrossRef]
29. Stein, E.M.; Laing, E.M.; Hall, D.B.; Hausman, D.B.; Kimlin, M.G.; Johnson, M.A.; Modlesky, C.M.; Wilson, A.R.; Lewis, R.D. Serum 25-hydroxyvitamin D concentrations in girls aged 4-8 y living in the southeastern United States. *Am. J. Clin. Nutr.* **2006**, *83*, 75–81. [CrossRef]
30. Zhai, L.; Liu, J.; Zhao, J.; Liu, J.; Bai, Y.; Jia, L.; Yao, X. Association of obesity with onset of puberty and sex hormones in Chinese girls: A 4-year longitudinal study. *PLoS ONE* **2015**, *10*, e0134656. [CrossRef]
31. Zhai, L.; Zhao, J.; Bai, Y.; Liu, L.; Zheng, L.; Jia, L.; Yao, X. Sexual development in prepubertal obese boys: A 4-year longitudinal study. *J. Pediatr. Endocrinol. Metab.* **2013**, *26*, 895–901. [CrossRef] [PubMed]
32. Foo, L.H.; Zhang, Q.; Zhu, K.; Ma, G.; Hu, X.; Greenfield, H.; Fraser, D.R. Low Vitamin D Status Has an Adverse Influence on Bone Mass, Bone Turnover, and Muscle Strength in Chinese Adolescent Girls. *J. Nutr.* **2009**, *139*, 1002–1007. [CrossRef] [PubMed]
33. Ward, K.A.; Das, G.; Berry, J.L.; Roberts, S.A.; Rawer, R.; Adams, J.E.; Mughal, Z. Vitamin D status and muscle function in post-menarchal adolescent girls. *J. Clin. Endocrinol. Metab.* **2009**, *94*, 559–563. [CrossRef] [PubMed]
34. Blakeley, C.E.; Van Rompay, M.I.; Schultz, N.S.; Sacheck, J.M. Relationship between muscle strength and dyslipidemia, serum 25(OH)D, and weight status among diverse schoolchildren: A cross-sectional analysis. *BMC Pediatr.* **2018**, *18*, 1–9. [CrossRef] [PubMed]
35. Frost, H.M. Bone's Mechanostat: A 2003 Update. *Anat. Rec.—Part A Discov. Mol. Cell. Evol. Biol.* **2003**, *275*, 1081–1101. [CrossRef]
36. Ceglia, L. Vitamin D and Its Role in Skeletal Muscle. *Curr. Opin. Clin. Nutr. Metab. Care* **2009**, *12*, 628–633. [CrossRef]
37. Cossio-Bolaños, M.; Lee-Andruske, C.; de Arruda, M.; Luarte-Rocha, C.; Almonacid-Fierro, A.; Gómez-Campos, R. Hand grip strength and maximum peak expiratory flow: Determinants of bone mineral density of adolescent students. *BMC Pediatr.* **2018**, *18*, 96. [CrossRef]
38. Foley, S.; Quinn, S.; Dwyer, T.; Venn, A.; Jones, G. Measures of childhood fitness and body mass index are associated with bone mass in adulthood: A 20-year prospective study. *J. Bone Miner. Res.* **2008**, *23*, 994–1001. [CrossRef]

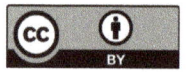

© 2019 by the authors. Licensee MDPI, Basel, Switzerland. This article is an open access article distributed under the terms and conditions of the Creative Commons Attribution (CC BY) license (http://creativecommons.org/licenses/by/4.0/).

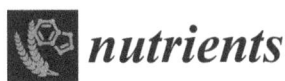

Article

May Young Elite Cyclists Have Less Efficient Bone Metabolism?

Marta Rapún-López [1], Hugo Olmedillas [2], Alejandro Gonzalez-Agüero [3,4,5,6], Alba Gomez-Cabello [3,5,6,7], Francisco Pradas de la Fuente [1], Luis A. Moreno [3,5,6,8], José A. Casajús [3,5,6,8] and Germán Vicente-Rodríguez [3,4,5,6,*]

1. Departamento de Expresión Musical, Plástica y Corporal, Facultad de Ciencias de la Salud y del Deporte, Universidad de Zaragoza, Huesca, C/Ronda Misericordia, 5, 22001 Huesca, Spain; mrapun@unizar.es (M.R.-L.); franprad@unizar.es (F.P.d.l.F.)
2. Department of Functional Biology, Universidad de Oviedo, Campus del Cristo B. Julián Clavería s/n, 33006 Asturias, Spain; olmedillashugo@uniovi.es
3. GENUD (Growth, Exercise, NUtrition and Development) Research Group, Universidad de Zaragoza, 50009 Zaragoza, Spain; alexgonz@unizar.es (A.G.-A.); agomez@unizar.es (A.G.-C.); lmoreno@unizar.es (L.A.M.); joseant@unizar.es (J.A.C.)
4. Department of Physiatry and Nursing, Faculty of Health and Sport Sciences (FCSD), University of Zaragoza, Ronda Misericordia 5, 22001 Huesca, Spain
5. Centro de Investigación Biomédica en Red de Fisiopatología de la Obesidad y Nutrición (CIBERObn), 28029 Madrid, Spain
6. Instituto Agroalimentario de Aragón (IA2), 50013 Zaragoza, Spain
7. Centro Universitario de la Defensa, 50090 Zaragoza, Spain
8. Department of Physiatry and Nursing, Faculty of Health Sciences, University of Zaragoza, Calle Domingo Miral, s/n, 50009 Zaragoza, Spain
* Correspondence: gervicen@unizar.es

Received: 10 April 2019; Accepted: 21 May 2019; Published: 26 May 2019

Abstract: The purpose of this work was to describe changes in metabolic activity in the bones of young male competitive cyclists (CYC) as compared with age-matched controls (CON) over a one-year period of study. Eight adolescent male cyclists aged between fourteen and twenty, and eight age-matched controls participated in this longitudinal study. Serum osteocalcin (OC), amino-terminal propeptide of type I procollagen (PINP), beta-isomerized C-telopeptides (β-CTx) and plasma 25 hydroxyvitamin D [25(OH)D], were investigated by an electrogenerated chemiluminescence immunoassay. Analysis of variance revealed no significant differences in formation and resorption markers between cyclists and controls. Within the groups, both CYC and CON showed decreased OC at −30% and −24%, respectively, and PINP where the figures were −28% and −30% respectively (all $p < 0.05$). However, only the CYC group showed a decrease in [25(OH)D], lower by 11% ($p < 0.05$). The similarity in the concentrations of markers in cyclists and controls seems to indicate that cycling does not modify the process of bone remodeling. The decrease in vitamin D in cyclists might be detrimental to their future bone health.

Keywords: cyclists; adolescence; bone turnover; osteocalcin; vitamin D

1. Introduction

Osteoporosis is a serious skeletal disease which continues to grow in our society, characterized by low bone mineral density (BMD) and microarchitectural deterioration of bone tissue, affected by the peak of bone mass obtained before 20 years of age [1]. People affected by osteoporosis present bone fragility and fracture risk, with a consequent deterioration in quality of life [2], and increased mortality [3]. Therefore, the prevention of the development of the disease is crucial and it should start during adolescence [4].

Several studies suggested that maximizing bone mineral acquisition during growth might reduce the risk of osteoporosis in later life [5–8]. Bone health and positive metabolic balance are influenced by genetic and environmental factors, including physical activity. Exercise during adolescence may contribute to the prevention of osteoporosis, although it needs to be a weight-bearing activity to be osteogenic [5,9]. In this sense, cycling may adversely affect bone mass during adolescence [10], and several studies have diagnosed osteopenia and osteoporosis in professional and master cyclists [11–13].

Bone development depends mainly on bone turnover, which includes bone formation and resorption [14], and may be estimated by different biochemical markers, osteocalcin (OC) and amino-terminal propeptide of type I procollagen (PINP) as markers of bone formation, and serum or urine beta-isomerized C-telopeptides (β-CTx) as a marker of bone resorption. The bone metabolism markers have been widely used to determinate the variations in the bone remodeling process as a consequence of physical activity [15–17], and indicate modeling and remodeling of bone tissue during pubertal growth and maturation [18].

Higher values of bone formation and resorption markers have been found in adolescent athletes [10,19], although similar results among athletes and controls have also been determined [20]. Additionally, it is important to know the vitamin D status because of the influence that this nutrient has on bone mass and bone loss [21]. Positive and direct associations between plasma 25 hydroxyvitamin D [25(OH)D] (active form of vitamin D) and bone mineral content (BMC) were previously described [21–24], however, there is a scarce amount of information on young cyclists, a population that may be at a higher risk due to their non-osteogenic sport participation.

Despite the importance of assessing bone metabolism in adolescents, there has been little research on the association between biochemical markers and sport participation, and most are cross-sectional studies. However, longitudinal studies may help us to understand how sport can influence bone metabolism, and how this is translated to bone development, which is crucial information to cyclists who seem to be at a higher risk of not achieving optimal peak bone mass [25,26].

The purpose of our longitudinal study was to measure the effect of cycling on bone metabolism in adolescent cyclists and to compare it to active age-matched peers.

2. Materials and Methods

2.1. Study Design

A one-year longitudinal design was used, with repeated measurements performed at the beginning and at the end of the season, in November and in October.

2.2. Ethics Statement

Written informed consent was obtained from parents and adolescents. The study was performed following the ethical guidelines of the Declaration of Helsinki 1961 (revision of Fortaleza 2013) and the Ethics Committee of Clinical Research from the Government of Aragón (CEICA; Spain) approved the study protocol. REF: CEICA: PI09/00063.

2.3. Participants

A total of eight young elite male road cyclists (CYC) from different cycling teams in Spain, and eight physically active controls (CON), recruited from secondary schools and colleges, agreed to participate in the study (Table 1). Cyclists and controls were excluded if they were aged over twenty-one, or if they were unhealthy, with any chronic disease, musculoskeletal condition, or bone fracture, if they regularly took medicines, or if they had other habits affecting bone development. One of the cyclists presented extreme values for most bone markers and was consequently deemed an outlier, and excluded.

Table 1. Descriptive characteristics of the sample. BMI, body mass index; SD, standard deviation.

	PRE				POST			
	Cyclists n = 7		Controls n = 8		Cyclists n = 7		Controls n = 8	
	Mean	SD	Mean	SD	Mean	SD	Mean	SD
Age (years)	16.3 ±	0.9	15.8 ±	1.5	17.6 ±	1.2	16.9 ±	1.5
Height (cm)	171.1 ±	7.5	173.3 ±	8	173.6 ±	8	174.5 ±	6.6
Weight (kg)	57 ±	5.8	66.1 ±	15.1	62.8 ±	6.6	67.1 ±	15.1
BMI (kg/m^2)	19.5 ±	1.7	22 ±	4.1	20.9 ±	1.8	22 ±	4.8
Years of cycling training (years)	2.6 ±	2.8			3.6 ±	2.8		
Hours of cycling training (h/week)	10.5 ±	7			13.5 ±	5.2		

BMI: Body mass index; SD: Standard deviation.

These young road cyclists were regular participants in regional competitions, and had trained under supervision for an average of 13.5 h per week (h/week) over a minimum of two and a maximum of seven years prior to the study. Control subjects were involved in recreational sports (rugby, tennis, handball, or football) for at least 2 h/week with occasional weekend matches, however, none of them cycled for more than one hour per week.

Subjects were asked to complete a medical and physical activity questionnaire, and to provide additional information in respect to physical activity, past injuries, medicines taken and known diseases.

2.4. Anthropometric Measurements

While the subjects were barefoot and clad in light indoor clothing, their body weight (kg) and height (cm) were measured with an electronic weighing scale (Type SECA 861; precision 100 g, range 0 to 150 kg) and a stadiometer (Type Seca 225; precision 0.1 cm, range 70 to 200 cm). Body mass index (BMI) was calculated as weight (kg) divided by height squared (m^2).

2.5. Blood Collection and Biochemical Analysis

Fasting blood samples (10 mL) were drawn at 8:00 a.m., after 10 h overnight, through an indwelling venous catheter placed in a forearm vein. Then, serum was separated and stored at −20 °C for later analysis. In order to avoid diurnal variations in plasma levels of total [25(OH)D], blood samples were obtained at the same time of the day [27].

2.6. Bone Turnover Markers

The concentrations of serum OC, PINP and β-CTx were determined by an electrogenerated chemiluminescence immunoassay using an Elecsys 2010 analyzer from Roche Diagnostics GmbH (Germany). The kits used were also purchased from Roche Diagnostics GmbH. The measuring range for serum osteocalcin was 0.50 µg/L to 300 µg/L (defined by the lower detection limit and the maximum of the calibration curve). Values below the detection limit were reported as <0.50 µg/L. Values above the measuring range were diluted with Elecsys Diluent Universal at a concentration below 60 µg/L. Osteocalcin presented coefficients of variation (CV) of 4.0% and 6.5% at 15.5 µg/L and 1.4% and 1.8% at 68.3 µg/L. The measurement range for total PINP in serum ran over from 5 µg/L to 1200 µg/L. Intra- and inter-assay CVs were 1.8% and 2.3% at 274 µg/L and 2.9% and 3.7% at 799 µg/L. Values below the detection limit were reported as <5 µg/L. Values above the measuring range of 1200 µg/L were diluted with Elecsys Diluent Universal at a recommended concentration of 1100 µg/L. Analytical sensitivity (the lower detection limit) was <5 µg/L. β-CTx had intra- and inter-assay CVs of 1.0% and 1.6% at 3.59 µg/L and 4.6% and 4.7% at 0.08 µg/L. The range for measurements was between 0.010 µg/L and 6.00 µg/L, the analytical sensitivity or lower detection limit was 0.01 µg/L, and the functional sensitivity was 0.07 µg/L.

2.7. Vitamin D Status

Plasma [25(OH)D] was analyzed by ELISA using a kit (Octeia® 25-Hydroxy vitamin D) from Immuno Diagnostic Systems (Germany) and measured with a Sunrise™ Photometer by Tecan (Mannheim, Germany). The sensitivity of this method is 5 nmol/L 25(OH)D and the variation was under 6%. The CV for the method was below 1%. The complete methodology has been described elsewhere [15].

2.8. Statistics

The normality of the data distribution was evaluated with the Kolmogorov–Smirnov test. All variables presented normal distributions, except PINP. Thus, this was logarithmically transformed although the original data are also reported.

The characteristics of the subjects were described using averages and standard deviation (SD) values for continuous variables. Independent t-tests were performed to evaluate differences between groups for descriptive variables. To determine how bone turnover markers and vitamin D status differed between groups, analyses of covariance (ANCOVAs) were applied, and adjusted for age. ANCOVAs for repeated measures ×2 (time) were performed between pre- and post-evaluation to determine the effects of cycling on bone metabolic markers and vitamin D status.

The probability value for the significance level was fixed at 0.05. Data were analyzed using the SPSS 19.0 statistical program (SPSS Incorporated, Chicago, IL, USA).

3. Results

Table 1 summarizes the descriptive characteristics of participants of the sample as a whole (cyclists and controls), before and after evaluation. The results showed no differences in any of the variables.

3.1. Bone Metabolism Markers and Vitamin D

Figure 1 shows the OC, PINP, β-CTx and the [25(OH)D] concentrations in cyclists (CYC) and controls (CON), before and after evaluation. No difference was observed between the groups for the markers or for 25(OH)D, either before or after evaluation (all $p > 0.05$).

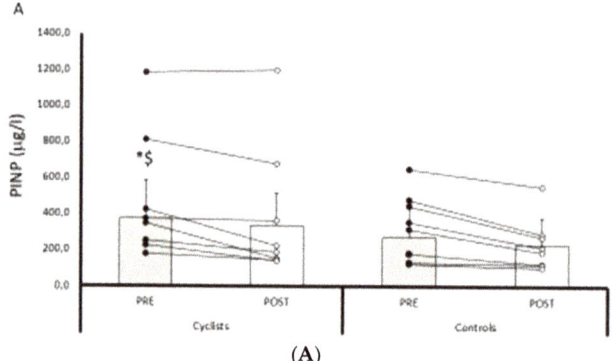

(A)

Figure 1. Cont.

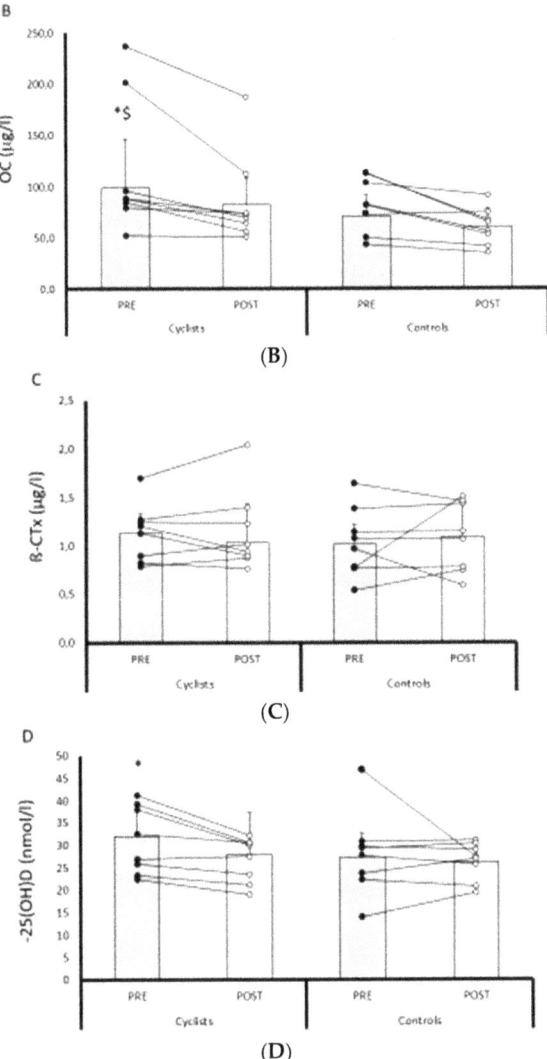

Figure 1. Panels (**A–D**) concentrations in cyclists ($n = 8$) and controls ($n = 8$), at pre- and post-evaluation. (**A**) Amino-terminal propeptide of type I precollagen (PINP). (**B**) Osteocalcin (OC). (**C**) beta-isomerized C-telopeptides (β-CTx). (**D**) Plasma 25 hydroxyvitamin D [25(OH)D]. Values are presented as the mean and SD. For final statistical analysis one cyclist has been removed (statistical outlier). The p values calculated with one-way analysis of covariance (ANCOVA), adjusting for age. * $p < 0.05$ compared to control group. $ $p < 0.05$ compared to cyclists group.

3.2. Changes within Group

Figure 1 shows intra-group results. With regard to bone metabolism, formation markers (OC and PINP) decreased in both the CYC and the CON groups (all $p < 0.05$). However, neither group showed changes in β-CTx (both $p > 0.05$). Nevertheless, [25(OH)D] decreased significantly in the CYC group ($p < 0.01$).

3.3. Group-by-Time Interactions

No group-by-time interactions were found in any parameters. This suggests that both groups evolved similarly (all $p > 0.05$).

4. Discussion

The results of this one-year longitudinal study showed similar decreases in bone formation markers for both the CYC and CON groups over time, just as had been described in previous long-term studies relating to bone turnover markers in young female athletes [20,28,29]. Thus, the results suggest that this trend seems to be similar in athletes of both sexes, and in accordance with the results recorded by García-Marco et al. [30] in a study with an adolescent population (aged between 12 and 17), which detected a decrease in markers as puberty progressed in both boys and girls. As previously noted, bone remodeling decreases with age independently of whatever sport may be practiced, so growth may perhaps mask the effects of physical activity at these ages. The relationship between bone metabolism markers and bone mineral parameters in children and adolescents is not clear. Hence, further studies are needed to determine the role of bone turnover markers and physical activity on bone mineral acquisition during puberty.

No differences were found between them, when adult cyclists and runners were investigated in one piece of research [13], and other authors have determined normal ranges of bone markers in a group of young cyclists [31]. However, adult cyclists presented lower values for bone alkaline phosphatase (BAP) as compared to triathletes, swimmers, and controls, but yielded similar values for OC and β-CTX in another study [16].

Although there has been no previous investigation of changes in bone metabolism markers in adolescent cyclists, some researchers have analyzed BMD and BMC amongst this population, finding that cyclists had lower values for both variables than the controls did [10,25]. Moreover, Olmedillas et al. [10] reported greater differences in BMC and BMD between cyclists and controls in adolescents over 17 years of age. Since bone mass can be defined as the net product of bone formation and bone resorption [14], the present results for bone metabolic markers cannot provide support for the lower bone mass described previously [10]. This may be because bone metabolism markers are not site-specific and reflect bone remodeling of the whole skeleton [32]. It is not clear how metabolic markers reflect bone changes during growth and this topic requires further research.

Although we have not found significant differences in bone remodeling markers between cyclists and controls, other researchers show that cycling compromises the acquisition of peak bone mass throughout life [12–14,25,26]. One possible explanation for these differences might be the limited number of participants in the two groups in this study. Longitudinal investigations with adolescent cyclists would be needed to gain an understanding of the causes of this decrease in bone mass, and to act to prevent osteoporosis in these subjects in the future. A conceivable hypothesis would be that, even with the same metabolic activity, metabolic efficiency may be compromised because of physiological or nutritional interactions [33–35]. For instance, a major finding in this work was that 25(OH)D decreased significantly in the CYC group, but not in the CON group. Vitamin D deficiency is associated with decreased bone mass, because it compromises calcium absorption and impairs bone accumulation [21]. A direct association between 25(OH)D and BMC has been described previously [22–24]. In children, vitamin D deficiency is associated with demineralized bones and with rickets [22], so an adequate consumption of vitamin D is essential in preventing this disease. Low intakes of vitamin D, relative to the recommended dietary allowance (RDA) in Spanish children were observed by Gómez-Bruton et al. [36]. In particular, active adolescents did not consume the amount of vitamin D set for their age group, with cyclists being the group farthest away from meeting the recommendations. On the basis of their results, these low intakes are of concern in cyclists, because they showed lower values of BMC and BMD than controls. It is possible that an insufficient intake of vitamin D is among the principal causes of decreased bone mass in adolescent cyclists, as previously described by Olmedillas and colleagues [10]. Potential diurnal variation in plasma levels of total [25(OH)D], due mainly to variations in plasma volume previously described [27], have been taken into consideration. Therefore, in our study, blood extractions were collected at the same time in the morning, under the same conditions for all participants in pre- and post-evaluation.

The main limitation of our study is a relatively small number of subjects, however, the practice level of the participants should be taken into account. These cyclists were training for at least the last two years for a mean time of 13.5 h/week and participating in competitions during this time. An additional issue, is the range of age of the participants (mean, 17 years), as it is a challenge for their trainers to maintain the adherence of this level of training for long periods with a high level of commitment. Actually, we enrolled 25 cyclists in the first evaluation, however, due to most of them abandoning the training and to specific abandonments of the study, the final sample is the one that is represented in this study. The study's principal strength is its longitudinal design (a one-year long-term design with two measurements in the season) and the specificity of the sample according to age and level of training. To date, there have been very few longitudinal studies that have analyzed the effects on biochemical markers in boys derived from practicing sport including cycling and gymnastics [37,38]. Further research, with dual energy X-ray absorptiometry (DXA) measurements and the assessment of a wider spectrum of bone osteoanabolic and catabolic parameters could provide a better understanding of the net process of bones.

5. Conclusions

The similar concentration of markers in cyclists and controls seems to indicate similar metabolic activity. As different levels of bone mass had previously been recorded in these cyclists, metabolic efficiency may have been compromised by other concurrent factors. Decreased vitamin D levels were, in fact, noted in the cyclists over this one-year period, which in the end could be detrimental to the future bone health of these individuals.

Author Contributions: Conceptualization, G.V.-R.; formal analysis, M.R.L. and F.P.d.l.F.; funding acquisition, G.V.-R.; investigation, A.G.-A., H.O. and A.G.-C.; methodology, A.G.-A., H.O. and A.G.-C.; project administration, G.V.-R.; resources, A.G.-C.; software, A.G.-A.; supervision, G.V.-R. and H.O.; visualization, M.R.L.; writing, M.R.L. and H.O.; writing—Review, J.A.C., G.V.-R., A.G.-A., H.O., A.G.-C., F.P.d.l.F. and L.A.M.

Funding: This study has been funded by: Ministerio de Ciencia e Innovación, Instituto de Salud Carlos III (DPS2008-06999). Presidencia del Gobierno de España, Consejo Superior de Deportes (21/UPB20/10). Fondo Europeo de Desarrollo Regional (MICINN-FEDER). GENUD Research Group, Gobierno de Aragón (SGI 216177).

Acknowledgments: The authors want to thank all the adolescents that participated in the study for their understanding and dedication to the project.

Conflicts of Interest: The authors declare no conflict of interest.

References

1. Bailey, D.A.; Faulkner, R.A.; McKay, H.A. Growth, physical activity, and bone mineral acquisition. *Exerc. Sport Sci. Rev.* **1996**, *24*, 233–266. [CrossRef]
2. Adachi, J.D.; Adami, S.; Gehlbach, S.; Anderson, F.A., Jr.; Boonen, S.; Chapurlat, R.D.; Compston, J.E.; Cooper, C.; Delmas, P.; Diez-Perez, A.; et al. Impact of prevalent fractures on quality of life: Baseline results from the global longitudinal study of osteoporosis in women. *Mayo Clin. Proc.* **2010**, *85*, 806–813. [CrossRef]
3. Haentjens, P.; Magaziner, J.; Colon-Emeric, C.S.; Vanderschueren, D.; Milisen, K.; Velkeniers, B.; Boonen, S. Meta-analysis: Excess mortality after hip fracture among older women and men. *Ann. Intern. Med.* **2010**, *152*, 380–390. [CrossRef]
4. Vlachopoulos, D.; Barker, A.R.; Williams, C.A.; Knapp, K.M.; Metcalf, B.S.; Gracia-Marco, L. Effect of a program of short bouts of exercise on bone health in adolescents involved in different sports: The PRO-BONE study protocol. *BMC Public Health* **2015**, *15*, 361. [CrossRef] [PubMed]
5. Dyson, K.; Blimkie, C.J.; Davison, K.S.; Webber, C.E.; Adachi, J.D. Gymnastic training and bone density in pre-adolescent females. *Med. Sci. Sports Exerc.* **1997**, *29*, 443–450. [PubMed]

6. Morris, F.L.; Naughton, G.A.; Gibbs, J.L.; Carlson, J.S.; Wark, J.D. Prospective ten-month exercise intervention in premenarcheal girls: Positive effects on bone and lean mass. *J. Bone Miner. Res.* **1997**, *12*, 1453–1462. [CrossRef] [PubMed]
7. Gracia-Marco, L.; Vicente-Rodriguez, G.; Valtuena, J.; Rey-Lopez, J.P.; Diaz Martinez, A.E.; Mesana, M.I.; Widhalm, K.; Ruiz, J.R.; Gonzalez-Gross, M.; Castillo, M.J.; et al. Bone mass and bone metabolism markers during adolescence: The HELENA Study. *Horm. Res. Paediatr.* **2010**, *74*, 339–350. [CrossRef]
8. Rizzoli, R.; Bonjour, J.P. Determinants of peak bone mass and mechanisms of bone loss. *Osteoporosis Int.* **1999**, *9* (Suppl. S2), S17–S23. [CrossRef]
9. Grimston, S.K.; Willows, N.D.; Hanley, D.A. Mechanical loading regime and its relationship to bone mineral density in children. *Med. Sci. Sports Exerc.* **1993**, *25*, 1203–1210. [CrossRef]
10. Olmedillas, H.; Gonzalez-Aguero, A.; Moreno, L.A.; Casajus, J.A.; Vicente-Rodriguez, G. Bone related health status in adolescent cyclists. *PLoS ONE* **2011**, *6*, e24841. [CrossRef]
11. Medelli, J.; Lounana, J.; Menuet, J.J.; Shabani, M.; Cordero-MacIntyre, Z. Is osteopenia a health risk in professional cyclists? *J. Clin. Densitom.* **2009**, *12*, 28–34. [CrossRef] [PubMed]
12. Nichols, J.F.; Palmer, J.E.; Levy, S.S. Low bone mineral density in highly trained male master cyclists. *Osteoporosis Int.* **2003**, *14*, 644–649.
13. Rector, R.S.; Rogers, R.; Ruebel, M.; Hinton, P.S. Participation in road cycling vs running is associated with lower bone mineral density in men. *Metabolism* **2008**, *57*, 226–232. [CrossRef]
14. Seibel, M.J. Biochemical markers of bone turnover: Part I: Biochemistry and variability. *Clin. Biochem. Rev.* **2005**, *26*, 97–122. [PubMed]
15. Brahm, H.; Strom, H.; Piehl-Aulin, K.; Mallmin, H.; Ljunghall, S. Bone metabolism in endurance trained athletes: A comparison to population-based controls based on DXA, SXA, quantitative ultrasound, and biochemical markers. *Calcif. Tissue Int.* **1997**, *61*, 448–454. [CrossRef]
16. Maimoun, L.; Mariano-Goulart, D.; Couret, I.; Manetta, J.; Peruchon, E.; Micallef, J.P.; Verdier, R.; Rossi, M.; Leroux, J.L. Effects of physical activities that induce moderate external loading on bone metabolism in male athletes. *J. Sports Sci.* **2004**, *22*, 875–883. [CrossRef]
17. Maimoun, L.; Galy, O.; Manetta, J.; Coste, O.; Peruchon, E.; Micallef, J.P.; Mariano-Goulart, D.; Couret, I.; Sultan, C.; Rossi, M. Competitive Season of Triathlon Does not Alter Bone Metabolism and Bone Mineral Status in Male Triathletes. *Int. J. Sports Med.* **2004**, *25*, 230–234.
18. Slemenda, C.W.; Peacock, M.; Hui, S.; Zhou, L.; Johnston, C.C. Reduced rates of skeletal remodeling are associated with increased bone mineral density during the development of peak skeletal mass. *J. Bone Miner. Res.* **1997**, *12*, 676–682. [CrossRef] [PubMed]
19. Chaari, H.; Zouch, M.; Denguezli, M.; Bouajina, E.; Zaouali, M.; Tabka, Z. A high level of volleyball practice enhances bone formation markers and hormones in prepubescent boys. *Biol. Sport* **2012**, *29*, 303–309. [CrossRef]
20. Lehtonen-Veromaa, M.; Mottonen, T.; Irjala, K.; Nuotio, I.; Leino, A.; Viikari, J. A 1-year prospective study on the relationship between physical activity, markers of bone metabolism, and bone acquisition in peripubertal girls. *J. Clin. Endocrinol. Metab.* **2000**, *85*, 3726–3732. [PubMed]
21. Cashman, K.D. Calcium intake, calcium bioavailability and bone health. *Br. J. Nutr.* **2002**, *87* (Suppl. S2), S169–S177. [CrossRef]
22. Holick, M.F. Sunlight and vitamin D for bone health and prevention of autoimmune diseases, cancers, and cardiovascular disease. *Am. J. Clin. Nutr.* **2004**, *80* (Suppl. S6), 1678S–1688S. [CrossRef]
23. Cranney, A.; Weiler, H.A.; O'Donnell, S.; Puil, L. Summary of evidence-based review on vitamin D efficacy and safety in relation to bone health. *Am. J. Clin. Nutr.* **2008**, *88*, 513S–519S. [CrossRef] [PubMed]
24. Valtuena, J.; Gracia-Marco, L.; Vicente-Rodriguez, G.; Gonzalez-Gross, M.; Huybrechts, I.; Rey-Lopez, J.P.; Mouratidou, T.; Sioen, I.; Mesana, M.I.; Martinez, A.E.; et al. Vitamin D status and physical activity interact to improve bone mass in adolescents. The HELENA Study. *Osteoporosis Int.* **2012**, *23*, 2227–2237. [CrossRef] [PubMed]
25. Gonzalez-Aguero, A.; Olmedillas, H.; Gomez-Cabello, A.; Casajus, J.A.; Vicente-Rodriguez, G. Bone Structure and Geometric Properties at the Radius and Tibia in Adolescent Endurance-Trained Cyclists. *Clin. J. Sport Med.* **2017**, *27*, 69–77. [CrossRef]
26. Olmedillas, H.; Gonzalez-Aguero, A.; Moreno, L.A.; Casajus, J.A.; Vicente-Rodriguez, G. Cycling and bone health: A systematic review. *BMC Med.* **2012**, *10*, 168. [CrossRef] [PubMed]

27. Rejnmark, L.; Lauridsen, A.L.; Vestergaard, P.; Heickendorff, L.; Andreasen, F.; Mosekilde, L. Diurnal rhythm of plasma 1,25-dihydroxyvitamin D and vitamin D-binding protein in postmenopausal women: Relationship to plasma parathyroid hormone and calcium and phosphate metabolism. *Eur. J. Endocrinol.* **2002**, *146*, 635–642. [CrossRef]
28. Nickols-Richardson, S.M.; O'Connor, P.J.; Shapses, S.A.; Lewis, R.D. Longitudinal bone mineral density changes in female child artistic gymnasts. *J. Bone Miner. Res.* **1999**, *14*, 994–1002. [CrossRef]
29. Maimoun, L.; Coste, O.; Mura, T.; Philibert, P.; Galtier, F.; Mariano-Goulart, D.; Paris, F.; Sultan, C. Specific bone mass acquisition in elite female athletes. *J. Clin. Endocrinol. Metab.* **2013**, *98*, 2844–2853. [CrossRef]
30. Gracia-Marco, L.; Ortega, F.B.; Jimenez-Pavon, D.; Rodriguez, G.; Valtuena, J.; Diaz-Martinez, A.E.; Gonzalez-Gross, M.; Castillo, M.J.; Vicente-Rodriguez, G.; Moreno, L.A. Contribution of bone turnover markers to bone mass in pubertal boys and girls. *J. Pediatr. Endocrinol. Metab.* **2011**, *24*, 971–974. [CrossRef] [PubMed]
31. Guillaume, G.; Chappard, D.; Audran, M. Evaluation of the bone status in high-level cyclists. *J. Clin. Densitom.* **2012**, *15*, 103–107. [CrossRef] [PubMed]
32. Eliakim, A.; Raisz, L.G.; Brasel, J.A.; Cooper, D.M. Evidence for increased bone formation following a brief endurance-type training intervention in adolescent males. *J. Bone Miner. Res.* **1997**, *12*, 1708–1713. [CrossRef]
33. Vicente-Rodriguez, G. How does exercise affect bone development during growth? *Sports Med.* **2006**, *36*, 561–569. [CrossRef]
34. Julian-Almarcegui, C.; Gomez-Cabello, A.; Huybrechts, I.; Gonzalez-Aguero, A.; Kaufman, J.M.; Casajus, J.A.; Vicente-Rodriguez, G. Combined effects of interaction between physical activity and nutrition on bone health in children and adolescents: A systematic review. *Nutr. Rev.* **2015**, *73*, 127–139. [CrossRef]
35. Vicente-Rodriguez, G.; Ezquerra, J.; Mesana, M.I.; Fernandez-Alvira, J.M.; Rey-Lopez, J.P.; Casajus, J.A.; Moreno, L.A. Independent and combined effect of nutrition and exercise on bone mass development. *J. Bone Miner. Metab.* **2008**, *26*, 416–424. [CrossRef] [PubMed]
36. Gomez-Bruton, A.; Gonzalez-Aguero, A.; Olmedillas, H.; Gomez-Cabello, A.; Matute-Llorente, A.; Julian-Almarcegui, C.; Casajus, J.A.; Vicente-Rodriguez, G. Do calcium and vitamin D intake influence the effect of cycling on bone mass through adolescence? *Nutr. Hosp.* **2013**, *28*, 1136–1139. [PubMed]
37. Vlachopoulos, D.; Barker, A.R.; Ubago-Guisado, E.; Fatouros, I.G.; Knapp, K.M.; Williams, C.A.; Gracia-Marco, L. Longitudinal Adaptations of Bone Mass, Geometry, and Metabolism in Adolescent Male Athletes: The PRO-BONE Study. *J. Bone Miner. Res.* **2017**, *32*, 2269–2277. [CrossRef]
38. Daly, R.M.; Rich, P.A.; Klein, R.; Bass, S. Effects of high-impact exercise on ultrasonic and biochemical indices of skeletal status: A prospective study in young male gymnasts. *J. Bone Miner. Res.* **1999**, *14*, 1222–1230. [CrossRef]

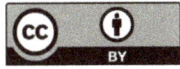

© 2019 by the authors. Licensee MDPI, Basel, Switzerland. This article is an open access article distributed under the terms and conditions of the Creative Commons Attribution (CC BY) license (http://creativecommons.org/licenses/by/4.0/).

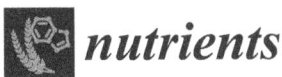

Article

Passive Commuting and Higher Sedentary Time Is Associated with Vitamin D Deficiency in Adult and Older Women: Results from Chilean National Health Survey 2016–2017

Patricio Solis-Urra [1,2,*], Carlos Cristi-Montero [2], Javier Romero-Parra [3], Juan Pablo Zavala-Crichton [4], Maria Jose Saez-Lara [5,6] and Julio Plaza-Diaz [6,7,8]

1. PROFITH "PROmoting FITness and Health through Physical Activity" Research Group, Department of Physical Education and Sport, Faculty of Sport Sciences, University of Granada, 18071 Granada, Spain
2. IRyS Research Group, School of Physical Education, Pontificia Universidad Católica de Valparaíso, Valparaiso 2374631, Chile; carlos.cristi.montero@gmail.com
3. Departamento de Ciencias Farmacéuticas, Facultad de Ciencias, Universidad Católica del Norte, Avda. Angamos 0610, Antofagasta 1270709, Chile; javier.romero@ucn.cl
4. Faculty of Education and Social Sciences, Universidad Andrés Bello, Viña del Mar 2531015, Chile; jzavala@unab.cl
5. Department of Biochemistry and Molecular Biology I, School of Sciences, University of Granada, 18071 Granada, Spain; mjsaez@ugr.es
6. Institute of Nutrition and Food Technology "José Mataix", Center of Biomedical Research, University of Granada, Avda. del Conocimiento s/n. Armilla, 18016 Granada, Spain; jrplaza@ugr.es
7. Department of Biochemistry and Molecular Biology II, School of Pharmacy, University of Granada, 18071 Granada, Spain
8. Instituto de Investigación Biosanitaria IBS.GRANADA, Complejo Hospitalario Universitario de Granada, 18014 Granada, Spain
* Correspondence: patricio.solis.u@gmail.com; Tel.: +34-6-4478-1297

Received: 26 December 2018; Accepted: 29 January 2019; Published: 31 January 2019

Abstract: The aim was to investigate the associations between different physical activity (PA) patterns and sedentary time (ST) with vitamin D deficiency (<12 ng/mL) in a large sample of Chilean women. In this cross-sectional study, the final sample included 1245 adult and 686 older women. The PA levels, mode of commuting, ST, and leisure-time PA were self-reported. Vitamin D deficiency was defined as <12 ng/mL and insufficiency as <20 ng/mL. A higher ST was associated with vitamin D deficiency (odds ratio (OR): 2.4, 95%: 1.6–4.3) in adults, and passive commuting was associated with vitamin D deficiency in older (OR: 1.7, 95%: 1.1–2.7). Additionally, we found a joint association in the high ST/passive commuting group in adults (OR: 2.8, 95%: 1.6–4.9) and older (OR: 2.8, 95%: 1.5–5.2) with vitamin D deficiency, in respect to low ST/active commuting. The PA levels and leisure-time PA were not associated with vitamin D deficiency. In conclusion, mode of commuting and ST seems important variables related to vitamin D deficiency. Promoting a healthy lifestyle appears important also for vitamin D levels in adult and older women. Further studies are needed to establish causality of this association and the effect of vitamin D deficiency in different diseases in this population.

Keywords: Vitamin D; females; exercise; sedentary lifestyle; nutrition; elderly

1. Introduction

Vitamin D was first characterized as a vitamin in the 20th century and nowadays it is recognized as a prohormone [1]. Vitamin D has two major forms, vitamin D_2 (ergocalciferol) and vitamin D_3 (cholecalciferol). The first is derived from plant sources, is not largely human-made, and added to foods, and the latter is synthesized in human skin and is consumed in diets via animal-based foods intake, mainly fish oils [1]. The active form of vitamin D generates a number of extraskeletal biological responses including inhibition of breast, colon, and prostate cancer cell progression; effects on the cardiovascular system; and protection against a number of autoimmune diseases including multiple sclerosis and inflammatory bowel disease [2].

Vitamin D is important in biological process related with women's health, such as fertility, pregnancy outcomes, and lactation at young age [3]. Some observational studies have revealed that a decrease in the vitamin D levels in women is related with reduced fertility [4], antenatal and postpartum depression [3]; as well high parathyroid hormone, the increasing risk of suffering sarcopenia and impaired glucose metabolism in the general population [5,6]. Moreover, supplementation with vitamin D probably might reduce the rate of falls but not risk of falling in older people [4,7]. Normal levels of vitamin D are associated to a low frequency of pathogenesis and neoplasm progressions, as well as hypertension, diabetes, immune disorders such as multiple sclerosis, musculoskeletal conditions [8,9], or bone mass status, especially in women [10]. Although vitamin D deficiency is rare in developed countries, subclinical forms occur, and they have public health relevance since low vitamin D concentrations are highly prevalent among population living in high latitudes, mainly indoors, and among those who are older or dark skinned [11]. Sunlight is the primary source of vitamin D [12], a very rough general estimation indicates that about 80% of vitamin D supply comes from skin ultraviolet-B-induced production, whereas only 20% comes from dietary intake; however, this varies considerably depending on different factors such as seasonal/sun exposure habits, latitude, nutrition/supplement intake or ethnicity [13].

In 2013, a review identified 243 studies related with vitamin D status in Caribbean and Latin American countries. The final analysis only included 28 studies with two major characteristics: small samples sizes and low national representativeness. Countries with available data have shown that vitamin D insufficiency was classified in the range of mild, moderate, or severe public health problem, and the only country with a nationally representative sample in this study was Mexico [14]. In Chile, a study conducted in 2007 with 555 post-menopausal women showed a vitamin D deficiency in 47.5% of the population, defined as less than 17 ng/mL [15]. Recommendations of normal levels of vitamin D in plasma are above of 30 ng/mL, and different cut-points have been used to classify insufficiency or deficiency, according the population [16,17]. For instance, recent data from the Chilean population showed that 80% of older subjects with a low-energy hip fracture have presented insufficient vitamin D levels (less than 20 ng/mL) [18]. Moreover, in healthy older populations, vitamin D values were very similar, 83% of women and 55.3% of men presented parameters below 20 ng/mL [19].

Regular physical activity (PA) and low sedentary time (ST) have significant benefits for health at all ages [20]. The principal recommendation is some PA is better than doing none [21]. The adult population (aged from 18–64 years) and older population (aged 65 years and above) should do 150 minutes of moderate-intensity PA throughout the week or at least 75 minutes of vigorous-intensity PA throughout the week, or an equivalent combination of moderate- and vigorous-intensity activity (e.g., walking, cycling, or doing sports) [20]. Globally, around 23% of adults aged from 18 and above, were not active enough in 2010 (men 20% and women 27%) [4,7,22–25]. Physical activity increase may be about general PA level, leisure PA, mode of commuting, organized sports, among others and independently reducing ST [20].

Previously, low serum vitamin D levels have been associated with lower PA level, gait speed, and balance. Vitamin D level below 30 ng/mL was not associated to an increased risk of fractures; however, a subgroup of women with serum vitamin D levels below 20 ng/mL showed an increased risk tendency of fractures, which may be associated to an inferior PA and postural stability [26]. Another report demonstrates that serum vitamin D concentrations below 20 ng/mL are associated to a poor physical performance, that is to say to a decreased physical performance in older men and women [27]. On the other hand, evidence shows that cycling is associated to high UV exposure, and thus, to high serum vitamin D levels compared to most other outdoors activities that are practiced, including walk [28,29]. It has been established that not all activities are equivalent regarding to sunlight exposure. Thus, whereas some patterns of PA have been associated with vitamin D levels, there is a lack of studies considering ST of mode of commuting. Interestingly, it is necessary to establish a relationship of the aforementioned according to the different population, since it has been shown that older people would be at risk [30]. Furthermore, a better understanding of the effects, according to the population, could help to provide valuable lifestyle recommendation.

Finally, data from general Chilean population regarding vitamin D levels are scarce, and associations with PA patterns and ST might be important factors in the status of vitamin D and maintenance of health [22]. Therefore, the aim of the present study was to investigate associations between self-reported PA patterns, ST, and different serum vitamin D levels in a large sample of Chilean adults and older women, adjusting for a number of potential confounders.

2. Material and Methods

2.1. Study Population

The 2016–2017 Chilean National Health Survey was a representative household survey with a stratified multistage probability sample of 6233 non-institutionalized participants over 14 years old from the 15 regions in Chile, both urban and rural. This survey represents the first, largest, and representative measurement of serum vitamin D levels in Chilean people. Sample size was calculated with a relative sampling error of less than 30%, and absolute sampling error of 2.6% to national level. The participation rate was 90.2%. Detailed information about the survey has been described elsewhere [31]. Vitamin D measurement was taken from a subsample of fertile age women (15 to 49 years) and older people. In this cross-sectional study were included those who have complete vitamin D measurement, valid response in PA questions and correct anthropometric parameters. Final sample was divided in adults ($\geq$18 to <65 years) and older ($\geq$65 years) groups, both for Chilean women. The ethics committee of the Pontificia Universidad Católica de Chile and the Chilean Ministry of Health approved the study protocol and ethical consent forms.

2.2. Survey and Sample

Standardized protocols were used and all investigators (nurses and research technicians) underwent joint training sessions prior to implementation of the survey. The fieldwork for this survey was conducted between August 2016 and March 2017; while blood samples and laboratory tests were made between September 2016 and February 2017.

2.3. Serum Vitamin D Levels

A nurse took venous blood samples in morning hours. Serum was extracted from 1 mL of total blood. Standardized liquid chromatography-tandem mass spectrometry (LC–MS/MS) method was used for measurement of 25(OH)-Vitamin D_3 for Chilean National Health Survey 2016–2017, which allows laboratories and surveys to compare 25(OH)-Vitamin D_3 measurements [32]. Vitamin D levels were categorized according two different criteria: (i) specific criteria for Chilean population according to the Health Ministry of Chile [33] of deficiency as <12 ng/mL [34], and (ii) internationally frequent cut-points used criteria corresponding to insufficiency of <20 ng/mL [16,17]. This method has better analytical specificity and sensitivity compared to immunoassay methods, and fixed analytical goals for imprecision ($\leq$10%) and bias ($\leq$5%) [35].

2.4. Physical Activity

The Global PA Questionnaire (GPAQ) (version 2) to measure PA was used. The physical active categories were defined according to standard criteria of the questionnaire. Those who had less of 600 metabolic equivalent of task (METS) per week were considered inactive and those who had 600 or more METS per week were considered active [36].

2.5. Leisure-Time Physical Activity

A question was made in the visit, the question was (i) *In the last month, Did you practice sport or did any PA out of work time, during 30 minutes or more each time*? The response options were: (i) Yes, three times a week or more; (ii) Yes, one or two times a week; (iii) Yes, less of four times per month; (iv) I do not practice sport. The responses then were categorized in "Yes" for those who exercise three times a week or more, and "no" for those who did not practice sport at least three times a week.

2.6. Commute Mode

A question was made in order to inquire the commute mode of every surveyed, (i) which is the mode of commuting that you use (at least one time per week?) The response options were: (i) drive a light car; (ii) drive a heavy car; (iii) light car passenger; (iv) heavy car passenger; (v) bicycle; (vi) walk; (vii) and other. The responses were categorized in "active commuting" for those had mode of commuting bicycle or walk, and "passive commuting" for the rest.

2.7. Sedentary Time

A question of the GPAQ to estimate ST was asked to every participant of the study. The question was (i) *How much time do you usually spend sitting or reclining on a typical day*? The participant had to respond in minutes and hours per day. This question was categorized according to low ST (<4 hours per day); middle ST ($\geq$4 and <8 hours per day); and high ST (>8 hours per day) [37].

2.8. Covariates

Socio-demographic data were collected for all participants, including age (years), menopausal status (yes/no), achieved education level (primary/secondary/beyond secondary), region (I to XV) and dairy consumption (three times a day or less, once each day, each two days, once a week, once a month or definitely never). Further, participants were asked according their sunlight exposure during the last week, (i) How much sunlight have you been exposed to in the last week? The responses were: (i) much; (ii) little.

2.9. Statistical Analysis

Data were presented as mean, standard deviation (SD), and percentages (%). Independent *t*-test and chi-square test were used to compare differences between adults and older women for continuous and categorical variables, respectively. Firstly, separated multivariable logistic regression model were employed to obtain odds ratio (OR) and confidence interval (CI 95%) in respect to different cut-points, adjusted by age (years), menopausal status (yes/no), achieved education level (primary/secondary/beyond secondary), region (I to XV), dairy consumption (three times a day or less, once each day, each two days, once a week, once a month or definitely never), and sunlight exposure (much/little). Finally, joint associations of ST and commute mode according to different criteria were tested. Here, ST was categorized as low ST (<4 hours per day) and high ST ($\geq$4 hours per day) and it was combined with active and passive commuting. Thus, low ST/active commuting was used as reference group, high ST/active commuting, low ST/passive commuting, high ST/active commuting were second, third, and fourth groups, respectively. The performed model was adjusted by the same covariates mentioned previously plus PA level (active/inactive). For the interpretation of odds ratio, the effect size cut points of 1.68, 3.47, and 6.71 were used, according to small, medium, and large effect size [38]. Analyses were performed using SPSS-IBM (Software, v.21.0 SPSS Inc., Chicago, IL, USA), and a value of $p < 0.05$ was considered statistically significant. The Figure 1 was performed using the ggplot2 package in R and Supplementary Materials Figure S1 with leaflet package.

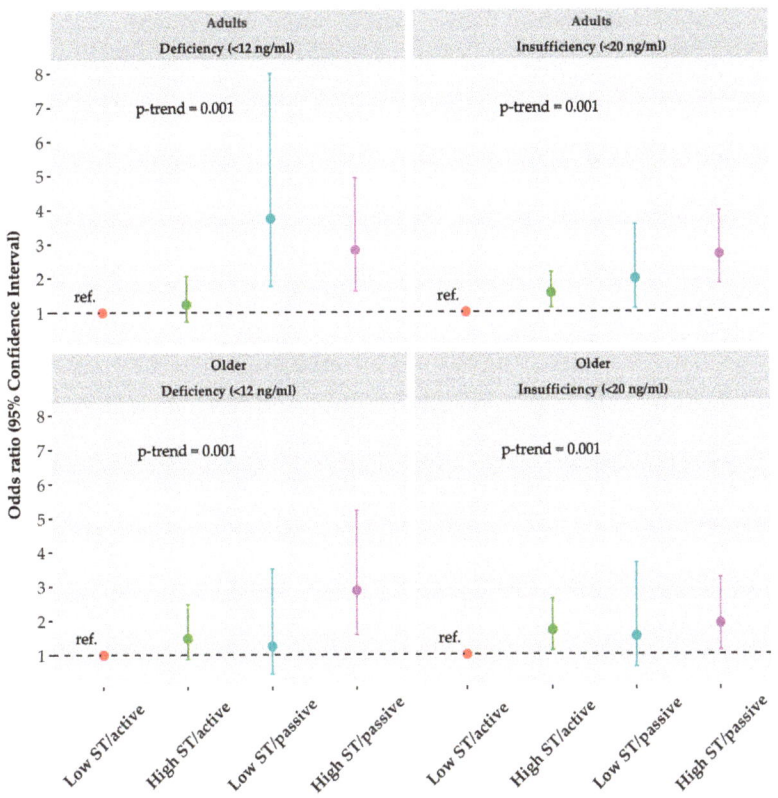

Figure 1. Odds ratio of the joint association between sedentary time (ST) and mode of commuting with different cut-points of vitamin D deficiency in adults and older women. The reference categories are groups with low ST (<4 hours/day) in combination with active commuting.

Figure 1 (bottom panels) shows joint OR for vitamin D deficiency for older women according the sedentary group and mode of commuting group. It can be appreciated from Figure 1 that for the cut-points of <12 ng/mL, compared to the reference group, the high ST/active group presents an OR of 1.476 (CI: 0.877–2.487, $p = 0.143$) the low ST/passive group presents an OR of 1.25 (CI: 0.444–3.514, $p = 0.673$) and high ST/passive group presents an OR of 2.875 (CI: 1.584–5.218, $p = 0.001$) for vitamin D deficiency. Furthermore, according to cut-points of <20 ng/mL, it can be appreciated in Figure 1 an OR of 1.712 9CI: 1.116–2.627, p: 0.014) for high ST/active, OR of 1.531 (CI: 0.638–3.676, $p = 0.34$) low ST/passive and OR of 1.905 (CI = 1.119–3.242, $p = 0.018$) high ST/active groups.

3. Results

The present study included only those who had a complete vitamin D measurement, valid responses in PA questions, and correct anthropometric measurements. The sample with serum vitamin D measurement was 2326. The final sample was divided into adults (≥ 18 years) and older (≥ 65 years) Chilean women groups. The final sample with complete data of physical activity patterns and covariates included was 1931 women. Table 1 shows descriptive characteristics of participants separated by group of age.

Table 1. Descriptive characteristic of the adults and older women.

Variables, Mean ± SD	Adults Women (1245)	Older Women (686)
Age (years)	35.4 ± 8.5	73.6 ± 6.6
Body mass index (kg/m^2)	29.2 ± 5.7	29.3 ± 5.3
Vitamin D levels (ng/mL)	20.2 ± 8.0	18 ± 8.5
Nutritional Status (n: %)		
Underweight	7 (0.6)	6 (0.9)
Normal weight	297 (23.9)	139 (20.3)
Overweight	455 (36.5)	245 (35.7)
Obese	486 (39.0)	296 (43.1)
Physical activity (n: %)		
Inactive	532 (42.7)	393 (57.3)
Active	713 (57.3)	293 (42.7)
Sedentary time (n: %)		
Low Sedentary time	868 (69.7)	508 (74.1)
Middle Sedentary time	260 (20.9)	138 (20.1)
High Sedentary time	117 (9.4)	40 (5.8)
Leisure-time physical activity (n: %)		
30 min, 3 times per week	153 (12.3)	34 (5.0)
Less than 30 min, 3 times per week	1092 (87.7)	652 (95.0)
Commute mode (n: %)		
Active Commuting	291 (23.4)	157 (22.9)
Passive Commuting	954 (76.6)	529 (77.1)
Educational Level (n: %)		
Primary	96 (7.7)	415 (60.4)
Secondary	725 (58.2)	224 (32.7)
Beyond secondary	424 (34.1)	47 (6.9)
Dairy consumption (n: %)		
Three times a day	84 (6.7)	46 (6.7)
Less than three times a day	79 (6.3)	55 (8)
Once a day	428 (34.4)	293 (42.7)
Every two days	223 (17.9)	124 (18.1)
At least once a week	242 (19.4)	104 (15.2)
At least once a month	73 (5.9)	22 (3.2)
Never	116 (9.3)	42 (6.1)
Menopausal status (n: %)		
Yes	48 (3.9)	693 (93.1)
No	1197 (96.1)	47 (6.9)
Vitamin D deficiency (<12 ng/mL) (n: %)		
<12 ng /mL	204 (16.4)	181 (26.4)
≥12 ng /mL	1041 (83.6)	505 (73.6)
Vitamin D insufficiency (<20 ng/mL) (n: %)		
<20 ng /mL	642 (51.6)	445 (64.9)
≥20 ng /mL	603 (48.4)	241 (35.1)
Sunlight exposure (n: %)		
Little	722 (58)	502 (73.2)
Much	523 (42)	184 (26.8)
Region (latitude *) (n: %)		
XV. Arica y Parinacota (−18.474)	94 (7.6)	30 (4.4)
I. Tarapacá (−20.213)	64 (5.1)	27 (3.9)
II. Antofagasta (−23.652)	57 (4.6)	23 (3.4)
III. Atacama (−27.366)	70 (5.6)	20 (2.9)
IV. Coquimbo (−29.953)	61 (4.9)	45 (6.6)
V. Valparaíso (−33.035)	125 (10)	85 (12.4)
XIII. Metropolitana (−33.456)	186 (14.9)	104 (15.2)
VI. L. Bdo. O'Higgins (−34.170)	74 (5.9)	33 (4.8)
VII. Maule (−35.426)	88 (7.1)	60 (8.7)
VIII. Bíobío (−36.826)	138 (11.1)	59 (8.6)
IX. La Araucanía (−38.739)	66 (5.3)	27 (3.9)
XIV. Los Ríos (−39.814)	56 (4.5)	48 (7)
X. Los Lagos (−41.469)	55 (4.4)	40 (5.8)
XI. Aysén (−45.575)	64 (5.1)	38 (5.5)
XII. Magallanes y Antártica (−53.154)	47 (3.8)	47 (6.9)

SD, standard deviation. * Coordinates have been calculated based on the world geodetic system (standard WGS84).

The anthropometric and nutritional values show similar results in both groups. The distribution of underweight, normal weight, overweight, and obese was the same for adult and older women. Vitamin D levels expressed as ng/mL were 20.2 for adult women and 18.0 for older women. Adult women exhibited higher vitamin D levels compared with older women, as well as higher PA patterns, leisure-time PA, educational level, and sunlight exposure. In contrast, ST, dairy consumption and menopausal status were lower in adult women compared to older population. Finally, the commute mode was similar in both groups. Table 2 shows the results of logistic regression analysis for each PA pattern according different cut-points and separated by adults and older women.

3.1. Adults

Table 2 (left side) shows the OR of vitamin D deficiency for adults. It can be seen that middle and high ST groups are associated with vitamin D deficiency (OR between 1.7 to 2.6, all $p < 0.001$) in both cut-points. Furthermore, Table 2 shows that passive commuting are also associated with vitamin D deficiency only for cut-points less than 20 ng/mL. PA level pattern and leisure-time PA pattern were not associated with vitamin D deficiency (all $p > 0.05$).

Figure 1 was constructed using two variables, ST and commute mode. These variables were categorized as low and high, and passive or active, respectively. The OR of the joint association between ST and mode of commuting was determined with different cut-points of vitamin D deficiency in adult women (Figure 1, upper panels) and older women (Figure 1, bottom panels). Reference categories were groups with low ST (<4 hours/day) in combination with active commuting. It can be appreciated from Figure 1 that for the cut-points of <12 ng/mL, compare to reference group, the high ST/active group presents OR of 1.231 (CI: 0.735–2.060, $p = 0.43$), the low ST/passive group presents OR of 3.754 (CI: 1.761–8.000, $p = 0.001$) and high ST/passive group presents OR of 2.821 (CI: 1.614–4.931, $p = <0.001$) for vitamin D deficiency. Furthermore, according to cut-points of <20 ng/mL, it can be appreciated an OR of 1.555 (CI: 1.120–2.158, $p = 0.008$), OR of 1.980 (CI: 1.102–3.558, $p = 0.022$) and OR of 2.689 (CI: 1.822–3.967, $p = <0.001$), for high ST/active, low ST/passive and high ST/active groups, respectively.

3.2. Older

Table 2 (right side) shows the OR of vitamin D deficiency for older women. Middle ST group shows a high vitamin D deficiency and high ST group showed a tendency association ($p = 0.004$ and 0,074, respectively) only in <12 ng/mL cut-points. Passive commuting is associated with vitamin D deficiency in both cut-points. PA level group and leisure-time PA group were not associated with vitamin D deficiency (all $p > 0.005$).

Table 2. Odds ratio for vitamin D deficiency according to different criteria for each physical activity pattern.

Outcome	Adults (1245)						Older (686)					
	OR	(<12 ng/mL) (95% CI)	p	OR	(<20 ng/mL) (95% CI)	p	OR	(<12 ng/mL) (95% CI)	p	OR	(<20 ng/mL) (95% CI)	p
Sedentary time												
Low sedentary time	1.0	Ref.		1.0	Ref.		1.0	Ref.		1.0	Ref.	
Middle sedentary time	2.4	1.6–3.6	<0.001	1.7	1.2–2.3	0.001	1.9	1.2–2.9	0.004	1.152	0.8–1.7	0.505
High sedentary time	2.6	1.6–4.3	<0.001	2.1	1.4–3.2	0.001	1.9	0.9–3.8	0.074	1.672	0.8–3.6	0.184
Physical activity level												
Active	1.0	Ref.		1.0	Ref.		1.0	Ref.		1.0	Ref.	
Inactive	0.9	0.7–1.3	0.6	1.0	0.8–1.3	0.795	1.2	0.8–1.7	0.393	1.2	0.9–1.7	0.207
Leisure-time physical activity												
30 min 3 times/week	1.0	Ref.		1.0	Ref.		1.0	Ref.		1.0	Ref.	
Less 30 min 3 times/week	1.0	0.8–1.3	0.795	1.1	0.7–1.5	0.717	1.2	0.5–2.9	0.644	1.3	0.6–2.6	0.502
Commuting												
Active commuting	1.0	Ref.		1.0	Ref.		1.0	Ref.		1.0	Ref.	
Passive commuting	1.1	0.7–1.6	0.755	1.5	1.2–2.0	0.003	1.7	1.1–2.7	0.020	1.7	1.1–2.4	0.007

OR: Odds ratio. CI: confidence interval. Results of binary regression logistic analysis adjust by age, region, dairy consumption, menopause, education level, and sunlight exposure. Significant values (<0.05) in bold.

4. Discussion

We examined the association between PA patterns and ST with vitamin D deficiency and insufficiency in a nationally representative sample of Chilean women. The results showed that passive commuting is associated with vitamin D deficiency and insufficiency in older women, whereas high ST is associated with vitamin D deficiency and insufficiency in adult women. Additionally, we identify a joint effect of high ST/passive commuting on vitamin D deficiency and insufficiency in both groups. The magnitude of the effect was between small to medium.

To our knowledge, this is the first study that analyzes how different patterns of PA and ST are related with vitamin D levels in Chilean population. Interestingly, active adult women and inactive older women shares the same value, as well as inactive adult women correspond to active older women, creating a mirror effect. The vitamin D levels expressed as ng/mL was 20.2 for adult women and 18.0 for older women. These results were similar to another study in a little sample of Chilean older people ($n = 57$ participants); the aforementioned study have reported that women presented lower levels than men 15.6 ± 5.8 and 19.2 ± 6.0 ng/mL, respectively.

In Europe, vitamin D insufficiency (<20 ng/mL) is present in 36.0% of younger and 24.4% of older participants [39], while there is a high variability between countries. Contrary, to our results, the prevalence of vitamin D insufficiency was higher in young people compared to older participants; an explanation given by the authors is that older population are healthier and quite more active than younger participants. These differences are connected, in some cases, to institutionalization factors, especially combined with concurrent health and mobility problems, such as reduced skin efficiency to produce endogenous vitamin D levels [40], poor dietary vitamin D intake as well poor general nutritional status [41]. Thus, the evidence is not conclusive regarding vitamin D levels according to age, since other risk factors have been identified as skin pigmentation, latitude, health status, vitamin D intake by fortified food or any behavior related to sunlight exposure such as the use of lighter-weight clothes, or indoor working [42–44].

Physical Activity has been proposed to be an important determinant of vitamin D status in Caucasian adults. Jerome et al. [45] showed that sedentary students possessed significantly lower vitamin D levels compared to trained athletes' students that live at high latitudes, even if these sedentary students had a higher vitamin D food intake. Furthermore, leisure-time PA has also been associated to vitamin D levels in cancer survivor patients; however, differences between outdoor and indoor PA were found [46]. In our sample, self-report PA levels, as well as leisure PA, were not associated to vitamin D deficiency or insufficiency. A previous study showed that people who practice mountain sports are associated to a lower risk of serum vitamin D deficiency, while this association was not observed for people who practice nautical sports [47]. Moreover, a previous study of US population reported similar results, although the association was strongest to PA measure by accelerometers than by self-report [48]. Therefore, this could be a reason of non-association in our data. Our data were self-reported and does not discriminate between outdoor or indoor physical activities, therefore the method of measure of PA, outdoor/indoor factor and the different population (cancer patients versus healthy women) could explain these findings.

Hibler was one of the first in to associate ST with serum vitamin D levels. Their results support that PA is positively associated to high vitamin D levels, nonetheless they do not show associations between ST and vitamin D levels [49]. Furthermore, it was not found in association with between ST and vitamin D levels in a Brazilian sample. These contradictory findings could be due to the differences between analyzed populations, since the Brazilian study considered adolescents and participants suffering colorectal adenoma [22,49]. On the other hand, no previous studies that correlate the commute mode with vitamin D deficiency or insufficiency were found, only some activities that increase the UV-light exposition. In this sense, our results provide valuable information that shows the beneficial effect of active commuting on vitamin D levels, since the commute mode has been related positively with better health [50], low type 2 diabetes risk [51], cancer, cardiovascular disease, and all-mortality causes [52].

The joint association between commute mode, ST, and serum vitamin D levels has not been studied. Physical Activity time and ST were jointly evaluated in the previous Chilean national health survey, in order to estimate cardiovascular risk. The active/low sedentary behavior group presented lower cardiovascular risk factors such as hypertension, obesity, and type 2 diabetes [53]. Collectively, active commuting changes were associated to better PA patterns [54]. Therefore, both active commuting as low ST could be an important strategy to increase serum vitamin D levels and avoid the deficiency, considering the arguments exposed above where PA pattern has been estimated as a determinant variable, specifically in postmenopausal women [55].

Vitamin D deficiency is related to musculoskeletal diseases such as rickets and osteomalacia, or several infectious and metabolic processes [56]. Thus, it has been recommended the increase of vitamin D intake [57]. Indeed, in a Chilean population it has been demonstrated the combined beneficial effect of vitamin D supplementation plus exercise on vitamin D serum levels, bone density and functional capacity [58]. Despite this, two recent systematic-reviews, shows that vitamin D supplementation do not have a significant effect on fracture incidence [59] and musculoskeletal health [60]. On the other hand, aging is associated to a progressive bone mass decrease, thus remain physically active is one of the main strategies to combat this continuous loss [13,61]. An alternative to PA is the active commuting, most prevalent behavior associated to active commuting in older population is walking; especially in this population, the benefits of active commuting represents the possibility of independence and autonomy [62,63]. That allows increased sunlight exposure, and therefore, a greater possibility of vitamin D absorption. These results could have important public health implications, since several health problems are associated to low vitamin D levels. In this sense, decrease ST and increase active commuting could be useful strategies against these problems.

The mechanism implicated in this relationship remains unclear, physical activity has been related to sun exposure and vitamin D levels. Nevertheless, this report, as well as other works, has found this same association regardless of sun exposure [47,64]. Another hypothesis is related to physical activity effect and bone metabolism, suggesting an interaction between calcium and vitamin D absorption [65]. Additionally, it has been proposed a close link between sedentary time and increase adiposity, since adiposity is related to decline vitamin D levels [66,67]. Hence, in light to support these hypotheses, more researches are needed.

Important strengths in this study include the population-based sampling method and the wide consideration of potential confounders. However, this study has some limitations. The principal limitation is that cross-sectional study design does not allow to draw causal relationships as was addressed above. Thus, it is not possible to establish whether PA can lead to a vitamin D deficiency or participants with vitamin D deficiency have less PA. Another limitation is about sunlight exposure; despite having considered a question about sunlight exposure, self-report nature and dichotomy response do not grant accurate information about the real amount exposure. On the other hand, the specific vitamin D intake estimation could not be obtained from the used questionnaire and PA questionnaires utilized in our paper often fail to provide sufficient detail on activity type, frequency, duration, and intensity, especially in older adults. Finally, another limitation was the lack of calorie measures of total energy, fat and sugar intake, which could not be obtained from the questionnaire used.

5. Conclusions

We found that high ST is associated with vitamin D deficiency in adult women as well as, passive commuting is associated with vitamin D deficiency. Moreover, there is a joint association of high ST/passive commuting on vitamin D deficiency and insufficiency in both groups. These novel results may add key information for public policy in Chile related to health system approach. In this sense, lifestyle recommendations are needed in order to establish specific recommendations, since the patterns of PA and ST could affect differentially vitamin D status according to age. Further research directions should establish the causal effect of PA and ST patterns, as well as establish the vitamin D deficiency implications in different pathologies in the studied Chilean population.

Supplementary Materials: The following are available online at http://www.mdpi.com/2072-6643/11/2/300/s1, Figure S1: Vitamin D levels of all survey participants along Chilean territory. Population from North of Chile exhibit higher serum vitamin D levels compared to the population from the south territory, being rather deficient for the latter. It is noteworthy, that no region's present population hold the recommended serum vitamin D levels, which is higher than 30 ng/mL.

Author Contributions: P.S.-U. and J.P.-D. conceived the hypothesis and conducted the statistical analyses; P.S.-U. and J.P.-D. drafted the manuscript; C.C.-M., J.R.-P, J.P.Z.-C., M.J.S.-L. critically revised the drafted manuscript. All authors took part in the interpretation of data, the drafting of the manuscript, and the critical revision of the manuscript.

Funding: P.S.-U. was supported by a grant from CONICYT/BECAS Chile/72180543. J.P.-D is part of University of Granada, Plan Propio de Investigación 2016, Excellence actions: Units of Excellence; Unit of Excellence on Exercise and Health (UCEES).

Acknowledgments: We thank all participants for their cooperation and the Chilean Health Ministry and Department of Public Health, The Pontificia Universidad Católica de Chile for designing and conducting the third National Health Survey 2016–2017.

Conflicts of Interest: The authors declare no conflict of interest.

References

1. Gil, Á.; Plaza-Díaz, J.; Mesa, M.D. Vitamin D: Classic and Novel Actions. *Ann. Nutr. Metab.* **2018**, *72*, 87–95. [CrossRef] [PubMed]
2. Holick, M.F. Vitamin D Deficiency. *N. Engl. J. Med.* **2007**, *357*, 266–281. [CrossRef] [PubMed]
3. Aghajafari, F.; Letourneau, N.; Mahinpey, N.; Cosic, N.; Giesbrecht, G. Vitamin D Deficiency and Antenatal and Postpartum Depression: A Systematic Review. *Nutrients* **2018**, *10*, 10. [CrossRef] [PubMed]
4. Pilz, S.; Zittermann, A.; Obeid, R.; Hahn, A.; Pludowski, P.; Trummer, C.; Lerchbaum, E.; Pérez-López, F.R.; Karras, S.N.; März, W. The Role of Vitamin D in Fertility and during Pregnancy and Lactation: A Review of Clinical Data. *Int. J. Environ. Res. Public Health* **2018**, *15*, 2241. [CrossRef] [PubMed]
5. Visser, M.; Deeg, D.J.H.; Lips, P. Low Vitamin D and High Parathyroid Hormone Levels as Determinants of Loss of Muscle Strength and Muscle Mass (Sarcopenia): The Longitudinal Aging Study Amsterdam. *J. Clin. Endocrinol. Metab.* **2003**, *88*, 5766–5772. [CrossRef] [PubMed]
6. Mathieu, S.-V.; Fischer, K.; Dawson-Hughes, B.; Freystaetter, G.; Beuschlein, F.; Schietzel, S.; Egli, A.; Bischoff-Ferrari, H.A. Association between 25-Hydroxyvitamin D Status and Components of Body Composition and Glucose Metabolism in Older Men and Women. *Nutrients* **2018**, *10*, 1826. [CrossRef] [PubMed]
7. Cameron, I.D.; Dyer, S.M.; Panagoda, C.E.; Murray, G.R.; Hill, K.D.; Cumming, R.G.; Kerse, N. Interventions for preventing falls in older people in care facilities and hospitals. *Cochrane Database Syst. Rev.* **2018**, *9*, CD005465. [CrossRef]
8. Zhang, R.; Naughton, D.P. Vitamin D in health and disease: Current perspectives. *Nutr. J.* **2010**, *9*, 65. [CrossRef]
9. Agostini, D.; Zeppa, S.D.; Lucertini, F.; Annibalini, G.; Gervasi, M.; Marini, C.F.; Piccoli, G.; Stocchi, V.; Barbieri, E.; Sestili, P. Muscle and Bone Health in Postmenopausal Women: Role of Protein and Vitamin D Supplementation Combined with Exercise Training. *Nutrients* **2018**, *10*, 1103. [CrossRef]
10. Mouratidou, T.; Vicente-Rodríguez, G.; Gracia-Marco, L.; Huybrechts, I.; Sioen, I.; Widhalm, K.; Valtueña, J.; González-Gross, M.; Moreno, L.A.; HELENA Study Group. Associations of Dietary Calcium, Vitamin D, Milk Intakes, and 25-Hydroxyvitamin D With Bone Mass in Spanish Adolescents: The HELENA Study. *J. Clin. Densitom.* **2013**, *16*, 110–117. [CrossRef]
11. Zgaga, L.; Theodoratou, E.; Farrington, S.M.; Agakov, F.; Tenesa, A.; Walker, M.; Knox, S.; Wallace, A.M.; Cetnarskyj, R.; McNeill, G.; et al. Diet, Environmental Factors, and Lifestyle Underlie the High Prevalence of Vitamin D Deficiency in Healthy Adults in Scotland, and Supplementation Reduces the Proportion That Are Severely Deficient. *J. Nutr.* **2011**, *141*, 1535–1542. [CrossRef] [PubMed]
12. Scragg, R.; Rahman, J.; Thornley, S. Association of sun and UV exposure with blood pressure and cardiovascular disease: A systematic review. *J. Steroid Biochem. Mole. Biol.* **2018**. [CrossRef] [PubMed]

13. Pilz, S.; März, W.; Cashman, K.D.; Kiely, M.E.; Whiting, S.J.; Holick, M.F.; Grant, W.B.; Pludowski, P.; Hiligsmann, M.; Trummer, C.; et al. Rationale and Plan for Vitamin D Food Fortification: A Review and Guidance Paper. *Front. Endocrinol.* **2018**, *9*, 373. [CrossRef] [PubMed]
14. Brito, A.; Cori, H.; Olivares, M.; Mujica, M.F.; Cediel, G.; De Romaña, D.L. Less than Adequate Vitamin D Status and Intake in Latin America and the Caribbean: A Problem of Unknown Magnitude. *Food Nutr. Bull.* **2013**, *34*, 52–64. [CrossRef] [PubMed]
15. Rodríguez, P.J.A.; Valdivia, C.G.; Trincado, M.P. Vertebral fractures, osteoporosis and vitamin D levels in Chilean postmenopausal women. *Rev. Méd. Chile* **2007**, *135*, 31–36.
16. Holick, M.F.; Binkley, N.C.; Bischoff-Ferrari, H.A.; Gordon, C.M.; Hanley, D.A.; Heaney, R.P.; Murad, M.H.; Weaver, C.M. Evaluation, Treatment, and Prevention of Vitamin D Deficiency: An Endocrine Society Clinical Practice Guideline. *J. Clin. Endocrinol. Metab.* **2011**, *96*, 1911–1930. [CrossRef]
17. Ross, A.C.; Taylor, C.L.; Yaktine, A.L.; Del Valle, H.B. (Eds.) *Dietary Reference Intakes for Calcium and Vitamin D*; National Academies Press: Washington, DC, USA, 2011.
18. Schweitzer, D.; Amenabar, P.P.; Botello, E.; Lopez, M.; Saavedra, Y.; Klaber, I. Vitamin d levels among chilean older subjects with low energy hip fracture. *Rev. Med. Chile* **2016**, *144*, 175–180. [CrossRef]
19. Carrasco, G.M.; De Dominguez, L.A.; Martinez, F.G.; Ihle, S.S.; Rojas, A.V.; Foradori, C.A.; Marin, L.P. Vitamin d levels in older healthy chilean adults and their association with functional performance. *Rev. Med. Chile* **2014**, *142*, 1385–1391.
20. Piercy, K.L.; Troiano, R.P.; Ballard, R.M.; Carlson, S.A.; Fulton, J.E.; Galuska, D.A.; George, S.M.; Olson, R.D. The Physical Activity Guidelines for Americans. *JAMA* **2018**, *320*, 2020–2028. [CrossRef]
21. Foster, C.; Moore, J.B.; Singletary, C.R.; Skelton, J.A. Physical activity and family-based obesity treatment: A review of expert recommendations on physical activity in youth. *Clin. Obes.* **2017**, *8*, 68–79. [CrossRef]
22. Da Silva, A.C.M.; Cureau, F.V.; De Oliveira, C.L.; Giannini, D.T.; Bloch, K.V.; Kuschnir, M.C.C.; Dutra, E.S.; Schaan, B.D.; De Carvalho, K.M.B. Physical activity but not sedentary time is associated with vitamin D status in adolescents: Study of cardiovascular risk in adolescents (ERICA). *Eur. J. Clin. Nutr.* **2018**, 1. [CrossRef] [PubMed]
23. Hill, R.L.; Heesch, K.C. *The Problem of Physical Inactivity Worldwide Among Older People*; Springer: Berlin, Germany, 2018; pp. 25–41.
24. Mañas, A.; Del Pozo-Cruz, B.; Guadalupe-Grau, A.; Marín-Puyalto, J.; Alfaro-Acha, A.; Rodriguez-Mañas, L.; García-García, F.J.; Ara, I. Reallocating Accelerometer-Assessed Sedentary Time to Light or Moderate- to Vigorous-Intensity Physical Activity Reduces Frailty Levels in Older Adults: An Isotemporal Substitution Approach in the TSHA Study. *J. Am. Med. Dir. Assoc.* **2018**, *19*, 185.e1–185.e6.
25. Warburton, D.E.; Bredin, S.S. Lost in Translation: What Does the Physical Activity and Health Evidence Actually Tell Us? In *Lifestyle in Heart Health and Disease*; Elsevier: Amsterdam, The Netherland, 2018; pp. 175–186.
26. Gerdhem, P.; Ringsberg, K.A.M.; Obrant, K.J.; Åkesson, K. Association between 25-hydroxy vitamin D levels, physical activity, muscle strength and fractures in the prospective population-based OPRA Study of Elderly Women. *Osteoporos. Int.* **2005**, *16*, 1425–1431. [CrossRef] [PubMed]
27. Wicherts, I.S.; Van Schoor, N.M.; Boeke, A.J.P.; Visser, M.; Deeg, D.J.H.; Smit, J.; Knol, D.L.; Lips, P. Vitamin D Status Predicts Physical Performance and Its Decline in Older Persons. *J. Clin. Endocrinol. Metab.* **2007**, *92*, 2058–2065. [CrossRef]
28. Van den Heuvel, E.G.H.M.; Van Schoor, N.; De Jongh, R.T.; Visser, M.; Lips, P. Cross-sectional study on different characteristics of physical activity as determinants of vitamin D status; inadequate in half of the population. *Eur. J. Clin. Nutr.* **2013**, *67*, 360–365. [CrossRef] [PubMed]
29. De Rui, M.; Toffanello, E.D.; Veronese, N.; Zambon, S.; Bolzetta, F.; Sartori, L.; Musacchio, E.; Corti, M.C.; Baggio, G.; Crepaldi, G.; et al. Vitamin D Deficiency and Leisure Time Activities in the Elderly: Are All Pastimes the Same? *PLoS ONE* **2014**, *9*, e94805. [CrossRef] [PubMed]
30. Van Schoor, N.M.; Lips, P. Worldwide vitamin D status. *Best Pract. Res. Clin. Endocrinol. Metab.* **2011**, *25*, 671–680. [CrossRef] [PubMed]
31. Encuesta nacional de salud. *Encuesta Nacional de Salud (e.N.S) 2016-2017. Primeros Resultados*; Encuesta Nacional de Salud: Santiago, Chile, 2018.
32. Vogeser, M.; Parhofer, K. Liquid Chromatography Tandem-mass Spectrometry (LC-MS/MS) - Technique and Applications in Endocrinology. *Exp. Clin. Endocrinol. Diabetes* **2007**, *115*, 559–570. [CrossRef]

33. Ministerio de Salud. *Results Report of Vitamin D*; MINSAL: Santiago, Chile, 2018.
34. Gatti, D.; El Ghoch, M.; Viapiana, O.; Ruocco, A.; Chignola, E.; Rossini, M.; Giollo, A.; Idolazzi, L.; Adami, S.; Grave, R.D.; et al. Strong relationship between vitamin D status and bone mineral density in anorexia nervosa. *Bone* **2015**, *78*, 212–215. [CrossRef]
35. Orces, C.H. Association between leisure-time aerobic physical activity and vitamin D concentrations among US older adults: The NHANES 2007–2012. *Aging Clin. Exp. Res.* **2018**, 1–9. [CrossRef]
36. Armstrong, T.; Bull, F. Development of the World Health Organization Global Physical Activity Questionnaire (GPAQ). *J. Public Health* **2006**, *14*, 66–70. [CrossRef]
37. Díaz-Martínez, X.; Steell, L.; Martínez, M.A.; Leiva, A.M.; Salas-Bravo, C.; Labraña, A.M.; Durán, E.; Cristi-Montero, C.; Livingstone, K.M.; Garrido-Méndez, Á.; et al. Higher levels of self-reported sitting time is associated with higher risk of type 2 diabetes independent of physical activity in Chile. *J. Public Health* **2017**, *40*, 501–507. [CrossRef] [PubMed]
38. Chen, H.; Cohen, P.; Chen, S. How Big is a Big Odds Ratio? Interpreting the Magnitudes of Odds Ratios in Epidemiological Studies. *Commun. Stat. Simul. Comput.* **2010**, *39*, 860–864. [CrossRef]
39. Manios, Y.; Moschonis, G.; Lambrinou, C.P.; Mavrogianni, C.; Tsirigoti, L.; Hoeller, U.; Roos, F.F.; Bendik, I.; Eggersdorfer, M.; Celis-Morales, C.; et al. Associations of vitamin D status with dietary intakes and physical activity levels among adults from seven European countries: The Food4Me study. *Eur. J. Nutr.* **2017**, *57*, 1357–1368. [CrossRef]
40. MacLaughlin, J.; Holick, M. Aging decreases the capacity of human skin to produce vitamin D3. *J. Clin. Investig.* **1985**, *76*, 1536–1538. [CrossRef] [PubMed]
41. Lips, P.; Van Ginkel, F.C.; Jongen, M.J.; Rubertus, F.; Van Der Vijgh, W.J.; Netelenbos, J.C. Determinants of vitamin D status in patients with hip fracture and in elderly control subjects. *Am. J. Clin. Nutr.* **1987**, *46*, 1005–1010. [CrossRef] [PubMed]
42. Hilger, J.; Friedel, A.; Herr, R.; Rausch, T.; Roos, F.; Wahl, D.A.; Pierroz, D.D.; Weber, P.; Hoffmann, K. A systematic review of vitamin D status in populations worldwide. *Br. J. Nutr.* **2013**, *111*, 23–45. [CrossRef]
43. Cashman, K.D.; Dowling, K.G.; Škrabáková, Z.; González-Gross, M.; Valtueña, J.; De Henauw, S.; Moreno, L.; Damsgaard, C.T.; Michaelsen, K.F.; Mølgaard, C.; et al. Vitamin D deficiency in Europe: Pandemic? *Am. J. Clin. Nutr.* **2016**, *103*, 1033–1044. [CrossRef]
44. Casey, C.; Woodside, J.V.; McGinty, A.; Young, I.S.; McPeake, J.; Chakravarthy, U.; Rahu, M.; Seland, J.; Soubrane, G.; Tomazzoli, L.; et al. Factors associated with serum 25-hydroxyvitamin D concentrations in older people in Europe: The EUREYE study. *Eur. J. Clin. Nutr.* **2018**, *1*. [CrossRef]
45. Jerome, S.P.; Sticka, K.D.; Schnurr, T.M.; Mangum, S.J.; Reynolds, A.J.; Dunlap, K.L. 25(oh)d levels in trained versus sedentary university students at 64 degrees north. *Int. J. Circumpolar Health* **2017**, *76*, 1314414. [CrossRef]
46. Yang, L.; Toriola, A.T. Leisure-time physical activity and circulating 25-hydroxyvitamin D levels in cancer survivors: A cross-sectional analysis using data from the US National Health and Nutrition Examination Survey. *BMJ Open* **2017**, *7*, e016064. [CrossRef] [PubMed]
47. Touvier, M.; Deschasaux, M.; Montourcy, M.; Sutton, A.; Charnaux, N.; Kesse-Guyot, E.; Assmann, K.E.; Fezeu, L.; Latino-Martel, P.; Druesne-Pecollo, N.; et al. Determinants of Vitamin D Status in Caucasian Adults: Influence of Sun Exposure, Dietary Intake, Sociodemographic, Lifestyle, Anthropometric, and Genetic Factors. *J. Investig. Dermatol.* **2015**, *135*, 378–388. [CrossRef] [PubMed]
48. Wanner, M.; Richard, A.; Martin, B.; Linseisen, J.; Rohrmann, S. Associations between objective and self-reported physical activity and vitamin D serum levels in the US population. *Cancer Causes Control* **2015**, *26*, 881–891. [CrossRef] [PubMed]
49. Hibler, E.A.; Molmenti, C.L.S.; Dai, Q.; Kohler, L.N.; Anderson, S.W.; Jurutka, P.W.; Jacobs, E.T. Physical activity, sedentary behavior, and vitamin D metabolites. *Bone* **2016**, *83*, 248–255. [CrossRef] [PubMed]
50. Andersen, L.B. Active commuting is beneficial for health. *BMJ* **2017**, *357*, 1740. [CrossRef] [PubMed]
51. Rasmussen, M.G.; Grøntved, A.; Blond, K.; Overvad, K.; Tjønneland, A.; Jensen, M.K.; Østergaard, L. Associations between Recreational and Commuter Cycling, Changes in Cycling, and Type 2 Diabetes Risk: A Cohort Study of Danish Men and Women. *PLoS Med.* **2016**, *13*, e1002076. [CrossRef] [PubMed]
52. Celis-Morales, C.A.; Lyall, D.M.; Welsh, P.; Anderson, J.; Steell, L.; Guo, Y.; Maldonado, R.; Mackay, D.F.; Pell, J.P.; Sattar, N.; et al. Association between active commuting and incident cardiovascular disease, cancer, and mortality: Prospective cohort study. *BMJ* **2017**, *357*, j1456. [CrossRef]

53. Cristi-Montero, C.; Steell, L.; Petermann, F.; Garrido-Méndez, A.; Díaz-Martínez, X.; Salas-Bravo, C.; Ramirez-Campillo, R.; Alvarez, C.; Rodriguez, F.; Aguilar-Farias, N.; et al. Joint effect of physical activity and sedentary behaviour on cardiovascular risk factors in Chilean adults. *J. Public Health* **2017**, *40*, 485–492. [CrossRef]
54. Foley, L.; Panter, J.; Heinen, E.; Prins, R.; Ogilvie, D. Changes in active commuting and changes in physical activity in adults: A cohort study. *Int. J. Behav. Nutr. Phys. Act.* **2015**, *12*, 161. [CrossRef]
55. Millen, A.E.; Wactawski-Wende, J.; Pettinger, M.; Melamed, M.L.; Tylavsky, F.A.; Liu, S.; Robbins, J.; Lacroix, A.Z.; LeBoff, M.S.; Jackson, R.D.; et al. Predictors of serum 25-hydroxyvitamin D concentrations among postmenopausal women: The Women's Health Initiative Calcium plus Vitamin D Clinical Trial. *Am. J. Clin. Nutr.* **2010**, *91*, 1324–1335. [CrossRef]
56. Muscogiuri, G. Vitamin D: Past, present and future perspectives in the prevention of chronic diseases. *Eur. J. Clin. Nutr.* **2018**, *72*, 1221–1225. [CrossRef] [PubMed]
57. Mayor, S. Public Health England recommends vitamin D supplements in autumn and winter. *BMJ* **2016**, *354*, 4061. [CrossRef] [PubMed]
58. Bunout, D.; Barrera, G.; Leiva, L.; Gattás, V.; De La Maza, M.P.; Avendaño, M.; Hirsch, S. Effects of vitamin D supplementation and exercise training on physical performance in Chilean vitamin D deficient elderly subjects. *Exp. Gerontol.* **2006**, *41*, 746–752. [CrossRef] [PubMed]
59. Zhao, J.-G.; Zeng, X.-T.; Wang, J.; Liu, L. Association Between Calcium or Vitamin D Supplementation and Fracture Incidence in Community-Dwelling Older Adults: A Systematic Review and Meta-analysis. *JAMA* **2017**, *318*, 2466–2482. [CrossRef] [PubMed]
60. Bolland, M.J.; Grey, A.; Avenell, A. Effects of vitamin D supplementation on musculoskeletal health: A systematic review, meta-analysis, and trial sequential analysis. *Lancet Diabetes Endocrinol.* **2018**, *6*, 847–858. [CrossRef]
61. Rodríguez-Gómez, I.; Mañas, A.; Losa-Reyna, J.; Rodríguez-Mañas, L.; Chastin, S.F.M.; Alegre, L.M.; García-García, F.J.; Ara, I. Associations between sedentary time, physical activity and bone health among older people using compositional data analysis. *PLoS ONE* **2018**, *13*, e0206013. [CrossRef] [PubMed]
62. O'hern, S.; Oxley, J. Understanding travel patterns to support safe active transport for older adults. *J. Transp. Health* **2015**, *2*, 79–85. [CrossRef]
63. Musselwhite, C.; Holland, C.; Walker, I. The role of transport and mobility in the health of older people. *J. Transp. Health* **2015**, *2*, 1–4. [CrossRef]
64. Kluczynski, M.A.; LaMonte, M.J.; Mares, J.A.; Wactawski-Wende, J.; Smith, A.W.; Engelman, C.D.; Andrews, C.A.; Snetselaar, L.G.; Sarto, G.E.; Millen, A.E.; et al. Duration of Physical Activity and Serum 25-hydroxyvitamin D Status of Postmenopausal Women. *Ann. Epidemiol.* **2011**, *21*, 440–449. [CrossRef]
65. Al-Musharaf, S.; Krishnaswamy, S.; Yusuf, D.S.; Alkharfy, K.M.; Al-Saleh, Y.; Al-Attas, O.S.; Alokail, M.S.; Moharram, O.; Sabico, S.; Al-Othman, A.; et al. Effect of physical activity and sun exposure on vitamin D status of Saudi children and adolescents. *BMC Pediatr.* **2012**, *12*, 92.
66. Wortsman, J.; Matsuoka, L.Y.; Chen, T.C.; Lu, Z.; Holick, M.F. Decreased bioavailability of vitamin D in obesity. *Am. J. Clin. Nutr.* **2000**, *72*, 690–693. [CrossRef] [PubMed]
67. Scott, D.; Blizzard, L.; Fell, J.; Ding, C.; Winzenberg, T.; Jones, G. A prospective study of the associations between 25-hydroxy-vitamin D, sarcopenia progression and physical activity in older adults. *Clin. Endocrinol.* **2010**, *73*, 581–587. [CrossRef] [PubMed]

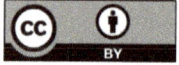

© 2019 by the authors. Licensee MDPI, Basel, Switzerland. This article is an open access article distributed under the terms and conditions of the Creative Commons Attribution (CC BY) license (http://creativecommons.org/licenses/by/4.0/).

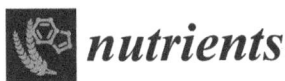

Article

Vitamin D and the Risk of Depression: A Causal Relationship? Findings from a Mendelian Randomization Study

Lars Libuda [1,*], Björn-Hergen Laabs [2], Christine Ludwig [1], Judith Bühlmeier [1], Jochen Antel [1], Anke Hinney [1], Roaa Naaresh [1], Manuel Föcker [3], Johannes Hebebrand [1], Inke R. König [2] and Triinu Peters [1]

[1] Department of Child and Adolescent Psychiatry, Psychosomatics and Psychotherapy, University Hospital Essen, University of Duisburg-Essen, 45147 Essen, Germany; christine.ludwig@lvr.de (C.L.); judith.buehlmeier@uni-due.de (J.B.); jochen.antel@uni-due.de (J.A.); Anke.hinney@uni-due.de (A.H.); roaanaaresh@gmail.com (R.N.); johannes.hebebrand@uni-due.de (J.H.); triinu.peters@uni-due.de (T.P.)
[2] Institut für Medizinische Biometrie und Statistik, Universität zu Lübeck, Universitätsklinikum Schleswig-Holstein, 23562 Lübeck, Germany; laabs@imbs.uni-luebeck.de (B.-H.L.); Inke.Koenig@imbs.uni-luebeck.de (I.R.K.)
[3] Department of Child and Adolescent Psychiatry, University of Münster, 48149 Münster, Germany; Manuel.Foecker@ukmuenster.de
* Correspondence: lars.libuda@uni-due.de; Tel.: +49-201-7227-343

Received: 5 April 2019; Accepted: 14 May 2019; Published: 16 May 2019

Abstract: While observational studies show an association between 25(OH)vitamin D concentrations and depressive symptoms, intervention studies, which examine the preventive effects of vitamin D supplementation on the development of depression, are lacking. To estimate the role of lowered 25(OH)vitamin D concentrations in the etiology of depressive disorders, we conducted a two-sample Mendelian randomization (MR) study on depression, i.e., "depressive symptoms" (DS, $n = 161,460$) and "broad depression" (BD, $n = 113,769$ cases and 208,811 controls). Six single nucleotide polymorphisms (SNPs), which were genome-wide significantly associated with 25(OH)vitamin D concentrations in 79,366 subjects from the SUNLIGHT genome-wide association study (GWAS), were used as an instrumental variable. None of the six SNPs was associated with DS or BD (all $p > 0.05$). MR analysis revealed no causal effects of 25(OH)vitamin D concentration, either on DS (inverse variance weighted (IVW); b = 0.025, SE = 0.038, $p = 0.52$) or on BD (IVW; b = 0.020, SE = 0.012, $p = 0.10$). Sensitivity analyses confirmed that 25(OH)vitamin D concentrations were not significantly associated with DS or BD. The findings from this MR study indicate no causal relationship between vitamin D concentrations and depressive symptoms, or broad depression. Conflicting findings from observational studies might have resulted from residual confounding or reverse causation.

Keywords: vitamin D; depression; depressive symptoms; Mendelian randomization

1. Introduction

Depressive disorders are the most common mental disorders worldwide, with more than 300 million people having been affected, in 2015 [1]. Considering that major depressive disorders (MDD) recently became the third leading cause of disability worldwide [1], effective preventive approaches are urgently needed. Interventions aiming at the prevention of mental disorders should ideally focus on youth, since the first onset of mental disorders is frequently seen during childhood/adolescence [2].

Diet as one modifiable lifestyle factor could be a target for such preventive interventions. Considering the increasing evidence for an inverse association between diet quality and mental disorders, it was recently claimed to consider "nutritional medicine as mainstream in psychiatry" [3].

At the same time, vitamin D deficiency was suggested to be linked with increased depressive symptoms [3]. In fact, a number of studies have confirmed a relationship between vitamin D levels and mental health already in childhood and adolescence. The majority of such studies focused on the autism spectrum disorders and ADHD [4]. The few observational studies on depression in adolescence seemed to confirm the suggested inverse association between 25(OH)vitamin D concentrations (recommended biomarker for vitamin D status), and depression or emotional problems [5–7]. However, findings from observational studies are not sufficient to draw conclusions on cause–effect relationships.

In childhood and adolescent depression, randomized controlled trials (RCTs)—the gold standard to imply causality—are currently missing [4,8]. In adults, RCTs have examined vitamin D supplementation effects on the course of an already existing depression, but meta-analyses of these studies have revealed conflicting results [9–11]. Furthermore, these RCTs have focused on the therapeutic effects, but have not examined a preventive role of vitamin D, prior to the development of depression. The few RCTs on preventive effects had only been conducted in postmenopausal women [12] or women older than 70 years [13], without showing any beneficial effects. Transferability of these results to the general population remains unclear. However, such preventive RCTs would require long-term interventions and follow-up periods of several years, to cover a critical time frame of disorder pathogenesis, and very large sample sizes, to provide sufficient statistical power. In contrast, two-sample Mendelian Randomization (MR) studies based on summary data from large-scale genome-wide association studies (GWAS) are a time-effective approach to examine the causal effect of an exposure (e.g., 25(OH)vitamin D concentration) on an outcome (e.g., depression), by using genetic markers as instrumental variables (IVs) [14]. The concept of MR studies implies a natural "quasi randomization", since the individual composition of alleles and, thus, of IVs are determined randomly at conception, resulting in a reduced risk of confounding [15]. Bias from reverse causation, another limitation of observational studies, is also precluded in MR studies, as the individual genotype is determined at conception, and cannot be modified by the outcome of interest [15].

Recently, a two-sample MR study was conducted which focused on the causal effects of 25(OH)vitamin D on MDD. Using data from the most recent MDD GWAS with 59,851 cases and 113,154 controls, this MR study did not reveal a causal association between 25(OH)vitamin D concentrations and the risk of MDD [16]. However, the phenotype of MDD does not completely cover the complex dimensional and transitional aspects in the etiology of depression, ranging from single depressive symptoms to a depressive syndrome, and finally a diagnosis of MDD or other subtypes of depressive disorders [17]. To include both the dimensional aspects of depression and different depression subtypes as outcomes, our two-sample MR study examined the effects of 25(OH)vitamin D concentrations on depressive symptoms (DS) and broad depression (BD), using summary-level data of the most recent large-scaled GWAS.

2. Materials and Methods

2.1. Data Sources for MR Analyses

This two-sample MR study relied on publicly available summary statistics of three different GWAS meta-analyses on 25(OH)vitamin D concentration [18], DS [19], and BD [20,21]. For the definition of the genetic instrument we used the most recent GWAS on serum 25(OH)vitamin D (i.e., the exposure in this MR analysis) from the SUNLIGHT consortium with 79,366 participants of European ancestry, including 31 studies from Europe, Canada, and USA [18]. The following studies were included in the SUNLIGHT GWAS: 1958 British Birth (1956BC), the Cardiovascular Health Study (CHS), the Framingham Heart Study (FHS), Gothenburg Osteoporosis and Obesity Determinants (GOOD), the Health, Aging, and Body Composition study (Health ABC), the Study of Indiana Women (Indiana), the Northern Finland Birth Cohort 1966 (NFBC), the Old Older Amish Study (OOA), the Rotterdam Study, the Twins UK registry, the Alpha-Tocopherol, Beta-Carotene Cancer Prevention Study (ATBC), the Atherosclerosis Risk in Communities Study (ARIC), the AtheroGene registry, B-vitamins for the Prevention of Osteoporotic Fractures (B-PROOF), Epidemiology of Diabetes Interventions and Complications (EDIC), the Case-Control Study for Metabolic Syndrome (GenMets), the Helsinki Birth Cohort Study (HBCS), the Health Professional Follow-Up Study (HPFS, nested coronary heart disease case-control study), the Invecchiare in Chianti Study (InChianti), the Cooperative Health Research in the region Augsburg (KORA), the Leiden Longevity Study (LLS), the Ludwigshafen Risk and Cardiovascular Health Study (LURIC), the Multi-Ethnic Study of Atherosclerosis (MESA), the Nijmegen Biomedische Studie (NBS), the Nurses' Health Study (NHS, nested breast cancer case-control study, and type2 diabetes case-control study), the Orkney Complex Disease Study (ORCADES), the Prostate, Lung, Colorectal, and Ovarian Cancer Screening Trial (PLCO), the PROspective Study of Pravastatin in the Elderly at Risk (PROSPER), the Study of Health in Pomerania (SHIP), the Scottish Colorectal Cancer Study (SOCCS), and the Cardiovascular Risk in Young Finns Study (YFS). The majority of these 31 studies used radioimmunoassay techniques, HPLC-MS, or LC-MS for the detection of serum 25(OH)vitamin D. Detailed information about ethical approvals of the respective studies, as well as the sample characteristics, are given in the supplementary files of the SUNLIGHT GWAS meta-analysis [18,22]. For our MR study we used independent single nucleotide polymorphisms (SNPs) of all six loci as genetic instruments, which were genome-wide significantly associated with the exposure of interest (i.e., serum 25-hydroxyvitamin D concentrations) [18]. The effect sizes of the six genetic variants on the exposure were derived from the publicly available summary statistics of the GWAS meta-analysis (Table 1). Overall, these six SNPs explained 2.8% of the variance of serum 25(OH)vitamin D concentrations [18].

Effect estimates of these six genetic instruments on the two outcomes DS and BD were obtained from the summary statistics of the two GWAS, including 161,460 individuals with European descent for DS [19] and 113,769 "white British" BD cases, along with 208,811 controls from the UK Biobank for BD [20,21]. The GWAS on DS [19] used data of the following cohorts: (1) UK Biobank (information about ethics: https://www.ukbiobank.ac.uk/wp-content/uploads/2011/05/EGF20082.pdf.) (2) GERA, Resource for Genetic Epidemiology Research on Adult Health and Aging; Subsample of the longitudinal cohort enrolled in the Kaiser Permanente Research Program on Genes, Environment, and Health (RPGEH) [23]. The institutional review boards of both, KPNC and the University of California San Francisco approved the project. (3) The Psychiatric Genetics Consortium (PGC) data on MDD [24] also relied on the GERA cohorts. The UK Biobank included people who were currently aged 40–69, participants of RPGEH were all adult (≥18 years old). Okbay et al. (2016) considered only persons with European ancestry (UK Biobank: "White-British" ancestry) and constructed a continuous phenotype for DS, by combining the responses to two questions about the experienced feelings of disinterest and feelings of depression with case-control data on MDD [19].

The GWAS on BD [20] used data from the UK Biobank study [25], which was conducted under the generic approval from the NHS National Research Ethics Service (approval letter dated 17th June 2011, Ref 11/NW/0382). According to the study protocol, the UK Biobank aimed to include 500,000 people from all over UK, who were currently aged 40–69 and were living within a reasonable travelling distance to an assessment center. While the study protocol of the UK Biobank (https://www.ukbiobank.ac.uk/wp-content/uploads/2011/11/UK-Biobank-Protocol.pdf) did not list any criterion for exclusion, Howard et al. excluded individuals which were not recorded as "white British" as well as the outliers (e.g., based on heterozygosity, shared relatedness of up to the third degree, etc.) [20]. Howard et al. defined BD via self-reported help-seeking behavior for non-specific mental health difficulties, which might reflect the beginning of a depressive episode [20]. They hypothesized that genetic variants identified in cohorts using self-reported measures of depression are known to be highly correlated with those obtained from cohorts using clinically diagnosed depression phenotypes, but at the same time offer the opportunity to analyze large cohorts rather than smaller studies with a clinically defined phenotype [20]. Accordingly, BD represents the broadest of the examined phenotypes in this GWAS, including different depression diagnoses (e.g., single episode depression, recurrent depressive disorder), which resulted in the largest number of, both, subjects for analysis and identified significant SNPs [20].

Using summary data of these three GWAS, two separate two-sample MR studies were conducted for BD and DS, including analyses of pleiotropy, sensitivity, and power.

2.2. Testing Mendelian Randomization Assumptions

MR studies require fulfillment of three core assumptions [15]: (1) The first assumption states that the selected genetic instrument has to be truly associated with the exposure of interest, i.e., 25(OH)vitamin D. By selecting our instrument based on large-scaled GWAS and focusing only on genome-wide significant SNPs for 25(OH)vitamin D, we ensured that this first assumption was fulfilled. (2) If there is an effect of the genetic instrument on the outcome, besides the effect of 25(OH)vitamin D, it ss no longer possible to distinguish between the effects in an MR study. Accordingly, the second assumption states that the genetic instrument has to be independent of the outcome, conditional on the exposure and confounders of the exposure–outcome association [26]. (3) The third assumption states that the genetic instrument must not be associated with any confounder of the exposure–outcome relationship. Assumptions 2 and 3 are difficult to test, because it also includes associations with unknown confounders. Therefore, we investigated whether there was horizontal pleiotropy, i.e., genetics had an effect on DS or BD, besides its effect on 25(OH)vitamin D, by estimating the coefficients of Egger's regression for MR, and checking whether the intercept was significantly unequal to zero.

2.3. Statistical Analysis

All tests were performed using the statistical software "R" version 3.5.2 (R Foundation for Statistical Computing, Vienna, Austria). Since the two outcomes were analyzed separately, the overall significance level of 0.05 was applied for each outcome, in order to control for multiple testing in the sense of a family-wise error rate.

To ensure that our analyses were not based on weak instruments, the F-statistics were computed. Following general recommendations, F-statistics above 10 indicate that the instruments were sufficiently strong. Given no evidence for horizontal pleiotropy, the summary data were analyzed for the single SNPs, as well as the combination of all SNPs as IV, using two MR methods (inverse variance weighted regression (IVW) and Egger's regression). Other MR methods (simple mode, weighted mode and weighted median) were applied, with similar results (not shown). To visualize the results, forest and scatter plots were used, which combined the results of single and multi SNP analyses. In the forest plots, the single SNP effect estimates were displayed beside the multi SNP effect estimates, with the corresponding 95% confidence intervals. In the scatter plots, the single SNP effects on the exposure were plotted against the single SNP effects on the outcome (with corresponding standard deviation in both directions) and the estimated regression lines of the multi SNP analyses were added.

To examine whether the analyses were driven by any single SNP, sensitivity analyses using a leave-one-out approach were conducted. For this purpose, all SNPs but one were analyzed, using the IVW regression. In general, if the analyses are not driven by one single SNP, the regression coefficients remain relatively stable. Finally, we estimated the power to detect a true causal effect of a relative difference between 1% and 20%, per 1 standard deviation in 25(OH)vitamin D, which corresponded to the odds ratio values between 0.8 and 1.2 in 0.01 steps, with the approach proposed by Brion et al. [27]. Results from our analysis of the German representative KiGGS study might give a crude impression on the standard deviation of 25(OH)vitamin D in a healthy sample. In this analysis, we observed a standard deviation of 25.0 nmol/l and 25.5 nmol/l, in boys and girls aged 3–17 years [5].

Table 1. Genome-wide significant single nucleotide polymorphisms (SNPs) for natural log-transformed 25(OH)vitamin D concentrations and their association with broad depression and depressive symptoms.

SNP	Chromosome	Gene	Effect/Reference Allele	AF *	Association with Natural Log-Transformed 25(OH)vitamin D			Association with Broad Depression			Association with Depressive Symptoms		
					Effect Estimate (Beta) #	SE	p	Effect Estimate (Beta)	SE	p	Effect Estimate (Beta)	SE	p
rs3755967	4	GC	T/C	0.28	−0.089	0.0023	4.74E-343	0.0012	0.0013	0.350	−0.001	0.004	0.731
rs10741657	11	CYP2R1	A/G	0.4	0.031	0.0022	2.05E-46	0.002	0.001	0.055	0.005	0.004	0.309
rs12785878	11	NADSYN1_DHCR7	T/G	0.75	0.036	0.0022	3.80E-62	−0.002	0.001	0.287	0.006	0.005	0.215
rs10745742	12	AMDHD1	T/C	0.4	0.017	0.0022	1.88E-14	0.001	0.001	0.412	0.000	0.004	0.976
rs8018720	14	SEC23A	C/G	0.82	−0.017	0.0029	4.72E-09	0.0003	0.0015	0.857	0.001	0.005	0.780
rs17216707	20	CYP24A1	T/C	0.79	0.026	0.0027	8.14E-23	0.0003	0.0015	0.862	−0.004	0.004	0.340

AF: allele frequency; SE: standard error; * information on allele frequency were derived from [18]. # Calculating e^(beta) gives the change in 25(OH)vitamin D in percentage. For instance, for SNP rs3755967, e^(−0.089) renders 0.91, meaning that carriage of the alternative allele reduces 25(OH)D by 9%.

3. Results

The information on the association of the six selected SNPs with 25(OH)vitamin D concentrations, DS, and BD are presented in Table 1. None of the six 25(OH)vitamin D-lowering alleles were either associated with DS or with BD. With F = 381.0103 the F-statistic indicated strong instrumental variables. The overall estimates, calculated by IVW or MR Egger, did not reveal associations between 25(OH)vitamin D concentrations and DS or BD (Table 2, Figures 1 and 2). Sensitivity analyses using the leave-one-out approach confirmed the lack of associations (Supplemental Tables S1 and S2). There was no evidence for pleiotropy either for DS (MR-Egger intercept: 0.0002; $p = 0.949$) or BD (MR-Egger intercept: −0.0001; $p = 0.886$). Power analyses revealed that our MR analyses had a 100% power to detect an OR of 1.1 for BD per 1 standard deviation decrease in natural-log transformed 25(OH)vitamin D (Supplemental Figure S1).

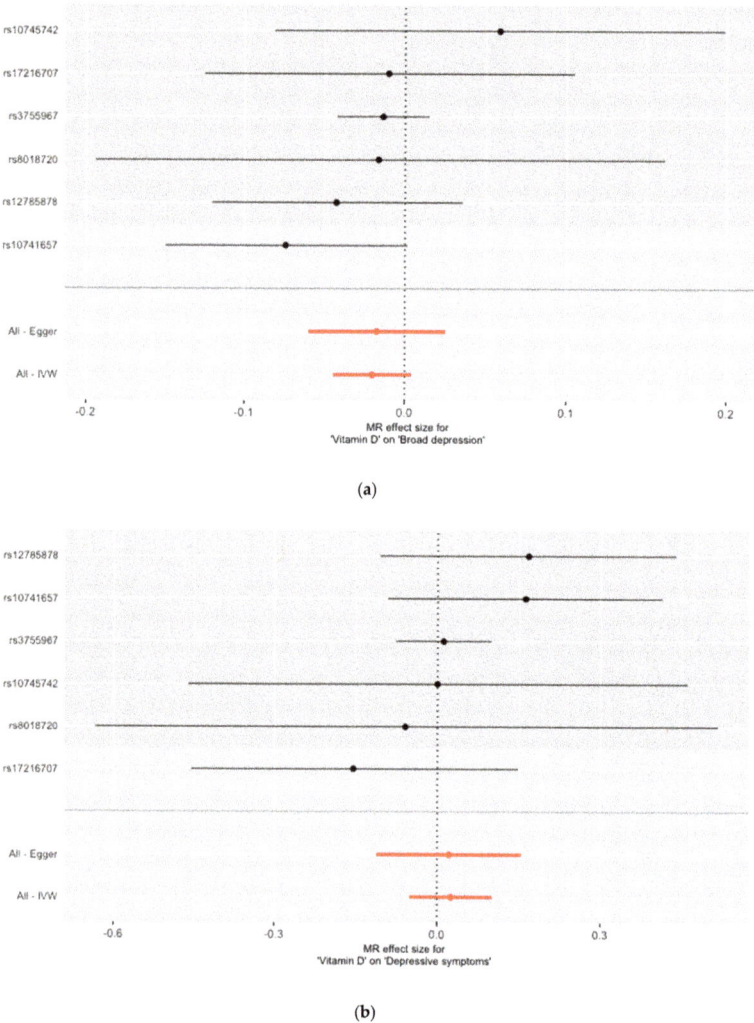

Figure 1. Results of the single and multi SNP analyses for the SNP effect of natural-log transformed 25(OH)vitamin D on (**a**) broad depression, and (**b**) depressive symptoms. The black lines visualize the results of single SNP analyses, the red lines visualize the results of the multi SNP analysis.

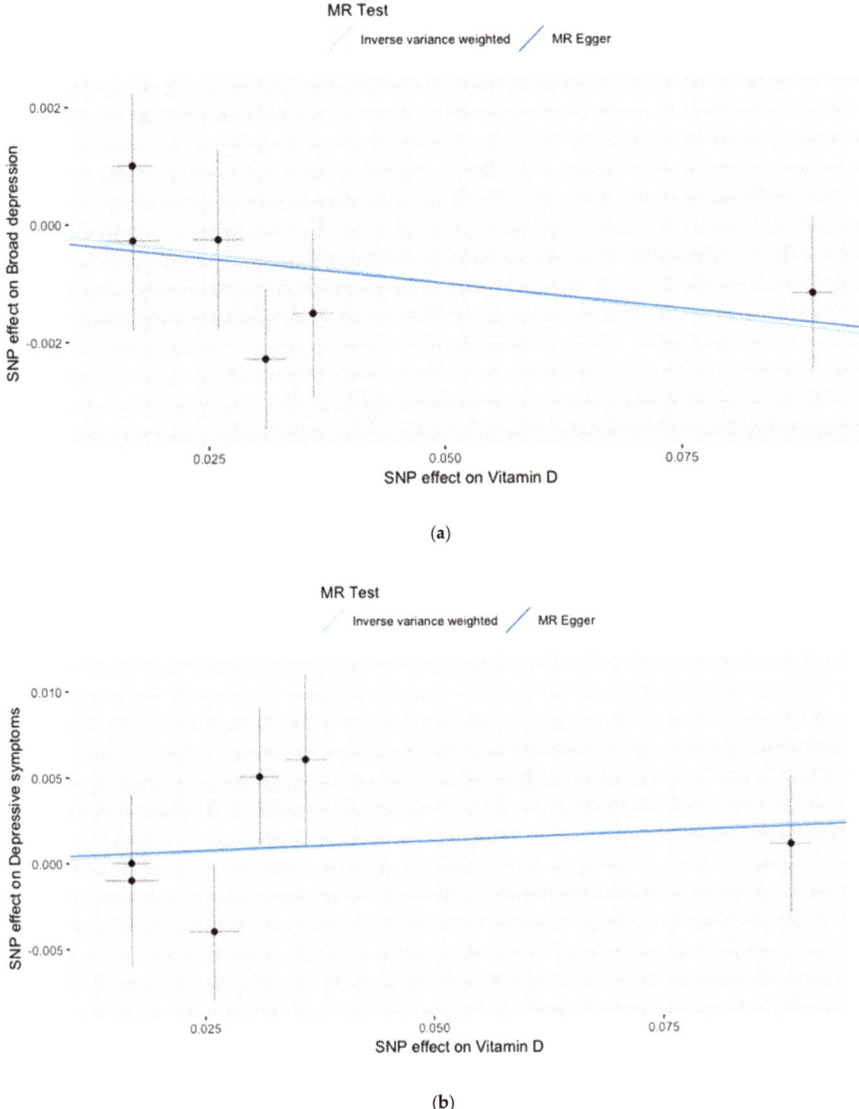

Figure 2. Results of the single and multi SNP analyses on the association between natural-log transformed 25(OH)vitamin D concentration and (**a**) broad depression and (**b**) depressive symptoms. A SNP effect of 0.025 means that carrying an alternative allele at this SNP was associated with an expected increase in the natural-log transformed 25(OH)D by 0.025; e^(beta) gives the change in 25(OH)vitamin D in percentage. Accordingly, a SNP effect of 0.025 was associated with an expected increase of 25(OH)D by 2.5% (e^0.025 = 1.025), while a SNP effect of 0.1 was associated with an expected increase of 25(OH)D by 10.5% (e^0.1 = 1.105).

Table 2. Results of the Mendelian Randomization analyses on the associations of natural-log transformed 25(OH)vitamin D concentrations with broad depression and depressive symptoms.

SNP	Association of 25(OH)vitamin D with Broad Depression			Association of 25(OH)vitamin D with Depressive Symptoms		
	Effect Estimate (Beta)	SE	p	Effect Estimate (Beta)	SE	p
rs3755967	−0.0136	0.0145	0.350	0.0112	0.0450	0.803
rs10741657	−0.0743	0.0386	0.055	0.1613	0.1290	0.211
rs12785878	−0.0424	0.0398	0.287	0.1667	0.1389	0.230
rs10745742	0.0586	0.0715	0.412	0.0000	0.2353	1.000
rs8018720	−0.0163	0.0907	0.857	−0.0588	0.2941	0.841
rs17216707	−0.0102	0.0587	0.862	−0.1538	0.1538	0.317
All—Inverse variance weighted (IVW)	−0.0202	0.0123	0.099	0.0246	0.0384	0.521
All—MR Egger	−0.0175	0.0217	0.464	0.0209	0.0674	0.772

SE: standard error; SNP: single nucleotide polymorphisms.

4. Discussion

Using data from the large-scaled GWAS in subjects from European descent, this MR study did not provide evidence for the suggested role of (genetically determined) 25(OH)vitamin D concentrations in the onset of DS or BD. Combined with the results from a previous MR study, based on a subsample of the data sets used for this current study, which showed no association with MDD, it might be hypothesized that raising of vitamin D concentrations seems to have no discernible preventive effect on the onset of depressive disorders in individuals of European descent.

In contrast to this conclusion, a meta-analysis of observational studies that compared the lowest and the highest category of vitamin D concentrations in adults, revealed an OR of 1.31 (95% confidence interval (CI) 1.0–1.71, $p = 0.05$) for depression derived from nine cross-sectional studies and a hazard ratio of 2.21 (95% CI 1.40–3.49, $p = 0.0007$) from three cohort studies [28]. We recently confirmed these findings in children using cross-sectional data of the representative KiGGS study in Germany, which illustrated an inverse association between 25(OH)vitamin D concentrations and emotional problems, measured by the Strengths and Difficulties Questionnaire (SDQ) [5]. A prospective analysis of the Avon longitudinal study for parents and children (ALSPAC) also seemed to indicate a preventive role of vitamin D in adolescence. While 25(OH)vitamin D concentrations at the age of 10 years were not associated with self-reported DS at the age of eleven years, long-term analyses revealed that those participants with 25(OH)D <50 nmol/l at ten years had a 20% increased risk of self-reported depressive symptoms at 14 years [7]. Overall, these associations from observational studies stand in contrast to the MR study on MDD [16], and stand also in contrast to our findings on DS and BD. As suggested by König and Del Greco, reverse causation and residual confounding should be considered as alternative explanations, if MR studies do not support findings from observational studies [15]. In fact, low vitamin D levels could well be a consequence of an already developing depression, e.g., in case of social withdrawal and reduced sunlight exposure (reverse causation). Residual confounding also seems reasonable considering that decreasing vitamin D concentrations were discussed to be a biomarker for impaired general health [29]. Accordingly, low vitamin D concentrations could be associated with a number of potential confounds, which hamper a complete adjustment in the statistical analyses of observational studies.

A limitation of our MR study was that the analyzed SNPs only explained 2.8% of the variance of vitamin D concentrations. Accordingly, the lacking association between the respective SNPs and the development of depression might be confounded by the weak effect of these genetic determinants on the vitamin D level (weak instrument bias). However, the F-Statistics indicated that the genetic instruments used were sufficiently strong.

The considered GWAS meta-analyses for vitamin D, DS, and BD for MR analysis were all restricted to individuals of European descent. Since our MR analysis relied on the provided information in the underlying GWAS meta-analyses, it was, for example, not possible to conduct stratified analyses for different countries, ethnicities, or age groups. Accordingly, the effects of vitamin D concentrations observed in this MR study might not be transferable to populations with other specific characteristics (e.g., ethnicity and age). Furthermore, horizontal pleiotropy, i.e., an association between the MR instrument and the outcome of interest via pathways other than the suggested exposure, is a general issue in MR studies and is a source of bias [14]. Although pleiotropy cannot be completely ruled out in our MR study, the MR Egger intercept revealed no indication of pleiotropy. Another limitation is that the statistical power only allowed the detection of OR > 1.1 per 1 standard deviation decrease in the natural-log transformed 25(OH)vitamin D with a statistical power of 100% (OR > 1.07 with 80% power). Accordingly, small preventive effects below this threshold could not completely be ruled out. Additionally, it must be kept in mind that DS and BD represent a broad definition of depression. As depression is a heterogenic disorder, vitamin D might still be effective in specific subtypes of depression. Finally, it has to be considered that vitamin D represents only one of numerous etiological factors in the complex etiological model of depression, including endocrinology, inflammation, and neurotransmission pathways [17]. At least, at the population level, the role of vitamin D in this process might be of minor importance.

5. Conclusions

This MR study did not support the suggested preventive role of 25(OH)vitamin D concentrations in the development of depression. Other health and lifestyle factors related to low 25(OH)vitamin D concentrations, such as insufficient sunlight exposure as a consequence of an already beginning depression, could explain the observed associations from observational studies.

Supplementary Materials: The following are available online at http://www.mdpi.com/2072-6643/11/5/1085/s1, Table S1: Sensitivity analyses using the leave-one-out approach on the association of natural-log transformed 25(OH)vitamin D concentrations with broad depression, Table S2: Sensitivity analyses using the leave-one-out approach on the association of natural-log transformed 25(OH)vitamin D concentrations with depressive symptoms. Figure S1. Calculated power to detect a true causal effect of a relative difference between 1% and 20% per 1 standard deviation in 25(OH)vitamin D.

Author Contributions: Conceptualization: L.L., J.H., I.R.K., and T.P.; methodology: B.-H.L., I.R.K., T.P., and L.L.; formal analysis: B.-H.L. and I.R.K.; writing—original draft preparation: L.L., B.-H.L., I.R.K., T.P., M.F., and J.H.; writing—review & editing: C.L., J.A., R.N., A.H., J.B., and L.L.; all authors revised it critically for important intellectual content, and approved the final version to be published.

Funding: We acknowledge the support from the Open Access Publication Fund of the University of Duisburg-Essen. A.H. was supported by the "Landesprogramm für Geschlechtergerechte Hochschulen–Programmstrang Förderung von Denominationen in der Genderforschung".

Conflicts of Interest: The authors declare no conflict of interest.

References

1. GBD 2015 Disease and Injury Incidence and Prevalence Collaborators. Global, regional, and national incidence, prevalence, and years lived with disability for 310 diseases and injuries, 1990–2015: A systematic analysis for the Global Burden of Disease Study 2015. *Lancet* **2016**, *388*, 1545–1602. [CrossRef]
2. Kessler, R.C.; Berglund, P.; Demler, O.; Jin, R.; Merikangas, K.R.; Walters, E.E. Lifetime prevalence and age-of-onset distributions of DSM-IV disorders in the National Comorbidity Survey Replication. *Arch Gen. Psychiatry* **2005**, *62*, 593–602. [CrossRef]
3. Sarris, J.; Logan, A.C.; Akbaraly, T.N.; Amminger, G.P.; Balanza-Martinez, V.; Freeman, M.P.; Hibbeln, J.; Matsuoka, Y.; Mischoulon, D.; Mizoue, T.; et al. Nutritional medicine as mainstream in psychiatry. *Lancet Psychiatry* **2015**, *2*, 271–274. [CrossRef]
4. Föcker, M.; Antel, J.; Ring, S.; Hahn, D.; Kanal, O.; Ozturk, D.; Hebebrand, J.; Libuda, L. Vitamin D and mental health in children and adolescents. *Eur. Child Adolesc. Psychiatry* **2017**, *26*, 1043–1066. [CrossRef] [PubMed]
5. Husmann, C.; Frank, M.; Schmidt, B.; Jöckel, K.H.; Antel, J.; Reissner, V.; Libuda, L.; Hebebrand, J.; Föcker, M. Low 25(OH)-vitamin D concentrations are associated with emotional and behavioral problems in German children and adolescents. *PLoS ONE* **2017**, *12*, e0183091. [CrossRef]
6. Schäfer, T.K.; Herrmann-Lingen, C.; Meyer, T. Association of circulating 25-hydroxyvitamin D with mental well-being in a population-based, nationally representative sample of German adolescents. *Qual. Life Res.* **2016**, *25*, 3077–3086. [CrossRef] [PubMed]
7. Tolppanen, A.M.; Sayers, A.; Fraser, W.D.; Lewis, G.; Zammit, S.; Lawlor, D.A. The association of serum 25-hydroxyvitamin D3 and D2 with depressive symptoms in childhood—A prospective cohort study. *J. Child Psychol. Psychiatry* **2012**, *53*, 757–766. [CrossRef] [PubMed]
8. Föcker, M.; Antel, J.; Grasemann, C.; Fuhrer, D.; Timmesfeld, N.; Ozturk, D.; Peters, T.; Hinney, A.; Hebebrand, J.; Libuda, L. Effect of an vitamin D deficiency on depressive symptoms in child and adolescent psychiatric patients—A randomized controlled trial: Study protocol. *BMC Psychiatry* **2018**, *18*, 57. [CrossRef]
9. Shaffer, J.A.; Edmondson, D.; Wasson, L.T.; Falzon, L.; Homma, K.; Ezeokoli, N.; Li, P.; Davidson, K.W. Vitamin D supplementation for depressive symptoms: A systematic review and meta-analysis of randomized controlled trials. *Psychosom. Med.* **2014**, *76*, 190–196. [CrossRef]

10. Spedding, S. Vitamin D and depression: A systematic review and meta-analysis comparing studies with and without biological flaws. *Nutrients* **2014**, *6*, 1501–1518. [CrossRef]
11. Vellekkatt, F.; Menon, V. Efficacy of vitamin D supplementation in major depression: A meta-analysis of randomized controlled trials. *J. Postgrad. Med.* **2018**. [CrossRef]
12. Bertone-Johnson, E.R.; Powers, S.I.; Spangler, L.; Larson, J.; Michael, Y.L.; Millen, A.E.; Bueche, M.N.; Salmoirago-Blotcher, E.; Wassertheil-Smoller, S.; Brunner, R.L.; et al. Vitamin D supplementation and depression in the women's health initiative calcium and vitamin D trial. *Am. J. Epidemiol.* **2012**, *176*, 1–13. [CrossRef]
13. Sanders, K.M.; Stuart, A.L.; Williamson, E.J.; Jacka, F.N.; Dodd, S.; Nicholson, G.; Berk, M. Annual high-dose vitamin D3 and mental well-being: Randomised controlled trial. *Br. J. Psychiatry* **2011**, *198*, 357–364. [CrossRef]
14. Zheng, J.; Baird, D.; Borges, M.C.; Bowden, J.; Hemani, G.; Haycock, P.; Evans, D.M.; Smith, G.D. Recent Developments in Mendelian Randomization Studies. *Curr. Epidemiol. Rep.* **2017**, *4*, 330–345. [CrossRef]
15. König, I.R.; Greco, F.M.D. Mendelian randomization: Progressing towards understanding causality. *Ann. Neurol.* **2018**, *84*, 176–177. [CrossRef] [PubMed]
16. Michaelsson, K.; Melhus, H.; Larsson, S.C. Serum 25-Hydroxyvitamin D Concentrations and Major Depression: A Mendelian Randomization Study. *Nutrients* **2018**, *10*, 1987. [CrossRef] [PubMed]
17. Stapelberg, N.J.C.; Neumann, D.L.; Shum, D.; Headrick, J.P. Health, pre-disease and critical transition to disease in the psycho-immune-neuroendocrine network: Are there distinct states in the progression from health to major depressive disorder? *Physiol. Behav.* **2019**, *198*, 108–119. [CrossRef] [PubMed]
18. Jiang, X.; O'Reilly, P.F.; Aschard, H.; Hsu, Y.H.; Richards, J.B.; Dupuis, J.; Ingelsson, E.; Karasik, D.; Pilz, S.; Berry, D.; et al. Genome-wide association study in 79,366 European-ancestry individuals informs the genetic architecture of 25-hydroxyvitamin D levels. *Nat. Commun.* **2018**, *9*, 260. [CrossRef]
19. Okbay, A.; Baselmans, B.M.; De Neve, J.E.; Turley, P.; Nivard, M.G.; Fontana, M.A.; Meddens, S.F.; Linner, R.K.; Rietveld, C.A.; Derringer, J.; et al. Genetic variants associated with subjective well-being, depressive symptoms, and neuroticism identified through genome-wide analyses. *Nat. Genet.* **2016**, *48*, 624–633. [CrossRef]
20. Howard, D.M.; Adams, M.J.; Shirali, M.; Clarke, T.K.; Marioni, R.E.; Davies, G.; Coleman, J.R.I.; Alloza, C.; Shen, X.; Barbu, M.C.; et al. Genome-wide association study of depression phenotypes in UK Biobank identifies variants in excitatory synaptic pathways. *Nat. Commun.* **2018**, *9*, 1470. [CrossRef]
21. Howard, D.M.; Adams, M.J.; Shirali, M.; Clarke, T.K.; Marioni, R.E.; Davies, G.; Coleman, J.R.I.; Alloza, C.; Shen, X.; Barbu, M.C.; et al. Addendum: Genome-wide association study of depression phenotypes in UK Biobank identifies variants in excitatory synaptic pathways. *Nat. Commun.* **2018**, *9*, 3578. [CrossRef]
22. Wang, T.J.; Zhang, F.; Richards, J.B.; Kestenbaum, B.; van Meurs, J.B.; Berry, D.; Kiel, D.P.; Streeten, E.A.; Ohlsson, C.; Koller, D.L.; et al. Common genetic determinants of vitamin D insufficiency: A genome-wide association study. *Lancet* **2010**, *376*, 180–188. [CrossRef]
23. Kvale, M.N.; Hesselson, S.; Hoffmann, T.J.; Cao, Y.; Chan, D.; Connell, S.; Croen, L.A.; Dispensa, B.P.; Eshragh, J.; Finn, A.; et al. Genotyping Informatics and Quality Control for 100,000 Subjects in the Genetic Epidemiology Research on Adult Health and Aging (GERA) Cohort. *Genetics* **2015**, *200*, 1051–1060. [CrossRef]
24. Major Depressive Disorder Working Group of the Psychiatric; Ripke, S.; Wray, N.R.; Lewis, C.M.; Hamilton, S.P.; Weissman, M.M.; Breen, G.; Byrne, E.M.; Blackwood, D.H.; Boomsma, D.I.; et al. A mega-analysis of genome-wide association studies for major depressive disorder. *Mol. Psychiatry* **2013**, *18*, 497–511. [CrossRef] [PubMed]
25. Sudlow, C.; Gallacher, J.; Allen, N.; Beral, V.; Burton, P.; Danesh, J.; Downey, P.; Elliott, P.; Green, J.; Landray, M.; et al. UK biobank: An open access resource for identifying the causes of a wide range of complex diseases of middle and old age. *PLoS Med.* **2015**, *12*, e1001779. [CrossRef]
26. Haycock, P.C.; Burgess, S.; Wade, K.H.; Bowden, J.; Relton, C.; Davey Smith, G. Best (but oft-forgotten) practices: The design, analysis, and interpretation of Mendelian randomization studies. *Am. J. Clin. Nutr.* **2016**, *103*, 965–978. [CrossRef] [PubMed]
27. Brion, M.J.; Shakhbazov, K.; Visscher, P.M. Calculating statistical power in Mendelian randomization studies. *Int. J. Epidemiol.* **2013**, *42*, 1497–1501. [CrossRef]

28. Anglin, R.E.; Samaan, Z.; Walter, S.D.; McDonald, S.D. Vitamin D deficiency and depression in adults: Systematic review and meta-analysis. *Br. J. Psychiatry* **2013**, *202*, 100–107. [CrossRef]
29. Autier, P.; Boniol, M.; Pizot, C.; Mullie, P. Vitamin D status and ill health: A systematic review. *Lancet Diabetes Endocrinol.* **2014**, *2*, 76–89. [CrossRef]

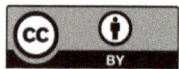

© 2019 by the authors. Licensee MDPI, Basel, Switzerland. This article is an open access article distributed under the terms and conditions of the Creative Commons Attribution (CC BY) license (http://creativecommons.org/licenses/by/4.0/).

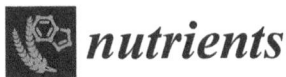

Article

Multiple Sclerosis Patients Show Lower Bioavailable 25(OH)D and 1,25(OH)$_2$D, but No Difference in Ratio of 25(OH)D/24,25(OH)$_2$D and FGF23 Concentrations

Mariska C Vlot [1,2,†], Laura Boekel [1,†], Jolijn Kragt [3], Joep Killestein [4], Barbara M. van Amerongen [5], Robert de Jonge [1], Martin den Heijer [2] and Annemieke C. Heijboer [1,6,*]

[1] Department of Clinical Chemistry, Endocrine Laboratory, Amsterdam University Medical Center, 1081 HV Amsterdam, The Netherlands; m.vlot@amsterdamumc.nl (M.C.V.); l.boekel@student.vu.nl (L.B.); r.dejonge1@amsterdamumc.nl (R.d.J.)
[2] Department of Internal Medicine, Amsterdam UMC, Amsterdam University medical Center, 1081 HV Amsterdam, The Netherlands; m.denheijer@amsterdamumc.nl
[3] Department of Neurology, Reinier de Graaf Gasthuis, 2625 AD Delft, The Netherlands; J.Kragt@rdgg.nl
[4] Department of Neurology, Amsterdam Neuroscience, MS Center Amsterdam, Amsterdam University Medical Center, 1081 HV, Amsterdam, The Netherlands; j.killestein@amsterdamumc.nl
[5] Department of Molecular Cell Biology and Immunology, Amsterdam University Medical Center, Vrije Universiteit Amsterdam, 1081 HV Amsterdam, The Netherlands; bmvanamerongen@gmail.com
[6] Department of Clinical Chemistry, Endocrine Laboratory, Amsterdam University Medical Center, 1105 AZ Amsterdam, The Netherlands
* Correspondence: a.heijboer@amsterdamumc.nl; Tel.: +31-205665940
† Both authors contributed equally.

Received: 10 October 2019; Accepted: 13 November 2019; Published: 15 November 2019

Abstract: Vitamin D (VitD) insufficiency is common in multiple sclerosis (MS). VitD has possible anti-inflammatory effects on the immune system. The ratio between VitD metabolites in MS patients and the severity of the disease are suggested to be related. However, the exact effect of the bone-derived hormone fibroblast-growth-factor-23 (FGF23) and VitD binding protein (VDBP) on this ratio is not fully elucidated yet. Therefore, the aim is to study differences in total, free, and bioavailable VD metabolites and FGF23 between MS patients and healthy controls (HCs). FGF23, vitD (25(OH)D), active vitD (1,25(OH)$_2$D), inactive 24,25(OH)$_2$D, and VDBP were measured in 91 MS patients and 92 HCs. Bioavailable and free concentrations were calculated. No difference in FGF23 ($p = 0.65$) and 25(OH)D/24.25(OH)$_2$D ratio ($p = 0.21$) between MS patients and HCs was observed. Bioavailable 25(OH)D and bioavailable 1.25(OH)$_2$D were lower ($p < 0.01$), while VDBP concentrations were higher in MS patients ($p = 0.02$) compared with HCs, specifically in male MS patients ($p = 0.01$). In conclusion, FGF23 and 25(OH)D/24.25(OH)$_2$D did not differ between MS patients and HCs, yet bioavailable VitD concentrations are of potential clinical relevance in MS patients. The possible immunomodulating role of VDBP and gender-related differences in the VD-FGF23 axis in MS need further study.

Keywords: multiple sclerosis; fibroblast growth factor 23; vitamin D metabolites; vitamin D binding protein

1. Introduction

Multiple sclerosis (MS) is a chronic, progressive disease of the central nervous system characterized by an inflammatory, demyelinating, and neurodegenerative process, which can result in varying levels of disability. Consequently, MS has a negative effect on the daily life of patients, resulting from fatigue, muscle weakness, and imbalance to immobility, which all negatively affect bone health [1–4]. Earlier studies showed that decreased bone mineral density (BMD) is prevalent already shortly after clinical onset even in physically active patients with MS [2,4–6]. Lower BMD combined with impaired mobility can result in an increased fracture risk in MS patients and accompanying disability and economic burden [7]. The specific aetiology of MS is still unknown, but strong evidence exists regarding viral, genetic, and immunological causes of the disease [8,9].

Vitamin D is thought to play a role in the pathogenesis of MS, as it is known that the prevalence of MS increases with latitude, which in turn is associated with lower serum concentrations of vitamin D (25(OH)D) [10,11]. Vitamin D possibly modulates T-lymphocyte subset differentiation and, therefore, a lower concentration is thought to lead to an increased risk of MS [12]. In line with this, associations between lower serum concentrations 25(OH)D and an increased risk of MS are shown in several studies [13–15]. As a result, vitamin D supplementation is often advised to MS patients, although contra-dictionary effects regarding the beneficial effects of increased 25(OH)D concentrations on, for example, the recurrence rate of relapses, deterioration of number of brain laesions, and improvement of disability are described [16–20]. Because of the potential role of vitamin D in MS, other vitamin D metabolites have been studied in MS patients. 25(OH)D needs to be metabolized to the biologically active 1.25(OH)$_2$D, and both metabolites are predominantly bound to their carrier vitamin D binding protein (VDBP). Previous research showed a higher plasma VDBP concentration in MS patients compared with healthy controls (HCs) [21]. VDBP is known to play an important role in the intracellular actin scavenging system by removing actin derived from damaged tissue and also promotes inflammation [22–26]. Polymorphisms of both VDBP and also of the vitamin D receptor (VDR) can result in a changed equilibrium between active and inactive vitamin D metabolites [24,27,28]. Interestingly, lower concentrations of the vitamin D metabolite 24.25(OH)$_2$D were associated with a higher grade of disability based on the Expanded Disability Status Scale (EDSS) score in MS patients [29]. Moreover, the ratio of 25(OH)D/24.25(OH)$_2$D was strongly inversely associated with brain parenchymal function [29].

A key player in vitamin D metabolism is the bone-derived hormone fibroblast growth factor 23 (FGF23), as it inhibits the enzyme 1-alpha hydroxylase and stimulates the enzyme 24-hydroxylase, resulting in the conversion of 25(OH)D into 24.25(OH)$_2$D instead of into 1.25(OH)$_2$D. We thus hypothesize that plasma FGF23 concentrations differ between MS patients and healthy controls.

The primary aim of this study is to further elucidate the vitamin D-FGF23 axis by measuring multiple D metabolites and FGF23 using accurate state-of-the art analytical methods in a well-defined cohort of MS patients and healthy controls. The second aim of our study is to assess bone turnover markers (BTMs) in our cohort MS patients and healthy controls and to study the possible associations of BTMs with vitamin D metabolites, as vitamin D deficiency is associated with increased bone turnover and lower bone mineral density [30–32]. Lastly, it is known that MS affects more women than men and that women have higher VDBP concentrations compared with men [13,21,33–36]. Therefore, possible gender-related differences of vitamin D metabolites and BTMs between MS patients and healthy controls will be studied.

2. Materials and Methods

2.1. Subjects and Study Protocol

The subjects and study protocol were described earlier by Kragt et al. [13]. Patients were eligible to participate in the study if they provided informed consent and were between 18 and 75 years of age. Three subtypes of MS were identified: relapsing-remitting MS (RRMS), secondary progressive MS (SPMS), and primary progressive MS (PPMS). Patients with all subtypes of MS were eligible to participate. In addition, patients with clinically isolated syndrome (CIS) were also included, which refers to a single episode of symptoms that are suggestive for MS. Patients were recruited between July and September 2003, to ensure that all blood samples were drawn during summer season. Patients were asked to bring a healthy control with them to the outpatient clinic if possible, preferably their partner in order to match the patients based on age and environmental factors. If a healthy control was lacking, hospital personnel volunteered to participate as controls. Patients were excluded if they were diagnosed with osteomalacia, hyperparathyroidism, hyperthyroidism, or hypercortisolism, or if they had been receiving glucocorticoid treatment in the previous three weeks (daily oral treatment or intravenous methylprednisolone treatment), anti-epileptic drugs, or vitamin D supplementation of more than 200 IU/day. The controls were excluded if they had MS or had a first-degree family member with MS. In addition, study participants were excluded in the case of suspicion of concomitant bone disease based on their laboratory results. All subjects gave their informed consent for inclusion before they participated in the study. The study was conducted in accordance with the Declaration of Helsinki, and the protocol was approved by the Medical Ethical Committee of the Amsterdam UMC, location VU University Medical Center (code 2003.029).

2.2. Measurements

2.2.1. General

The functional disability of MS patients was evaluated using the Expanded Disability Status Scale (EDSS) [37]. EDSS quantifies disability in MS patients, which ranges from 0 to 10, with higher scores representing higher levels of disability. Blood samples were collected before 00:00 and after an overnight fast. Samples were collected in 2003 and stored (both as serum and EDTA plasma in several aliquots) in minus 80 degrees Celsius. Analyses were performed in 2011 (parathyroid hormone (PTH), alkaline phosphatase (ALP), albumin, calcium, phosphate, estimated glomerular filtration rate (eGFR)) and in 2017 (25(OH)D, 24.25(OH)$_2$D, 1.25(OH)$_2$D, VDBP, FGF23, c-terminal telopeptide (CTX), osteocalcin, procollagen type 1 N-terminal propeptide (P1NP)) in the various aliquots.

2.2.2. Vitamin D Metabolites

In the current study, 25(OH)D and 24.25(OH)$_2$D were measured in serum using a dedicated isotope dilution liquid chromatography-tandem mass spectrometry (ID-LC-MS/MS) [38]. Total serum concentrations of 25(OH)D were calculated by the sum of 25(OH)D$_2$ and 25(OH)D$_3$. For 25(OH)D$_2$, the lower limit of quantitation (LLOQ) was 0.36 nmol/L and the inter-assay coefficient of variation (CV) was 6%. For 25(OH)D$_3$, LLOQ was 1.19 nmol/L and the inter-assay CV was 6%. For 24.25(OH)$_2$D, LLOQ was 0.12 nmol/L and the inter-assay CV was 5% [37,39]. A two-dimensional isotope dilution ultra-pressure liquid chromatography tandem mass spectrometry (2D ID-UPLC-MS/MS) was used to measure serum 1.25(OH)$_2$D with an LLOQ of 3.4 pmol/L and inter-assay CV of 11% [40]. It is of note that, in the earlier study of Kragt et al., a radioimmunoassay was used for the measurement of 25(OH)D and 1.25(OH)$_2$D [13], but the concentrations shown in the current study are obtained using an LC-MS/MS method. VDBP was measured using a polyclonal ELISA (Immundiagnostik AG) with a LLOQ of 2.2 µg/L and an inter-assay CV of <13%.

2.2.3. Free and Bioavailable Vitamin D Metabolites

Vitamin D metabolites bound to protein are not biologically active, whereas the unbound hormones are. Free 25(OH)D was calculated using equations and affinity constants according to Malmstroem et al. [41] and free 1.25(OH)$_2$D was calculated using equations and affinity constants according to Bikle et al. [42]. Bioavailable 25(OH)D and 1.25(OH)$_2$D were calculated using equations adapted from Vermeulen et al. [43] and the supplement of Powe et al. [44].

2.2.4. Bone Turnover Markers (BTMs)

FGF23 was measured in EDTA plasma using a c-terminal immunoassay (Immutopics) with an LLOQ of 20 RU/mL and inter-assay CV of <10% [45]. CTX and P1NP were measured in EDTA plasma using an immunoassay (Cobas, Roche Diagnostics, Almere, The Netherlands), with an LLOQ of 10 ng/L and inter-assay CV of <6.5% for CTX and an LLOQ of 5 µg/L and inter-assay CV of <8% for P1NP, respectively. Osteocalcin was measured in EDTA plasma using an immunometric-assay (Biosource, Nivelles, Belgium) with an LLOQ of 0.4 nmol/L and inter-assay CV of 8–15%.

2.2.5. Other Measurements

PTH was measured in EDTA plasma using an immunoassay (Architect, Abbott Diagnosher, Chicago, IL, USA) with an LLOQ 0.5 pmol/L and inter-assay CV of <9%. ALP, eGFR, calcium, phosphate, and albumin were measured in heparin plasma using the chemistry module of the Cobas (Roche Diagnostics).

2.3. Statistical Analysis

Baseline characteristics between MS patients and healthy controls were compared using a Student's t-test or chi-square test. The Mann–Whitney U test was used in the case of non-parametric variables. To detect differences between patients and controls in biochemical indices of the vitamin D metabolites and BTMs, the Mann–Whitney U test was used as well. In addition, separate analyses for men and women were performed. Lastly, correlations between serum vitamin D metabolites, BTMs, and EDSS were calculated using Spearman correlations owing to non-parametric variables. All statistical analyses were carried out using SPSS software, version 23.0.

3. Results

3.1. General

A total of 213 participants were eligible to be included in this study. After applying the in- and exclusion criteria, a total of 30 participants were excluded; see Figure 1. The final study population that was included in the analyses consisted of 183 participants based on 91 MS patients and 92 healthy controls. Table 1 summarizes the baseline characteristics of all participants. In total, 61% of the MS patients were female. Relapsing remitting MS was the most predominant subtype of MS (57%).

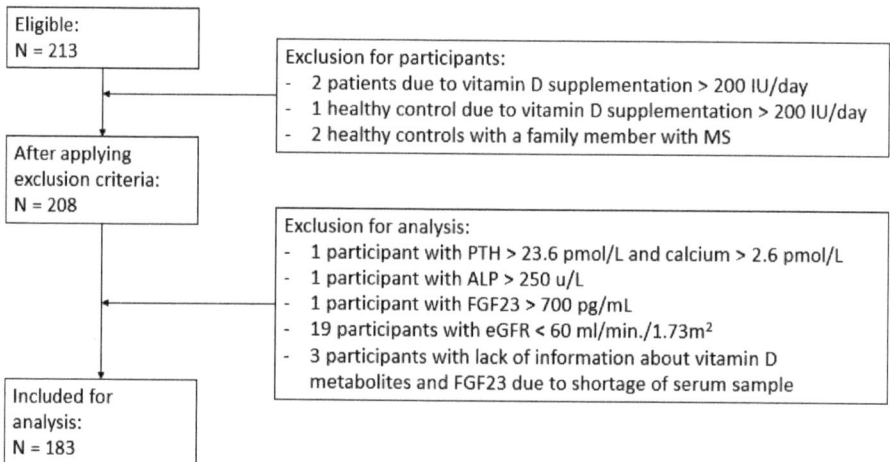

Figure 1. Flow chart of study population selection. PTH = parathyroid hormone, ALP = alkaline phosphatase, eGFR = estimated glomerular filtration rate FGF23 = fibroblast growth factor 23, MS = multiple sclerosis.

Table 1. Baseline characteristics, vitamin D metabolites, FGF23, and bone turnover markers of multiple sclerosis (MS) patients and controls displayed as median with corresponding interquartile range (IQR), unless specified otherwise, of MS patients and controls.

	Patients (n = 91)	Controls (n = 92)	p Value [a]	Reference Range
Age, yr (mean ± SD)	45 ± 11	42 ± 11	0.30	
Female of total population (%)	67	41	<0.01 *	
Postmenopausal of total population (%)	34	16	0.04 *	
Caucasian (%)	98	95	0.44	
eGFR, mL/min/1.73m^2 (median, IQR)	71 (66–81)	71 (67–78)	0.42	>60
MS subtype (%)				
RRMS	57			
SPMS	24	n.a.		
PPMS	14			
CIS	1			
Disease duration, yr (median, IQR)	10 (5–16)	n.a.		
EDSS (median, IQR)	4 (3–6)	n.a.		
Use of vitamin D supplements [b], (%)	40	14	<0.01 *	
Use of using disease modifying therapy, (%)	32	n.a.		
Total 25(OH)D, nmol/L	75 (59–93)	77 (67–98)	0.06 #	>50
Total 1.25(OH)$_2$D, pmol/L	105 (74–143)	99 (79–133)	0.57	59–159
25(OH)D$_2$, nmol/L	1.1 (0.8–1.5)	1.2 (0.9–1.5)	0.66	
25(OH)D$_3$, nmol/L	73 (58–92)	76 (66–96)	0.05 #	
24.25(OH)D, nmol/L	6.5 (4.4–9.0)	7.1 (5.4–9.6)	0.08 #	0.4–8.9
Free 25(OH)D (* 10^{-2}), nmol/L	1.2 (1.0–1.5)	1.4 (1.2–1.7)	<0.01 *	
Albumin bound 25(OH)D, nmol/L	4.5 (3.5–5.6)	5.1 (4.1–6.1)	<0.01 *	
Bioavailable 25(OH)D, nmol/L	4.5 (3.5–5.6)	5.1 (4.1–6.1)	<0.01 *	
Free 1.25(OH)$_2$D (* 10^{-1}), pmol/L	2.0 (2.2–2.8)	2.5 (0.2–3.1)	<0.01 * #	
Albumin bound 1.25(OH)$_2$D, pmol/L	7.3 (5.7–9.1)	8.4 (6.7–9.9)	<0.01 *	
Bioavailable 1.25(OH)$_2$D, pmol/L	7.5 (5.9–9.4)	8.6 (7.0–10.2)	<0.01 *	
Ratio total 25(OH)D/24.25(OH)$_2$D	11.2 (9.9–13.6)	11.4 (9.5–12.9)	0.21	10–33
VDBP, µg/L	408 (374–445)	388 (361–427)	0.02 * #	200–550
Albumin, g/L	42 (39–44)	42 (40–43)	0.86	35–52
Calcium, mmol/L	2.4 (2.3–2.4)	2.4 (2.3–2.4)	0.73	2.2–2.6
Corrected calcium, mmol/L	2.3 (2.3–2.4)	2.3 (2.3–2.4)	0.81	
FGF23, RU/mL	88 (72–113)	89 (69–106)	0.65	<125
PTH, pmol/L	5.2 (4.0–6.6)	5.3 (3.8–6.7)	0.94	<10
Phosphate, mmol/L	1.0 (0.9–1.1)	0.8 (0.8–0.9)	<0.01 *	0.7–1.4
CTX, ng/L	256 (183–379)	307 (212–418)	0.10	<580
P1NP, µg/L	37 (27–54)	39 (29–56)	0.37	22–87
ALP, U/L	74 (53–89)	67 (56–79)	0.14	<115
Osteocalcin, nmol/L	1.5 (1.1–2.1)	1.5 (1.1–2.0)	0.99	0.4–4.0

eGFR = estimated glomerular filtration rate, RRMS = relapsing remitting MS, SPMS = secondary progressive MS, PPMS = primary progressive MS, CIS = clinically isolated syndrome, SP + R = secondary progressive + remitting, EDSS = Expanded Disability Status Scale, VDBP = vitamin D binding protein, PTH = parathyroid hormone, ALP = alkaline phosphatase, FGF23 = fibroblast growth factor 23, CTX = c-terminal telopeptide, P1NP = procollagen type 1 N-terminal propeptide. [a] p values of Student's t-test, chi-square test, or Mann–Whitney U test. [b] Maximum allowed dose of vitamin D supplements was 200 IU/day. * Bold, significance level $p \leq 0.05$. # Significant difference between male and female; details can be found in Table 2.

3.2. Vitamin D Metabolites, FGF23, and Bone Turnover Markers

Biochemical indices of vitamin D metabolism and bone turnover of the study population are displayed in Table 1. Again, it is of note that, in contrast to the earlier study of Kragt et al., current 25(OH)D and 1.25(OH)$_2$D measurements are reported based on the ID-LC-MS/MS measurements [13]. Overall, no significant difference between total serum concentrations of 25(OH)D ($p = 0.06$) was found between MS patients and the healthy controls. MS patients had significant lower serum concentrations of free, albumin bound, and bioavailable 25(OH)D and 1.25(OH)$_2$D compared with healthy controls ($p < 0.01$). In addition, MS patients had higher concentrations of phosphate and VDBP compared with controls, whereas no significant differences in BTMs were found. Plasma FGF23 concentrations did not differ between MS patient and the healthy controls ($p = 0.65$) (Figure 2).

Table 2 shows the significant results of separate analyses for men and women. In contrast to male patients, female MS patients had lower serum concentrations of total 25(OH)D, 25(OH)D$_3$, 24.25(OH)$_2$D, free 25(OH)D, and free 1.25(OH)$_2$D compared with healthy female controls ($p = 0.04$). Male MS patients had higher serum concentrations of VDBP compared with male controls ($p = 0.01$). No other significant differences were found between male MS patients and healthy male controls. Regarding BTMs, no significant differences were found between males and females (data not shown). Lastly, EDSS scores did not differ between male and female MS patients ($p = 0.77$, data not shown).

Table 2. Vitamin D metabolites of MS patients and controls stratified for gender, only shown in the case of significant differences between male and females, displayed as median with corresponding interquartile range (IQR).

	Men (n = 84)			Women (n = 99)		
	Patients (n = 30)	Controls (n = 54)	p values [a]	Patients (n = 61)	Controls (n = 38)	p values [a]
Total 25(OH)D, nmol/L	74 (56–97)	75 (66–90)	0.62	77 (60–90)	88 (68–106)	0.02 *
25(OH)D$_3$, nmol/L	73 (55–96)	74 (64–89)	0.64	75 (58–89)	86 (67–104)	0.01 *
24.25(OH)$_2$D, nmol/L	6.5 (4.5–8.8)	6.9 (5.4–8.7)	0.48	6.5 (4.4–9.1)	7.1 (5.6–11.0)	0.04 *
Free 25(OH)D (* 10^{-2}), nmol/L	0.013 (0.010–0.017)	0.014 (0.012–0.017)	0.17	0.012 (0.010–0.015)	0.013 (0.011–0.017)	0.03 *
Free 1.25(OH)$_2$D (* 10^{-1}), pmol/L	0.23 (0.17–0.30)	0.25 (0.22–0.31)	0.18	0.21 (0.17–0.27)	0.24 (0.21–0.31)	0.03 *
Phosphate, mmol/L	1.0 (0.9–1.0)	0.8 (0.8–0.9)	<0.01 *	1.0 (0.9–1.1)	0.8 (0.8–0.9)	<0.01 *

VDBP = vitamin D binding protein, PTH = parathyroid hormone. [a] p values of Mann–Whitney U test are shown as medians with interquartile ranges in parentheses. * bold significance level $p \leq 0.05$.

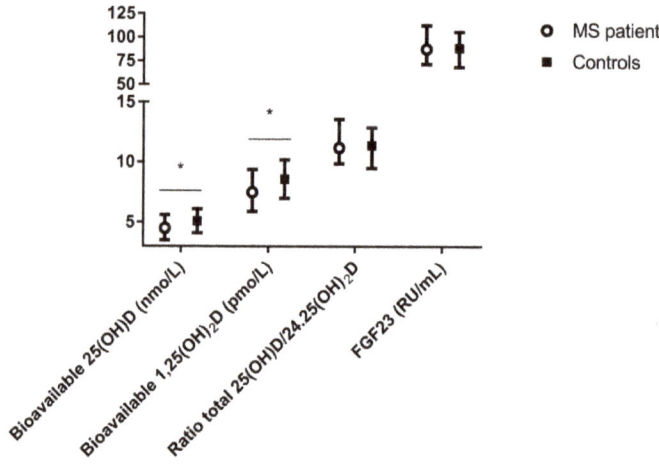

Figure 2. Vitamin D metabolites and FGF23 in MS patients versus healthy controls, * $p \leq 0.05$.

3.3. Associations

3.3.1. Associations between Vitamin D Metabolites, FGF23, Bone Turnover Markers, and EDSS in MS Patients

In MS patients, all vitamin D metabolites correlated strongly with each other (all $r > 0.77$; $p < 0.01$, data not shown). EDSS showed negative correlations with bioavailable 1.25(OH)$_2$D, bioavailable 25(OH)D, and 24.25(OH)$_2$D (r −0.30, $p < 0.01$; r −0.30, $p < 0.01$; and r −0.23, $p = 0.03$, respectively). No correlations between EDSS and FGF23 or BTMs in MS patients were found (data not shown).

As shown in Table 3, FGF23 correlated positively with serum 25(OH)D and serum 24.25(OH)$_2$D (r 0.22, $p = 0.04$ and r 0.22, $p = 0.04$, respectively), and CTX correlated negatively with serum 24.25(OH)$_2$D and 25(OH)D (r −0.31, $p < 0.01$ and r −0.23, $p = 0.03$, respectively) in MS patients. Phosphate showed a positive correlation with osteocalcin (r 0.22, p 0.04). Negative correlations for osteocalcin with 1.25(OH)$_2$D, and P1NP with 24.25(OH)$_2$D, were observed in MS patients only (r −0.24, $p = 0.02$ and r −0.25, $p = 0.02$, respectively), as were positive correlations of the ratio between total serum 25(OH)D and 24.25(OH)$_2$D with P1NP and CTX (r 0.27, $p = 0.01$ and r 0.31, $p < 0.01$, respectively). In addition, in MS patients, ALP showed a positive correlation with osteocalcin, CTX, and P1NP (r 0.36, $p < 0.01$; r 0.44, $p < 0.01$; and r 0.43, $p < 0.01$, respectively); P1NP showed a positive correlation with osteocalcin and CTX (r 0.75, $p < 0.01$ and r 0.74, $p < 0.01$, respectively); and CTX correlated positively with osteocalcin (r 0.67, $p < 0.01$).

Table 3. Correlation between vitamin D metabolites, bone turnover markers (BTMs), and EDSS in MS patients.

N = 90	ALP	FGF23	Osteocalcin	CTX	P1NP	EDSS
Free 1.25(OH)$_2$D	r −0.03 p 0.78	r 0.10 p 0.33	r 0.01 p 0.95	r −0.10 p 0.33	r −0.07 p 0.54	**r −0.28** **p 0.01**
Bioavailable 1.25(OH)$_2$D	r −0.04 p 0.71	r 0.10 p 0.33	r 0.04 p 0.72	r −0.06 p 0.59	r −0.03 p 0.77	**r −0.30** **$p < 0.01$**
Total 1.25(OH)$_2$D	r −0.12 p 0.25	r −0.05 p 0.65	**r −0.24** **p 0.02**	r −0.09 p 0.41	r −0.19 p 0.08	r −0.08 p 0.47
Free 25(OH)D	r −0.02 p 0.82	r 0.10 p 0.34	r 0.01 p 0.93	r −0.10 p 0.36	r −0.06 p 0.57	**r −0.28** **p 0.01**
Bioavailable 25(OH)D	r −0.03 p 0.77	r 0.11 p 0.33	r 0.05 p 0.66	r −0.05 p 0.67	r −0.02 p 0.84	**r −0.30** **$p < 0.01$**
Total 25(OH)D	r −0.16 p 0.14	**r 0.22** **p 0.04**	r −0.12 p 0.28	**r −0.23** **p 0.03**	r −0.19 p 0.08	**r −0.23** **p 0.03**
24.25(OH)D	r −0.20 p 0.06	**r 0.22** **p 0.04**	r −0.16 p 0.14	**r −0.31** **$p < 0.01$**	**r −0.25** **p 0.02**	**r −0.22** **p 0.04**
Ratio 25(OH)D/24.25(OH)$_2$D	r 0.18 p 0.09	r −0.13 p 0.23	r 0.16 p 0.13	**r 0.31** **$p <0.01$**	**r 0.27** **p 0.01**	r 0.10 p 0.34
PTH	r 0.09 p 0.40	r −0.04 p 0.69	r −0.04 p 0.97	r 0.04 p 0.69	r −0.08 p 0.46	r 0.16 p 0.13
Phosphate	r 0.10 p 0.35	r 0.03 p 0.78	**r 0.22** **p 0.04**	r 0.13 p 0.24	r 0.16 p 0.15	r −0.03 p 0.76

ALP = alkaline phosphatase, FGF23 = fibroblast growth factor 23, CTX = c-terminal telopeptide, P1NP = procollagen type 1 N-terminal propeptide, EDSS = Expanded Disability Status Scale, PTH = parathyroid hormone. Bold text indicates a significance level of $p \leq 0.05$. r: Spearman correlation coefficient.

3.3.2. Associations Based on Gender of MS Patients

Looking at gender differences, in female MS patients, the same correlations were found as described above, except for the correlations of FGF23 with serum 25(OH)D and 24.25(OH)$_2$D (r 0.12, $p = 0.37$ and r 0.10, $p = 0.44$, respectively). In male MS patients, however, FGF23 correlated positively with total (r 0.50, $p < 0.01$), free (r 0.43, $p = 0.02$), and bioavailable 25(OH)D (r 0.43, $p = 0.02$); free (r 0.43, p 0.02) and bioavailable 1.25(OH)$_2$D (r 0.43, p 0.02); and 24.25(OH)$_2$D (r 0.46, $p = 0.01$), respectively. Furthermore, EDSS showed negative correlations with CTX (r −0.53, $p < 0.01$), P1NP (r −0.48, $p < 0.01$), and osteocalcin (r −0.40, p 0.03) in male MS patients only.

3.3.3. Associations in Healthy Controls

Lastly, in healthy controls, similar correlations of osteocalcin, CTX, and P1NP were found (data not shown). FGF23 correlated significantly with serum 1.25(OH)$_2$D (r −0.35, $p < 0.01$; data not shown), and CTX correlated significantly with serum 25(OH)D (r −0.24, $p = 0.05$; data not shown). In addition, PTH showed a positive correlation with ALP (r 0.21, p 0.04; data not shown) and phosphate showed a negative correlation with P1NP (r −0.27, p 0.03; data not shown) in the healthy control group.

4. Discussion

This study examined differences in total, free, and bioavailable vitamin D, FGF23 and bone turnover markers in patients with MS compared with healthy controls and possible gender differences. Although positive correlations between FGF23 and total 25(OH)D and 24.25(OH)$_2$D in MS patients were seen, no differences in plasma FGF23 concentrations between MS patients and healthy controls were observed. No differences between serum concentrations of BTMs in MS patients and healthy controls were found. Yet, we did observe a negative correlation between CTX and total 25(OH)D and 24.25(OH)$_2$D. EDSS showed negative correlations with bioavailable 1.25(OH)2D, bioavailable 25(OH)D, and 24.25(OH)2D. We found gender differences in vitamin D metabolism: serum concentrations of total 25(OH)D, 25(OH)D$_3$, 24.25(OH)$_2$D, free 25(OH)D, and free 1.25(OH)$_2$D were lower in female MS patients compared with female healthy controls. Serum concentrations of VDBP were higher in male MS patients compared with healthy male controls.

The main aim of this study was to further elucidate the vitamin D-FGF23 axis by measuring multiple D metabolites and FGF23 using accurate state-of-the art analytical methods in a well-defined cohort of MS patients versus healthy controls. We confirmed the finding of an earlier study that the serum 24.25(OH)$_2$D concentration is negatively correlated with EDSS [29]. Although we found a significant positive correlation between FGF23 and 25(OH)D and 24.25(OH)$_2$D, we did not observe a difference in FGF23 concentration between MS patients and healthy controls. A previous study described comparable plasma concentrations of FGF23 in MS patients compared with healthy controls as well [46], although two other studies found higher serum concentrations of FGF23 in MS patients compared with healthy controls [47,48]. However, the latter study was performed in patients with RRMS only and these differences were found during autumn (September–November) and winter time, respectively. Therefore, seasonal effects or the use of different FGF23 assays measuring either intact or c-term FGF23 could have resulted in these different findings. We found a higher phosphate concentration in MS patients; nevertheless, no differences in PTH or eGFR compared with healthy controls were found. Lastly, no correlations between FGF23 and 1.25(OH)$_2$D or EDSS were found in MS patients, which is in line with two other recent studies [46,48]. Summarized, these findings do not support our hypothesis that FGF23 differs between MS patients and healthy controls.

Regarding the various vitamin D metabolites, we found similar concentrations of 25(OH)D and 1.25(OH)$_2$D between MS patients and healthy controls, as some showed earlier [13,49,50], whereas others found lower serum concentrations of 25(OH)D or 1.25(OH)$_2$D in MS patients compared with healthy controls, respectively [15,51–57]. These differences between studies might be caused by differences in sample size, analysis of both male and female participants in different seasons of the year, use of different assays to measure vitamin D and its metabolites, and possible VDBP polymorphisms [24,27,28]. In addition, a number of studies did report a relationship between lower serum concentrations of 1,25(OH)$_2$D and an increased risk of MS [51,52]. Furthermore, our study showed that MS patients were using supplementation of vitamin D more often compared with their healthy controls. However, the maximal supplementation dosage was <200 IU of vitamin D per day, of which no clinical relevant effect on the vitamin D metabolites is expected, as a higher supplementation dosage is normally advised [18,19,29]. Moreover, controls had similar baseline concentrations of 25(OH)D.

As suggested in recent studies, bioavailable 25(OH)D might be preferred above total 25(OH)D as a marker for vitamin D status, and might thus be a better marker of mineral metabolism [58–62]. The sum of the albumin bound fraction of 25(OH)D plus the freely circulating 25(OH)D results in the bioavailable 25(OH)D, which can be calculated similarly for bio-available 1.25(OH)$_2$D, respectively [58,60]. In the circulation, VDBP and albumin bind over 99% of the 25(OH)D and 1.25(OH)$_2$D [60], whereas the binding affinity of vitamin D to albumin is much lower than the binding affinity to VDBP [63]. We found lower serum concentrations of both free and bioavailable 25(OH)D and 1.25(OH)$_2$D, respectively, in MS patients compared with healthy controls, in contrast to comparable serum concentrations of total 25(OH)D and 1.25(OH)$_2$D between MS patients and healthy controls. In contrast to our findings, Behrens et al. found no difference in free and bioavailable 25(OH)D between MS patients and controls, yet 1.25(OH)$_2$D was not measured in this study [64]. However, their study included patients with CIS only (not yet diagnosed with MS), used non-parametrical statistical tests, and a de-seasonalized concentration of vitamin D was calculated afterwards. Our study measured summer concentrations of vitamin D only and included all subtypes of MS, which may explain the different findings.

The second aim of our study was to assess BTMs in MS patients versus healthy controls and to study the possible associations of BTMs with vitamin D metabolites, as vitamin D deficiency is associated with increased bone turnover [32]. Our study did not show any differences between BTMs and FGF23 in MS patients and their healthy controls. This finding is in line with earlier studies, where similar serum concentrations of CTX, P1NP, or osteocalcin between MS patients and healthy controls were found, and similar concentrations of cross-linked N terminal telopeptide type 1 collagen (NTX) and bone ALP in newly diagnosed MS patients and healthy controls were found [18,32,65–67]. The current study shows that, despite differences in vitamin D metabolites, bone turnover in MS patients seems to not be affected compared with healthy controls.

Lastly, possible gender-related differences of vitamin D metabolites and BTMs between MS patients and healthy controls were studied; as known, MS affects more women than men and, in general, women have higher VDBP concentrations compared with men [13,21,33–36]. Indeed, our study showed more female MS patients, of which the largest part was post-menopausal. Further analyses based on pre- or postmenopausal status was not possible because of small groups. Our study showed lower total and free 25(OH)D, free 1.25(OH)$_2$D, and 24.25(OH)$_2$D only in female MS patients compared with healthy female controls, but no difference in this respect between male MS patients compared with healthy men. No differences between FGF23 in male and female MS patients were found. Interestingly, in our study, VDBP was higher in MS patients compared with controls, but after further analysis, this difference was found in male MS patients only. An earlier study found that serum VDBP concentrations were higher in MS patients compared with healthy controls as well; however, this study included both female and males [21]. In contrast, other studies showed no difference in VDBP concentrations between MS patients and controls [64,68]. The differences between VDBP concentrations in the various studies could be the result of variation between numbers of male and female patients and controls included in these studies or by using either a polyclonal or monoclonal assay. It is known that VDBP can affect inflammatory processes [22,23,25,26,61,69,70]. As we found higher VDBP in male MS patients, in the presence of a similar EDSS score as in female MS patients, this suggests a possible modulating effect of VDBP in male MS patients. It was shown before that higher concentrations of VDBP restrict the uptake of free vitamin D metabolites and reduce anti-inflammatory responses of immune cells [71–74]. Moreover, VDBP can act as a chemotactic cofactor, which enhances chemotaxis of neutrophils and macrophages by complement factor C5a [23]. These macrophages are known to contribute to laesion formation and axonal damage [22,26]. Previous experimental studies showed that T-lymphocytes, glia cells, and neurons express 1-α-hydroxlyase and VDR, which enables them to convert 25(OH)D to 1.25(OH) [75–77]. Normally, in the central nervous system, focal inflammation is initiated by auto-reactive T-helper cells type 1 (Th 1) and T-helper cells type 17 (Th 17) [78]. The activated vitamin D is thought to induce anti-inflammatory effects in glia cells and neurons and affects vitamin D responsive genes in T-helper cells [76,79–82], thereby inhibiting pro-inflammatory T-helper cell activity (Th1 and Th 17) and promoting anti-inflammatory T-helper cell activity (Th2 and regulatory T-cells) [51,83]. However, whether vitamin D affects the T-cell response also depends on concentrations of VDBP [84,85]. On the basis of these studies, the elevated concentrations of VDBP found in our study strengthen the pro-inflammatory role of VDBP in enhancing neuronal damage in MS.

Lastly, EDSS scores were comparable between male and female MS patients, which is consistent with previous research [86,87]. In female MS patients, however, EDSS showed negative correlations with free and bioavailable 1.25(OH)$_2$D; free, bioavailable, and total 25(OH)D; and 24.25(OH)$_2$D, which is in line with earlier studies, which reported a negative correlation between EDSS and 1.25(OH)$_2$D or 25(OH)D, respectively [46,88]. In contrast, in male MS patients, negative correlations between EDSS and CTX, P1NP, and osteocalcin were observed, which differs from previous studies, which found no correlations between EDSS and BTMs or only a positive correlation between EDSS and CTX [67,89].

The strengths of this study are the relative large study population and the broad spectrum of vitamin D metabolites, FGF23, and BTMs that was measured. Accurate and well-standardized LC-MS/MS assays were used to measure vitamin D metabolites. In addition, to minimize seasonal changes known to affect vitamin D metabolism [48], only blood samples drawn during summertime were used. There are also some possible limitations of this study. First, owing to the cross-sectional study design, the described differences between MS patients and controls in serum concentrations of vitamin D metabolites are not necessarily causal. In addition, 97% of our study population is Caucasian, which reduces the generalizability of the results, as it is known that vitamin D metabolism differs between races [53]. Moreover, our study was not primarily designed to study gender difference, so the differences we found in this respect should be studied further in other cohorts. No data on fractures were available. Lastly, dual energy X-ray absorptiometry (DXA) scans were not available to compare vitamin D metabolites and bone turnover markers with BMD.

5. Conclusions

In conclusion, this study provides additional knowledge of vitamin D-FGF 23 axis and bone turnover markers in MS patients compared with healthy controls, as well as gender-related differences. Similar serum concentrations of total 25(OH)D and 1.25(OH)$_2$D in MS patients and healthy controls were found. Furthermore, no differences in plasma FGF23 concentrations and other bone turnover markers between MS patients and healthy controls were observed. The ratio total 25(OH)D/ 24.25(OH)$_2$D did not differ between MS patients and healthy controls. However, this study suggested a relevant gender difference as serum concentrations of total 25(OH)D, 24.25(OH)$_2$D, free 25(OH)D, and free 1.25(OH)$_2$D were lower in female MS patients compared with female healthy controls, while serum concentrations of VDBP were higher in male MS patients compared with male controls. This study thus shows that only a total 25(OH)D measurement probably does not reflect all changes in vitamin D metabolism in MS patients. The exact role of VDBP and its polymorphisms in MS needs further studies. Finally, given the high incidence of reduced bone mineral density and the still partially unknown mechanisms that affect bone turnover in MS patients [66], further studies should be performed to evaluate the relationship between change in the vitamin D-FGF23 axis, BMD, and fracture risk in both male and female MS patients.

Author Contributions: Authors' role: Study design: M.C.V., L.B., J.K. (Jolijn Kragt), M.d.H., and A.C.H.; Data collection: M.C.V., L.B., and J.K. (Jolijn Kragt); Data analysis: M.C.V. and L.B.; Drafting manuscript: M.C.V. and L.B.; Revising manuscript content: M.C.V., L.B., J.K. (Jolijn Kragt), J.K. (Joep Killestein), B.M.v.A., R.d.J., M.d.H., and A.C.H.; Approving final version of manuscript: A.C.H. A.C.H. takes responsibility for the integrity of the data analysis.

Funding: This research received no external funding.

Conflicts of Interest: The authors declare no conflict of interest.

References

1. Gupta, S.; Ahsan, I.; Mahfooz, N.; Abdelhamid, N.; Ramanathan, M.; Weinstock-Guttman, B. Osteoporosis and Multiple Sclerosis: Risk Factors, Pathophysiology, and Therapeutic Interventions. *CNS Drugs* **2014**, *28*, 731–742. [CrossRef]
2. Holmøy, T.; Kampman, M.T.; Smolders, J. Vitamin D in multiple sclerosis: Implications for assessment and treatment. *Expert Rev. Neurother.* **2012**, *12*, 1101–1112. [CrossRef]
3. Huang, Z.; Qi, Y.; Du, S.; Chen, G.; Yan, W. BMI levels with MS Bone mineral density levels in adults with multiple sclerosis: A meta-analysis. *Int. J. Neurosci.* **2015**, *125*, 904–912. [CrossRef]
4. Nieves, J.; Cosman, F.; Herbert, J.; Shen, V.; Lindsay, R. High prevalence of vitamin D deficiency and reduced bone mass in multiple sclerosis. *Neurology* **1994**, *44*, 1687. [CrossRef] [PubMed]
5. Moen, S.M.; Celius, E.G.; Sandvik, L.; Nordsletten, L.; Eriksen, E.F.; Holmøy, T. Low bone mass in newly diagnosed multiple sclerosis and clinically isolated syndrome. *Neurology* **2011**, *77*, 151–157. [CrossRef] [PubMed]

6. Steffensen, L.H.; Mellgren, S.I.; Kampman, M.T. Predictors and prevalence of low bone mineral density in fully ambulatory persons with multiple sclerosis. *J. Neurol.* **2010**, *257*, 410–418. [CrossRef] [PubMed]
7. Dobson, R.; Ramagopalan, S.; Giovannoni, G.; Bazelier, M.T.; De Vries, F. Risk of fractures in patients with multiple sclerosis: A population-based cohort study. *Neurology* **2012**, *79*, 1934–1935. [CrossRef] [PubMed]
8. Thompson, A.J.; Baranzini, S.E.; Geurts, J.; Hemmer, B.; Ciccarelli, O. Multiple sclerosis. *Lancet* **2018**, *391*, 1622–1636. [CrossRef]
9. Tobore, T.O. Towards a Comprehensive Etiopathogenetic and Pathophysiological Theory of Multiple Sclerosis. *Int. J. Neurosci.* **2019**, 1–41. [CrossRef]
10. Acheson, E.D.; Bachrach, C.A.; Wright, F.M. Some comments on the relationship of the distribution of multiple sclerosis to latitude, solar radiation, and other variables. *Acta Psychiatr. Scand.* **1960**, *35*, 132–147. [CrossRef]
11. Kurtzke, J.F. Geography in multiple sclerosis. *J. Neurol.* **1977**, *215*, 1–26. [CrossRef] [PubMed]
12. Hemmer, B.; Kerschensteiner, M.; Korn, T. Role of the innate and adaptive immune responses in the course of multiple sclerosis. *Lancet Neurol.* **2015**, *14*, 406–419. [CrossRef]
13. Kragt, J.; Van Amerongen, B.; Killestein, J.; Dijkstra, C.; Uitdehaag, B.; Polman, C.; Lips, P. Higher levels of 25-hydroxyvitamin D are associated with a lower incidence of multiple sclerosis only in women. *Mult. Scler. J.* **2009**, *15*, 9–15. [CrossRef] [PubMed]
14. Munger, K.L.; Levin, L.I.; Hollis, B.W.; Howard, N.S.; Ascherio, A. Serum 25-Hydroxyvitamin D Levels and Risk of Multiple Sclerosis. *JAMA* **2006**, *296*, 2832–2838. [CrossRef]
15. Soilu-Hänninen, M.; Airas, L.; Mononen, I.; Heikkilä, A.; Viljanen, M.; Hänninen, A. 25-Hydroxyvitamin D levels in serum at the onset of multiple sclerosis. *Mult. Scler. J.* **2005**, *11*, 266–271. [CrossRef]
16. Berezowska, M.; Coe, S.; Dawes, H. Effectiveness of Vitamin D Supplementation in the Management of Multiple Sclerosis: A Systematic Review. *Int. J. Mol. Sci.* **2019**, *20*, 1301. [CrossRef]
17. Fitzgerald, K.C.; Munger, K.L.; Köchert, K.; Arnason, B.G.W.; Comi, G.; Cook, S.; Goodin, D.S.; Filippi, M.; Hartung, H.-P.; Jeffery, D.R.; et al. Association of Vitamin D Levels With Multiple Sclerosis Activity and Progression in Patients Receiving Interferon Beta-1b. *JAMA Neurol.* **2015**, *72*, 1458–1465. [CrossRef]
18. Holmøy, T.; Lindstrøm, J.C.; Eriksen, E.F.; Steffensen, L.H.; Kampman, M.T. High dose vitamin D supplementation does not affect biochemical bone markers in multiple sclerosis—A randomized controlled trial. *BMC Neurol.* **2017**, *17*, 67. [CrossRef]
19. Jagannath, V.A.; Filippini, G.; Di Pietrantonj, C.; Asokan, G.V.; Robak, E.W.; Whamond, L.; Robinson, S.A. Vitamin D for the management of multiple sclerosis. *Cochrane Database Syst. Rev.* **2018**, *9*, CD008422. [CrossRef]
20. Sintzel, M.B.; Rametta, M.; Reder, A.T. Vitamin D and Multiple Sclerosis: A Comprehensive Review. *Neurol. Ther.* **2018**, *7*, 59–85. [CrossRef]
21. Rinaldi, A.O.; Sanseverino, I.; Purificato, C.; Cortese, A.; Mechelli, R.; Francisci, S.; Salvetti, M.; Millefiorini, E.; Gessani, S.; Gauzzi, M.C. Increased Circulating Levels of Vitamin D Binding Protein in MS Patients. *Toxins* **2015**, *7*, 129–137. [CrossRef] [PubMed]
22. Abdul-Majid, K.-B.; Stefferl, A.; Bourquin, C.; Lassmann, H.; Linington, C.; Olsson, T.; Kleinau, S.; Harris, R.A. Fc receptors are critical for autoimmune inflammatory damage to the central nervous system in experimental autoimmune encephalomyelitis. *Scand. J. Immunol.* **2002**, *55*, 70–81. [CrossRef] [PubMed]
23. Binder, R.; Kress, A.; Kan, G.; Herrmann, K.; Kirschfink, M. Neutrophil priming by cytokines and vitamin D binding protein (Gc-globulin): Impact on C5a-mediated chemotaxis, degranulation and respiratory burst. *Mol. Immunol.* **1999**, *36*, 885–892. [CrossRef]
24. Gauzzi, M.C. Vitamin D-binding protein and multiple sclerosis: Evidence, controversies, and needs. *Mult. Scler. J.* **2018**, *24*, 1526–1535. [CrossRef]
25. Vasconcellos, C.; Lind, S. Coordinated inhibition of actin-induced platelet aggregation by plasma gelsolin and vitamin D-binding protein. *Blood* **1993**, *82*, 3648–3657. [CrossRef]
26. Vogel, D.Y.; Vereyken, E.J.; Glim, J.E.; Heijnen, P.D.; Moeton, M.; Van Der Valk, P.; Amor, S.; Teunissen, C.E.; Van Horssen, J.; Dijkstra, C.D. Macrophages in inflammatory multiple sclerosis lesions have an intermediate activation status. *J. Neuroinflamm.* **2013**, *10*, 35. [CrossRef]
27. Bermúdez-Morales, V.H.; Fierros, G.; Lopez, R.L.; Martínez-Nava, G.; Flores-Aldana, M.; Flores-Rivera, J.; Hernández-Girón, C. Vitamin D receptor gene polymorphisms are associated with multiple sclerosis in Mexican adults. *J. Neuroimmunol.* **2017**, *306*, 20–24. [CrossRef]

28. Langer-Gould, A.; Lucas, R.M.; Xiang, A.H.; Wu, J.; Chen, L.H.; Gonzales, E.; Haraszti, S.; Smith, J.B.; Quach, H.; Barcellos, L.F. Vitamin D-Binding Protein Polymorphisms, 25-Hydroxyvitamin D, Sunshine and Multiple Sclerosis. *Nutrients* **2018**, *10*, 184. [CrossRef]
29. Weinstock-Guttman, B.; Zivadinov, R.; Qu, J.; Cookfair, D.; Duan, X.; Bang, E.; Bergsland, N.; Hussein, S.; Cherneva, M.; Willis, L.; et al. Vitamin D metabolites are associated with clinical and MRI outcomes in multiple sclerosis patients. *J. Neurol. Neurosurg. Psychiatry* **2011**, *82*, 189–195. [CrossRef]
30. Bischoff-Ferrari, H.A.; Dietrich, T.; Orav, E.; Dawson-Hughes, B. Positive association between 25-hydroxy vitamin d levels and bone mineral density: A population-based study of younger and older adults. *Am. J. Med.* **2004**, *116*, 634–639. [CrossRef]
31. Holick, M.F. Vitamin D deficiency. *N. Engl. J. Med.* **2007**, *357*, 266–281. [CrossRef] [PubMed]
32. Jorde, R.; Stunes, A.K.; Kubiak, J.; Joakimsen, R.; Grimnes, G.; Thorsby, P.M.; Syversen, U. Effects of vitamin D supplementation on bone turnover markers and other bone-related substances in subjects with vitamin D deficiency. *Bone* **2019**, *124*, 7–13. [CrossRef] [PubMed]
33. Bolland, M.J.; Grey, A.B.; Ames, R.W.; Horne, A.M.; Mason, B.H.; Wattie, D.J.; Gamble, G.D.; Bouillon, R.; Reid, I.R. Age-, gender-, and weight-related effects on levels of 25-hydroxyvitamin D are not mediated by vitamin D binding protein. *Clin. Endocrinol.* **2007**, *67*, 259–264. [CrossRef] [PubMed]
34. Spach, K.M.; Hayes, C.E. Vitamin D3 confers protection from autoimmune encephalomyelitis only in female mice. *J. Immunol.* **2005**, *175*, 4119–4126. [CrossRef] [PubMed]
35. Woolmore, J.; Stone, M.; Pye, E.; Partridge, J.; Boggild, M.; Young, C.; Jones, P.; Fryer, A.; Hawkins, C.; Strange, R.; et al. Studies of associations between disability in multiple sclerosis, skin type, gender and ultraviolet radiation. *Mult. Scler. J.* **2007**, *13*, 369–375. [CrossRef]
36. Yang, M.; Qin, Z.; Zhu, Y.; Li, Y.; Qin, Y.; Jing, Y.; Liu, S. Vitamin D-binding Protein in Cerebrospinal Fluid is Associated with Multiple Sclerosis Progression. *Mol. Neurobiol.* **2013**, *47*, 946–956. [CrossRef]
37. Meyer-Moock, S.; Feng, Y.-S.; Maeurer, M.; Dippel, F.-W.; Kohlmann, T. Systematic literature review and validity evaluation of the Expanded Disability Status Scale (EDSS) and the Multiple Sclerosis Functional Composite (MSFC) in patients with multiple sclerosis. *BMC Neurol.* **2014**, *14*, 58. [CrossRef]
38. Dirks, N.F.; Vesper, H.W.; Van Herwaarden, A.E.; Ouweland, J.M.V.D.; Kema, I.P.; Krabbe, J.G.; Heijboer, A.C. Various calibration procedures result in optimal standardization of routinely used 25(OH)D ID-LC-MS/MS methods. *Clin. Chim. Acta* **2016**, *462*, 49–54. [CrossRef]
39. Dirks, N.F.; Ackermans, M.T.; De Jonge, R.; Heijboer, A.C. Reference values for 24,25-dihydroxyvitamin D and the 25-hydroxyvitamin D/24,25-dihydroxyvitamin D ratio. *Clin. Chem. Lab. Med.* **2019**, *57*, e259–e261. [CrossRef]
40. Dirks, N.F.; Martens, F.; Vanderschueren, D.; Billen, J.; Pauwels, S.; Ackermans, M.T.; Endert, E.; Heijer, M.D.; Blankenstein, M.A.; Heijboer, A.C. Determination of human reference values for serum total 1,25-dihydroxyvitamin D using an extensively validated 2D ID-UPLC–MS/MS method. *J. Steroid Biochem. Mol. Boil.* **2016**, *164*, 127–133. [CrossRef]
41. Malmstroem, S.; Rejnmark, L.; Imboden, J.B.; Shoback, D.M.; Bikle, D.D. Current Assays to Determine Free 25-Hydroxyvitamin D in Serum. *J. AOAC Int.* **2017**, *100*, 1323–1327. [CrossRef] [PubMed]
42. Bikle, D.D.; Siiteri, P.K.; Ryzen, E.; Haddad, J.; Gee, E. Serum Protein Binding of 1,25-Dihydroxyvitamin D: A Reevaluation by Direct Measurement of Free Metabolite Levels. *J. Clin. Endocrinol. Metab.* **1985**, *61*, 969–975. [CrossRef] [PubMed]
43. Vermeulen, A.; Verdonck, L.; Kaufman, J.M. A Critical Evaluation of Simple Methods for the Estimation of Free Testosterone in Serum. *J. Clin. Endocrinol. Metab.* **1999**, *84*, 3666–3672. [CrossRef] [PubMed]
44. Powe, C.E.; Ricciardi, C.; Berg, A.H.; Erdenesanaa, D.; Collerone, G.; Ankers, E.; Wenger, J.; Karumanchi, S.A.; Thadhani, R.; Bhan, I. Vitamin D–Binding Protein Modifies the Vitamin D–Bone Mineral Density Relationship. *J. Bone Miner. Res.* **2011**, *26*, 1609–1616. [CrossRef]
45. Heijboer, A.C.; Levitus, M.; Vervloet, M.G.; Lips, P.; Wee, P.M.T.; Dijstelbloem, H.M.; Blankenstein, M.A. Determination of fibroblast growth factor 23. *Ann. Clin. Biochem. Int. J. Lab. Med.* **2009**, *46*, 338–340. [CrossRef]
46. Emami Aleagha, M.S.; Siroos, B.; Allameh, A.; Shakiba, S.; Ranji-Burachaloo, S.; Harirchian, M.H. Calcitriol, but not FGF23, increases in CSF and serum of MS patients. *J. Neuroimmunol.* **2018**, *328*, 89–93. [CrossRef]

47. Ellidag, H.Y.; Yilmaz, N.; Kurtulus, F.; Aydin, O.; Eren, E.; Inci, A.; Dolu, S.; Ince, F.D.A.; Giray, Ö.; Yaman, A. The Three Sisters of Fate in Multiple Sclerosis: Klotho (Clotho), Fibroblast Growth Factor-23 (Lachesis), and Vitamin D (Atropos). *Ann. Neurosci.* **2016**, *23*, 155–161. [CrossRef]
48. Stein, M.S.; Ward, G.J.; Butzkueven, H.; Kilpatrick, T.J.; Harrison, L.C. Dysequilibrium of the PTH-FGF23-vitamin D axis in relapsing remitting multiple sclerosis; a longitudinal study. *Mol. Med.* **2018**, *24*, 27. [CrossRef]
49. Barnes, M.; Bonham, M.; Robson, P.; Strain, J.; Lowe-Strong, A.; Eaton-Evans, J.; Ginty, F.; Wallace, J.; Robson, P. Assessment of 25-hydroxyvitamin D and 1,25-dihydroxyvitamin D3 concentrations in male and female multiple sclerosis patients and control volunteers. *Mult. Scler. J.* **2007**, *13*, 670–672. [CrossRef]
50. Soilu-Hänninen, M.; Laaksonen, M.; Laitinen, I.; Erälinna, J.-P.; Lilius, E.-M.; Mononen, I. A longitudinal study of serum 25-hydroxyvitamin D and intact parathyroid hormone levels indicate the importance of vitamin D and calcium homeostasis regulation in multiple sclerosis. *J. Neurol. Neurosurg. Psychiatry* **2008**, *79*, 152–157. [CrossRef]
51. Correale, J.; Ysrraelit, M.C.; Gaitán, M.I. Immunomodulatory effects of Vitamin D in multiple sclerosis. *Brain* **2009**, *132*, 1146–1160. [CrossRef] [PubMed]
52. Duan, X.; Weinstock-Guttman, B.; Wang, H.; Bang, E.; Li, J.; Ramanathan, M.; Qu, J. Ultrasensitive Quantification of Serum Vitamin D Metabolites Using Selective Solid-Phase Extraction Coupled to Microflow Liquid Chromatography and Isotope-Dilution Mass Spectrometry. *Anal. Chem.* **2010**, *82*, 2488–2497. [CrossRef] [PubMed]
53. Gelfand, J.M.; Cree, B.A.C.; McElroy, J.; Oksenberg, J.; Green, R.; Mowry, E.M.; Miller, J.W.; Hauser, S.L.; Green, A.J. Vitamin D in African Americans with multiple sclerosis. *Neurology* **2011**, *76*, 1824–1830. [CrossRef] [PubMed]
54. Lucas, R.M.; Ponsonby, A.-L.; Dear, K.; Valery, P.C.; Pender, M.P.; Taylor, B.V.; Kilpatrick, T.; Dwyer, T.; Coulthard, A.; Chapman, C.; et al. Sun exposure and vitamin D are independent risk factors for CNS demyelination. *Neurology* **2011**, *76*, 540–548. [CrossRef] [PubMed]
55. Ozgocmen, S.; Bulut, S.; Ilhan, N.; Gulkesen, A.; Ardicoglu, O.; Ozkan, Y. Vitamin D deficiency and reduced bone mineral density in multiple sclerosis: Effect of ambulatory status and functional capacity. *J. Bone Miner. Metab.* **2005**, *23*, 309–313. [CrossRef]
56. Shaygannejad, V.; Golabchi, K.; Haghighi, S.; Dehghan, H.; Moshayedi, A. A Comparative Study of 25 (OH) Vitamin D Serum Levels in Patients with Multiple Sclerosis and Control Group in Isfahan, Iran. *Int. J. Prev. Med.* **2010**, *1*, 195–201.
57. Van der Mei, I.A.; Ponsonby, A.L.; Dwyer, T.; Blizzard, L.; Taylor, B.V.; Kilpatrick, T.; Butzkueven, H.; McMichael, A.J. Vitamin D levels in people with multiple sclerosis and community controls in Tasmania, Australia. *J. Neurol.* **2007**, *254*, 581–590.
58. Bhan, I.; Powe, C.E.; Berg, A.H.; Ankers, E.; Wenger, J.B.; Karumanchi, S.A.; Thadhani, R.I. Bioavailable vitamin D is more tightly linked to mineral metabolism than total vitamin D in incident hemodialysis patients. *Kidney Int.* **2012**, *82*, 84–89. [CrossRef]
59. Bikle, D.D.; Gee, E.; Halloran, B.; Haddad, J.G. Free 1,25-dihydroxyvitamin D levels in serum from normal subjects, pregnant subjects, and subjects with liver disease. *J. Clin. Investig.* **1984**, *74*, 1966–1971. [CrossRef]
60. Bikle, D.D.; Gee, E.; Halloran, B.; Kowalski, M.A.; Ryzen, E.; Haddad, J.G. Assessment of the Free Fraction of 25-Hydroxyvitamin D in Serum and Its Regulation by Albumin and the Vitamin D-Binding Protein. *J. Clin. Endocrinol. Metab.* **1986**, *63*, 954–959. [CrossRef]
61. Jassil, N.K.; Sharma, A.; Bikle, D.; Wang, X. Vitamin d binding protein and 25-hydroxyvitamin d levels: Emerging clinical applications. *Endocr. Pract.* **2017**, *23*, 605–613. [CrossRef] [PubMed]
62. Kim, H.-J.; Ji, M.; Song, J.; Moon, H.-W.; Hur, M.; Yun, Y.-M. Clinical Utility of Measurement of Vitamin D-Binding Protein and Calculation of Bioavailable Vitamin D in Assessment of Vitamin D Status. *Ann. Lab. Med.* **2017**, *37*, 34–38. [CrossRef] [PubMed]
63. Mendel, C.M. Rates of dissociation of sex steroid hormones from human sex hormone-binding globulin: A reassessment. *J. Steroid Biochem. Mol. Boil.* **1990**, *37*, 251–255. [CrossRef]
64. Behrens, J.R.; Rasche, L.; Gieß, R.M.; Pfuhl, C.; Wakonig, K.; Freitag, E.; Deuschle, K.; Bellmann-Strobl, J.; Paul, F.; Ruprecht, K.; et al. Low 25-hydroxyvitamin D, but not the bioavailable fraction of 25-hydroxyvitamin D, is a risk factor for multiple sclerosis. *Eur. J. Neurol.* **2016**, *23*, 62–67. [CrossRef] [PubMed]

65. McKenna, M.J.; Murray, B.; Lonergan, R.; Segurado, R.; Tubridy, N.; Kilbane, M.T. Analysing the effect of multiple sclerosis on vitamin D related biochemical markers of bone remodelling. *J. Steroid Biochem. Mol. Boil.* **2018**, *177*, 91–95. [CrossRef] [PubMed]
66. Moen, S.M.; Celius, E.G.; Sandvik, L.; Brustad, M.; Nordsletten, L.; Eriksen, E.F.; Holmøy, T. Bone Turnover and Metabolism in Patients with Early Multiple Sclerosis and Prevalent Bone Mass Deficit: A Population-Based Case-Control Study. *PLoS ONE* **2012**, *7*, e45803. [CrossRef]
67. Štěpán, J.J.; Havrdova, E.K.; Tyblova, M.; Horakova, D.; Tichá, V.; Nováková, I.; Zikán, V. Markers of bone remodeling predict rate of bone loss in multiple sclerosis patients treated with low dose glucocorticoids. *Clin. Chim. Acta* **2004**, *348*, 147–154. [CrossRef]
68. Niino, M.; Sato, S.; Fukazawa, T.; Masaki, K.; Miyazaki, Y.; Matsuse, D.; Yamasaki, R.; Takahashi, E.; Kikuchi, S.; Kira, J.-I. Decreased serum vitamin D levels in Japanese patients with multiple sclerosis. *J. Neuroimmunol.* **2015**, *279*, 40–45. [CrossRef]
69. Disanto, G.; Ramagopalan, S.V.; Para, A.E.; Handunnetthi, L. The emerging role of vitamin D binding protein in multiple sclerosis. *J. Neurol.* **2011**, *258*, 353–358. [CrossRef]
70. Kułakowska, A.; Tarasiuk, J.; Kapica-Topczewska, K.; Chorąży, M.; Pogorzelski, R.; Kulczyńska-Przybik, A.; Mroczko, B.; Bucki, R. Pathophysiological implications of actin-free Gc-globulin concentration changes in blood plasma and cerebrospinal fluid collected from patients with Alzheimer's disease and other neurological disorders. *Adv. Clin. Exp. Med.* **2018**, *27*, 1075–1080. [CrossRef]
71. Adams, J.S.; Ren, S.; Liu, P.T.; Chun, R.F.; Lagishetty, V.; Gombart, A.F.; Borregaard, N.; Modlin, R.L.; Hewison, M. Vitamin d-directed rheostatic regulation of monocyte antibacterial responses. *J. Immunol.* **2009**, *182*, 4289–4295. [CrossRef] [PubMed]
72. Chun, R.F.; Lauridsen, A.L.; Suon, L.; Zella, L.A.; Pike, J.W.; Modlin, R.L.; Martineau, A.R.; Wilkinson, R.J.; Adams, J.; Hewison, M. Vitamin D-binding protein directs monocyte responses to 25-hydroxy- and 1,25-dihydroxyvitamin D. *J. Clin. Endocrinol. Metab.* **2010**, *95*, 3368–3376. [CrossRef] [PubMed]
73. Liu, P.T.; Stenger, S.; Li, H.; Wenzel, L.; Tan, B.H.; Krutzik, S.R.; Ochoa, M.T.; Schauber, J.; Wu, K.; Meinken, C.; et al. Toll-Like Receptor Triggering of a Vitamin D-Mediated Human Antimicrobial Response. *Science* **2006**, *311*, 1770–1773. [CrossRef] [PubMed]
74. Zella, L.A.; Shevde, N.K.; Hollis, B.W.; Cooke, N.E.; Pike, J.W. Vitamin D-binding protein influences total circulating levels of 1,25-dihydroxyvitamin D3 but does not directly modulate the bioactive levels of the hormone in vivo. *Endocrinology* **2008**, *149*, 3656–3667. [CrossRef] [PubMed]
75. De la Fuente, A.G.; Errea, O.; van Wijngaarden, P.; Gonzalez, G.A.; Kerninon, C.; Jarjour, A.A.; Lewis, H.J.; Jones, C.A.; Nait-Oumesmar, B.; Zhao, C.; et al. Vitamin D receptor-retinoid X receptor heterodimer signaling regulates oligodendrocyte progenitor cell differentiation. *J. Cell Biol.* **2015**, *211*, 975–985. [CrossRef]
76. Kongsbak, M.; Von Essen, M.R.; Levring, T.B.; Schjerling, P.; Woetmann, A.; Ødum, N.; Bonefeld, C.M.; Geisler, C. Vitamin D-binding protein controls T cell responses to vitamin D. *BMC Immunol.* **2014**, *15*, 35. [CrossRef]
77. Yamamoto, E.; Jørgensen, T.N. Immunological effects of vitamin D and their relations to autoimmunity. *J. Autoimmun.* **2019**, *100*, 7–16. [CrossRef]
78. Bar-Or, A. The Immunology of Multiple Sclerosis. *Semin. Neurol.* **2008**, *28*, 29–45. [CrossRef]
79. Brown, J.; Bianco, J.I.; McGrath, J.J.; Eyles, D.W. 1,25-dihydroxyvitamin D3 induces nerve growth factor, promotes neurite outgrowth and inhibits mitosis in embryonic rat hippocampal neurons. *Neurosci. Lett.* **2003**, *343*, 139–143. [CrossRef]
80. Neveu, I.; Naveilhan, P.; Baudet, C.; Brachet, P.; Metsis, M. 1,25-Dihydroxyvitamin D3 regulates NT-3, NT-4 but not BDNF mRNA in astrocytes. *NeuroReport* **1994**, *6*, 124–126. [CrossRef]
81. Neveu, I.; Naveilhan, P.; Jehan, F.; Baudet, C.; Wion, D.; De Luca, H.F.; Brachet, P. 1,25-Dihydroxyvitamin D3 regulates the synthesis of nerve growth factor in primary cultures of glial cells. *Mol. Brain Res.* **1994**, *24*, 70–76. [CrossRef]
82. Smolders, J.; Schuurman, K.G.; Van Strien, M.E.; Melief, J.; Hendrickx, D.; Hol, E.; Van Eden, C.; Luchetti, S.; Huitinga, I. Expression of Vitamin D Receptor and Metabolizing Enzymes in Multiple Sclerosis–Affected Brain Tissue. *J. Neuropathol. Exp. Neurol.* **2013**, *72*, 91–105. [PubMed]
83. Smolders, J.; Damoiseaux, J. Vitamin D as a T-cell Modulator in Multiple Sclerosis. *Vitam. Horm.* **2011**, *86*, 401–428. [PubMed]

84. Chun, R.F.; Peercy, B.E.; Orwoll, E.S.; Nielson, C.M.; Adams, J.S.; Hewison, M. Vitamin D and DBP: The free hormone hypothesis revisited. *J. Steroid Biochem. Mol. Biol.* **2014**, *144 Pt A*, 132–137. [CrossRef]
85. Delanghe, J.R.; Speeckaert, R.; Speeckaert, M.M. Behind the scenes of vitamin D binding protein: More than vitamin D binding. *Best Pract. Res. Clin. Endocrinol. Metab.* **2015**, *29*, 773–786. [CrossRef]
86. Casetta, I.; Riise, T.; Nortvedt, M.W.; Economou, N.T.; De Gennaro, R.; Fazio, P.; Cesnik, E.; Govoni, V.; Granieri, E. Gender differences in health-related quality of life in multiple sclerosis. *Mult. Scler. J.* **2009**, *15*, 1339–1346. [CrossRef]
87. Rojas, J.I.; Sánchez, F.; Patrucco, L.; Miguez, J.; Funes, J.; Cristiano, E. Structural sex differences at disease onset in multiple sclerosis patients. *Neuroradiol. J.* **2016**, *29*, 368–371. [CrossRef]
88. Niedziela, N.; Pierzchała, K.; Zalejska-Fiolka, J.; Niedziela, J.T.; Romuk, E.; Torbus-Paluszczak, M.; Adamczyk-Sowa, M. Assessment of Biochemical and Densitometric Markers of Calcium-Phosphate Metabolism in the Groups of Patients with Multiple Sclerosis Selected due to the Serum Level of Vitamin D3. *BioMed Res. Int.* **2018**, *2018*, 9329123. [CrossRef]
89. Terzi, T.; Terzi, M.; Tander, B.; Cantürk, F.; Onar, M. Changes in bone mineral density and bone metabolism markers in premenopausal women with multiple sclerosis and the relationship to clinical variables. *J. Clin. Neurosci.* **2010**, *17*, 1260–1264. [CrossRef]

© 2019 by the authors. Licensee MDPI, Basel, Switzerland. This article is an open access article distributed under the terms and conditions of the Creative Commons Attribution (CC BY) license (http://creativecommons.org/licenses/by/4.0/).

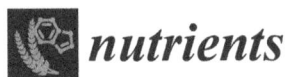

Article

The Effect of Vitamin D Supplementation on its Metabolism and the Vitamin D Metabolite Ratio

Vito Francic [1,†], Stan R. Ursem [2,†], Niek F. Dirks [2], Martin H. Keppel [3], Verena Theiler-Schwetz [1], Christian Trummer [1], Marlene Pandis [1], Valentin Borzan [1], Martin R. Grübler [1], Nicolas D. Verheyen [4], Winfried März [5], Andreas Tomaschitz [6], Stefan Pilz [1], Annemieke C. Heijboer [2] and Barbara Obermayer-Pietsch [1,*]

1. Division of Endocrinology and Diabetology, Endocrinology Lab Platform, Department of Internal Medicine, Medical University of Graz, 8036 Graz, Austria; vito.francic@medunigraz.at (V.F.); verena.schwetz@medunigraz.at (V.T.-S.); christian.trummer@medunigraz.at (C.T.); marlene.pandis@medunigraz.at (M.P.); valentin.borzan@medunigraz.at (V.B.); martin.gruebler@gmx.net (M.R.G.); stefan.pilz@chello.at (S.P.)
2. Department of Clinical Chemistry, Endocrine Laboratory, Amsterdam Gastroenterology & Metabolism, Vrije Universiteit Amsterdam and University of Amsterdam, Amsterdam UMC, 1105 Amsterdam, The Netherlands; s.ursem@amsterdamumc.nl (S.R.U.); n.dirks@amsterdamumc.nl (N.F.D.); a.heijboer@amsterdamumc.nl (A.C.H.)
3. Department of Laboratory Medicine, Paracelsus Medical University Salzburg, 5020 Salzburg, Austria; keppel.martin@gmail.com
4. Division of Cardiology, Department of Internal Medicine, Medical University of Graz, 8036 Graz, Austria; nicolas.verheyen@medunigraz.at
5. Synlab Academy, Synlab Holding Germany GmbH, 68163 Mannheim, Germany; Winfried.Maerz@synlab.com
6. Health Center Trofaiach-Gössgrabenstrasse, 8739 Trofaiach, Austria; andreas.tomaschitz@gmx.at
* Correspondence: barbara.obermayer@medunigraz.at; Tel.: +43 316 385 80253
† These authors contributed equally to this work.

Received: 25 September 2019; Accepted: 11 October 2019; Published: 21 October 2019

Abstract: 25-hydroxyvitamin D (25(OH)D) is commonly measured to assess vitamin D status. Other vitamin D metabolites such as 24,25-dihydroxyvitamin D (24,25(OH)$_2$D) provide additional insights into vitamin D status or metabolism. Earlier studies suggested that the vitamin D metabolite ratio (VMR), calculated as 24,25(OH)$_2$D/25(OH)D, could predict the 25(OH)D increase after vitamin D supplementation. However, the evidence for this additional value is inconclusive. Therefore, our aim was to assess whether the increase in 25(OH)D after supplementation was predicted by the VMR better than baseline 25(OH)D. Plasma samples of 106 individuals (25(OH)D < 75 nmol/L) with hypertension who completed the Styrian Vitamin D Hypertension Trial (NC.T.02136771) were analyzed. Participants received vitamin D (2800 IU daily) or placebo for 8 weeks. The treatment effect (ANCOVA) for 25(OH)D$_3$, 24,25(OH)$_2$D$_3$ and the VMR was 32 nmol/L, 3.3 nmol/L and 0.015 (all $p < 0.001$), respectively. Baseline 25(OH)D$_3$ and 24,25(OH)$_2$D$_3$ predicted the change in 25(OH)D$_3$ with comparable strength and magnitude. Correlation and regression analysis showed that the VMR did not predict the change in 25(OH)D$_3$. Therefore, our data do not support routine measurement of 24,25(OH)$_2$D$_3$ in order to individually optimize the dosage of vitamin D supplementation. Our data also suggest that activity of 24-hydroxylase increases after vitamin D supplementation.

Keywords: vitamin D metabolites; vitamin D supplementation; vitamin D metabolite ratio; randomized controlled trial; 24,25-dihydroxy vitamin D

1. Introduction

Vitamin D plays an essential role in calcium and phosphate homeostasis [1]. Vitamin D status is most commonly assessed by determining the 25-hydroxyvitamin D (25(OH)D) concentration in serum or plasma. However, several other vitamin D-related metabolites can be measured to provide a better understanding of individual vitamin D status and metabolism. Among them, 24,25(OH)$_2$D has emerged as a metabolite with potentially high utility [2].

In the kidneys, 25(OH)D is converted by 1-alpha-hydroxylase (CYP27B1) into 1,25-dihydroxyvitamin D (1,25(OH)$_2$D; also called active vitamin D or calcitriol) (Figure 1). 1,25(OH)$_2$D can bind to the vitamin D receptor (VDR) with high affinity. The subsequent signaling results in an increase in serum calcium and phosphate concentrations, mainly mediated by an increased intestinal uptake. In addition, 1,25(OH)$_2$D has effects on the parathyroid gland, kidneys and bones, all resulting in an increase in serum calcium and phosphate concentrations [1]. Furthermore, 1,25(OH)2D has major effects on modulating the immune system, which might be relevant for the treatment of autoimmune diseases, infections, cancer and cardiovascular diseases [3]. An excess of both 1,25(OH)$_2$D and/or 25(OH)D lead to their catabolism by the enzyme 24-hydroxylase (CYP24A1). This results in the formation of metabolites 1,24,25(OH)$_2$D and 24,25(OH)$_2$D, respectively [4]. It is still unclear whether 24,25(OH)$_2$D has a physiological role in humans [5].

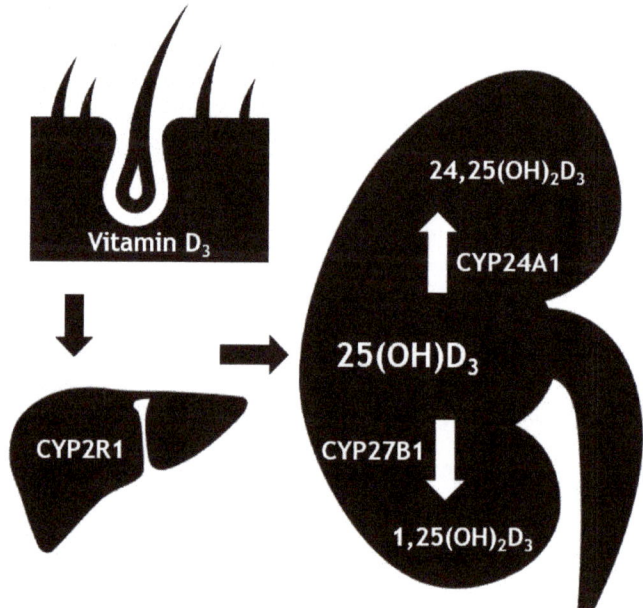

Figure 1. Metabolism of vitamin D. Vitamin D$_3$ (cholecalciferol) is produced in the skin when exposed to sunlight. The hepatic enzyme CYP2R1 then converts this into 25(OH)D$_3$ (calcifediol). In the kidneys, 25(OH)D$_3$ can be converted into the active form, 1,25(OH)$_2$D$_3$ (calcitriol), by CYP27B1 (1-α-hydroxylase). In the kidneys, CYP24A1 (24-hydroxylase) can catabolize the 25(OH)D$_3$ into 24,25(OH)$_2$D$_3$.

Using an LC-MS/MS method, 25(OH)D and 24,25(OH)$_2$D can be measured simultaneously, which allows for determination of the 24,25(OH)$_2$D/25(OH)D ratio, also known as the vitamin D metabolite ratio (VMR) [2]. The VMR is an indicator of CYP24A1 activity and thereby of vitamin D catabolism. It is currently used for diagnosing idiopathic infantile hypercalcemia, a rare genetic disorder in which a mutation in CYP24A1 results in severe hypercalcemia and suppressed parathyroid hormone (PTH) levels [5]. The VMR may also reflect vitamin D receptor (VDR) activity since CYP24A1 expression is upregulated in response to 1,25(OH)$_2$D [2].

In recent years, there has been an increasing interest in the use of the VMR when assessing vitamin D status. For example, it has been postulated to better reflect vitamin D deficiency [6]. In addition, it has been speculated that the ratio could provide useful information regarding bone health [7]. Interestingly, several studies show that the VMR can predict the change seen in 25(OH)D after vitamin D supplementation, although results are inconclusive [6,8–11]. The CYP24A1 activity could be partially responsible for the individual differences seen in the effect of vitamin D supplementation on serum levels of 25(OH)D. Theoretically, if CYP24A1 activity is a major predictor of the effect of vitamin D supplementation, the VMR could be used to personalize the treatment dosage. At present, 25(OH)D concentrations at the start of supplementation, as well as BMI, age, ethnicity and genetic background have been most commonly studied in regard to predicting the response to vitamin D supplementation, and studies involving 1,25(OH)$_2$D, 24,25(OH)$_2$D, free and bioavailable 25(OH)D and the VMR are scarce [12].

Therefore, we set out to determine whether baseline VMR measurements can predict changes in vitamin D-related metabolite levels after vitamin D supplementation. To that extent, we measured 25(OH)D$_3$, 1,25(OH)$_2$D and 24,25(OH)$_2$D$_3$ in a randomized clinical trial of patients (25(OH)D < 75 nmol/L) receiving vitamin D supplementation [13]. We hypothesized that measurements of baseline VMR would be advantageous over baseline 25(OH)D measurements for the prediction of the change in 25(OH)D upon supplementation.

2. Materials and Methods

2.1. Study Cohort

The present post-hoc analysis was conducted in adults (>18 years old) with 25(OH)D levels <75 nmol/L and hypertension, who completed the randomized, placebo-controlled Styrian Vitamin D Hypertension Trial (NC.T.02136771). The participants of this trial were treated with either placebo or 2800 IU daily of vitamin D$_3$ (Oleovit D$_3$, Fresenius Kabi, Graz, Austria) for 8 weeks. A total of 188 study participants completed the original study and sufficient material for analysis from both study visits was available for 106 of these subjects. The details regarding the study, including inclusion and exclusion criteria, can be found in the publication of the original study by Pilz et al. [13].

Study participants provided written informed consent. The study complied with the Declaration of Helsinki and was approved by the ethics committee of the Medical University of Graz, Austria.

2.2. Measurements

For the original study by Pilz et al, the 25(OH)D levels were determined with the ChemiLuminescence assay (IDS-iSYS 25-hydroxyvitamin D assay; Immunodiagnostic Systems Ltd., Boldon, UK) on an IDS-iSYS multidiscipline automated analyser [13]. The intra- and inter-assay CVs were 6.2% and 11.6%, respectively.

In the present study, 25(OH)D$_3$ and 24,25(OH)$_2$D$_3$ were measured in plasma samples by isotope dilution liquid chromatography-tandem mass spectrometry at the Endocrine Laboratory of the Amsterdam UMC, as described previously [14]. For 25(OH)D$_3$, the lower limit of quantitation (LLOQ) was 1.2 nmol/L and the inter- and intra-assay coefficients of variation (CV) were 6% and 3%, respectively. For 24,25(OH)$_2$D$_3$, the LLOQ was 0.1 nmol/L and the inter- and intra-assay coefficients of variation (CV) were 9% and 5%, respectively. 25(OH)D$_2$ was also measured, but as the concentrations were all very low (<7.9 nmol/L) and supplementation was given as vitamin D$_3$, these data were not taken into account in this paper. In order to calculate the VMR and as it is the golden standard, the LC/MS-MS method was used for the current study. Using this method, 7 subjects had 25(OH)D levels >75 nmol/L at baseline. Measurements of other study parameters have been described previously [13].

To calculate free and biologically available 25(OH)D$_3$ we used the equations from Powe et al. [15].

2.3. Statistical Analysis

Continuous data following a normal distribution are reported as means with standard deviations (SD). Variables with a skewed distribution are shown as medians with interquartile ranges. Categorical variables are shown as percentages of observations. Groups at baseline were compared using the unpaired Students t-test, the Mann–Whitney U test or the chi-squared test. Skewed variables were log transformed before being used in parametric analyses.

The changes from baseline for $25(OH)D_3$, $1,25(OH)_2D$ and $24,25(OH)_2D_3$ in the vitamin-D-treated group were calculated as the difference between the value at the final study visit and the value at baseline. They are depicted as $\Delta 25(OH)D_3$, $\Delta 1,25(OH)_2D$ and $\Delta 24,25(OH)_2D_3$. The VMR was calculated as the ratio between $24,25(OH)_2D_3$ and $25(OH)D_3$.

Analysis of covariance (ANCOVA) was used to calculate the treatment effects with adjustment for baseline values. Pearson correlation analysis was used to determine the strength of associations between vitamin-D-related parameters and $\Delta 25(OH)D_3$, $\Delta 1,25(OH)_2D$, as well as $\Delta 24,25(OH)_2D_3$. Bonferroni correction was applied to account for multiple testing. Univariate linear regression analysis was used to determine the relation between $\Delta 25(OH)D_3$ and baseline $25(OH)D_3$, $24,25(OH)_2D_3$ and VMR.

Using the LC/MS-MS method, 7 subjects had $25(OH)D$ levels >75 nmol/L at baseline. Therefore, we explored whether inclusion of these subjects had an effect on the analyses. In addition, we also investigated whether the inclusion of only subjects with $25(OH)D$ levels <50 nmol/L at baseline would affect the analyses.

If outliers were detected in the analyses by the software, defined as cases with standardized residuals greater than 3 standard deviations for ANCOVA analyses or as cases with values higher or lower than 1.5*IQR (interquartile range) for correlation analyses, they were removed and the analysis repeated to determine their potential effect on the analysis. In the case of Pearson correlation analyses, one extreme outlier was removed ($25(OH)D > 4\times SD$ at baseline) because of its significant effect on all of the analyses. This is marked in the results section. If the outliers had no significant effect on the analysis, the results including the outliers are reported. A p-value < 0.05 was considered statistically significant. All analyses were performed using S.P.SS version 25 (S.P.SS, Chicago, IL, USA).

3. Results

The baseline characteristics of study participants can be found in Table 1. There were no differences between the placebo and vitamin-D-treated groups in any of the parameters at baseline.

Table 1. Baseline characteristics.

Parameter	All (n = 106)	Placebo (n = 54)	Vitamin D (n = 52)	p-value
Age (years)	62.0 (51.3–68.7)	64.8 (50.8–70.2)	59.6 (52.4–66.6)	0.318
Body mass index (kg/m^2)	30.0 ± 5.4	29.7 ± 5.9	30.3 ± 4.9	0.562
Gender (% female)	57	57	56	0.865
$24,25(OH)_2D_3$ (nmol/L)	3.5 ± 1.6	3.4 ± 1.5	3.6 ± 1.5	0.419
$25(OH)D_3$ (nmol/L)	48 ± 18	46 ± 19	49 ± 18	0.401
VMR ((nmol/L)/(nmol/L))	0.073 ± 0.017	0.072 ± 0.018	0.073 ± 0.017	0.768
PTH (pmol/L)	5.5 (4.1–6.7)	5.5 (4.0–6.7)	5.3 (4.1–6.7)	0.779
$1,25(OH)_2D$ (pmol/L)	126 ± 53	118 ± 52	133 ± 52	0.142
Serum phosphate (mmol/L)	0.94 ± 0.17	0.96 ± 0.17	0.92 ± 0.16	0.282
Serum calcium (mmol/L)	2.26 (2.21–2.33)	2.26 (2.21–2.34)	2.26 (2.20–2.33)	0.773
eGFR (mL/min/1.73m^2)	72 ± 17	69 ± 16	74 ± 18	0.152
24h urinary calcium excretion (mmol/24h)	3.30 (1.90–5.00)	2.95 (1.83–4.78)	3.70 (2.10–6.30)	0.222
Calculated free $25(OH)D_3$ (pmol/L)	15 (9–21)	12 (8–21)	17 (11–20)	0.153
Vitamin D binding protein (μg/mL)	247.1 ± 109.5	254.8 ± 110.6	239.3 ± 109.0	0.772
Calculated bioavailable $25(OH)D_3$ (nmol/L)	5.9 (3.9–8.2)	5.2 (3.2–8.5)	6.6 (4.1–8.0)	0.149
$1,25(OH)_2D /25(OH)D_3$ ((nmol/L)/(nmol/L))	0.0023 (0.0019–0.0036)	0.0027 (0.0018–0.0039)	0.0028 (0.0021–0.0035)	0.753
$1,25(OH)_2D /24,25(OH)_2D_3$ ((nmol/L)/(nmol/L))	0.036 (0.025–0.05)	0.036 (0.024–0.051)	0.035 (0.026–0.050)	0.893

The calculated treatment effects after vitamin D supplementation are depicted in Table 2. We observed significant treatment effects for all included vitamin-D-related parameters. For $25(OH)D_3$, the treatment effect was 32 nmol/L (95% CI: 26 to 39; $p < 0.001$), for $1,25(OH)_2D$ 26 pmol/L (9 to 42; $p = 0.003$), for $24,25(OH)_2D_3$ 3.3 nmol/L (2.7 to 3.9; $p < 0.001$), for the VMR 0.015 (nmol/L)/(nmol/L)

(0.010–0.019; $p < 0.001$), for calculated free 25(OH)D$_3$ 12 pmol/L (6 to 18; $p < 0.001$), for calculated bioavailable 25(OH)D$_3$ 4.66 nmol/L (2.63 to 6.68; $p < 0.001$), for the 1,25(OH)$_2$D/25(OH)D$_3$ ratio −0.0010 (nmol/L)/(nmol/L) (−0.0013 to −0.0006; $p < 0.001$) and for the 1,25(OH)$_2$D/24,25(OH)$_2$D$_3$ ratio −0.020 (nmol/L)/(nmol/L) (−0.026 to −0.015; $p < 0.001$). In the subgroup of subjects with 25(OH)D$_3$ levels below 50 nmol/L, the treatment effects and p-values were comparable for all parameters.

Table 2. Analysis of covariance (ANCOVA) analysis for the effect of vitamin D or placebo treatment on vitamin-D-related parameters.

Parameter	Group	Baseline	Follow-up	Treatment Effect (95% CI)	p-value
25(OH)D$_3$ (nmol/L)	Placebo, $n=54$	46 ± 19	45 ± 20	32 (26 to 39)	<0.001
	Vitamin D, $n=52$	49 ± 18	79 ± 19		
1,25(OH)$_2$D (pmol/L)	Placebo, $n=52$	118 ± 52	114 ± 39	26 (9 to 42)	0.003
	Vitamin D, $n=52$	133 ± 52	150 ± 63		
24,25(OH)$_2$D$_3$ (nmol/L)	Placebo, $n=54$	3.4 ± 1.5	3.3 ± 1.8	3.3 (2.7 to 3.9)	<0.001
	Vitamin D, $n=52$	3.6 ± 1.6	6.8 ± 1.7		
VMR	Placebo, $n=54$	0.072 ± 0.018	0.071 ± 0.017	0.015 (0.010 to 0.020)	<0.001
	Vitamin D, $n=52$	0.073 ± 0.017	0.087 ± 0.018		
Calculated free 25(OH)D$_3$ (pmol/L)*	Placebo, $n=53$	12 (8–21)	12 (8–18)	12 (6 to 18)	<0.001
	Vitamin D, $n=51$	17 (11–20)	21 (17–31)		
Calculated bioavailable 25(OH)D$_3$ (nmol/L) *	Placebo, $n=53$	5.22 (3.15–8.51)	4.99 (2.95–6.83)	4.66 (2.63 to 6.68)	<0.001
	Vitamin D, $n=51$	6.60 (4.10–8.02)	8.69 (6.58–12.51)		
1,25(OH)$_2$D/ 25(OH)D$_3$ *	Placebo, $n=52$	0.0027 (0.0018–0.0039)	0.0026 (0.0019–0.0036)	−0.0010 (−0.0013 to −0.0006)	<0.001
	Vitamin D, $n=52$	0.0028 (0.0021–0.0035)	0.0019 (0.0014–0.0026)		
1,25(OH)$_2$D /24,25(OH)$_2$D$_3$ *	Placebo, $n=52$	0.036 (0.024–0.051)	0.037 (0.026–0.052)	−0.020 (−0.026 to −0.015)	<0.001
	Vitamin D, $n=52$	0.035 (0.026–0.050)	0.022 (0.016–0.028)		

* Log-transformed parameters.

The overall correlation between 25(OH)D$_3$ and 24,25(OH)$_2$D$_3$ at baseline was r = 0.815, $p < 0.001$. Results of the regression analyses of the Δ25(OH)D$_3$ in the vitamin-D-supplemented group are shown in Figure 2. The slope of the linear regression, p-values and R^2 values are highly similar for baseline 25(OH)D$_3$ and 24,25(OH)$_2$D$_3$. The VMR, however, could not predict the increase in 25(OH)D$_3$ concentration. The results of the correlation analyses in the vitamin-D-treated group are summarized in Table 3. None of the vitamin-D-related parameters correlated significantly with Δ25(OH)D$_3$ or Δ1,25(OH)$_2$D after Bonferroni correction. Also, in the subgroup of subjects with 25(OH)D levels below 50 nmol/L, none of the parameters correlated significantly with Δ25(OH)D$_3$ or Δ1,25(OH)$_2$D after Bonferroni correction. For Δ25(OH)D$_3$, a trend was seen for baseline 25(OH)D$_3$ and baseline 24,25(OH)$_2$D$_3$ (r = −0.388, p = 0.056 and r = −0.374, p = 0.056). This trend with Δ25(OH)D$_3$ was also observed for calculated free 25(OH)D$_3$ and calculated bioavailable 25(OH)D$_3$ (r = −0.373, p = 0.056 and r = −0.375, p = 0.056). Δ24,25(OH)$_2$D$_3$ was significantly associated with baseline 25(OH)D$_3$, 24,25(OH)$_2$D$_3$, calculated free 25(OH)D$_3$ and calculated bioavailable 25(OH)D$_3$ (r = −0.562, $p < 0.001$; r = −0.476, p = 0.003; r = −0.382, p = 0.048 and r = −0.393, p = 0.032, respectively), but not with other parameters. In the subgroup of subjects with 25(OH)D$_3$ levels below 50 nmol/L, none of the parameters correlated significantly with Δ24,25(OH)$_2$D$_3$ after Bonferroni correction.

Correlation analyses after adjustment for gender, age, BMI, PTH, eGFR, serum phosphate and serum calcium showed that none of the vitamin-D-related parameters were significantly associated with Δ25(OH)D$_3$ or Δ1,25(OH)$_2$D after Bonferroni correction (Table A1). However, when corrected for the above-mentioned parameters, only baseline 25(OH)D$_3$ was still significantly associated with Δ24,25(OH)$_2$D$_3$ (r = −0.657, p = 0.008). In the subgroup of subjects with 25(OH)D$_3$ levels below 50 nmol/L, none of the parameters correlated significantly with Δ25(OH)D$_3$, Δ1,25(OH)$_2$D or Δ24,25(OH)$_2$D$_3$ after Bonferroni correction.

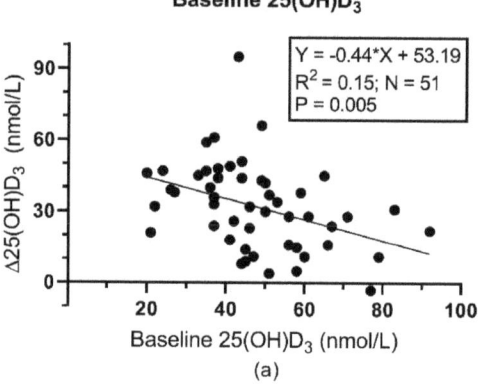
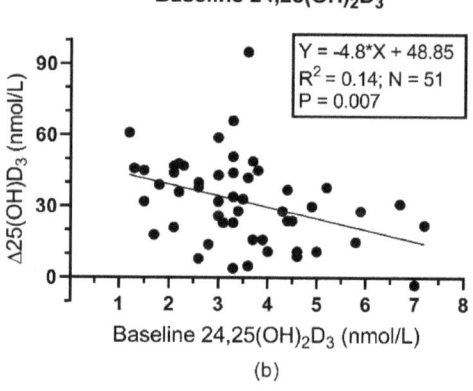
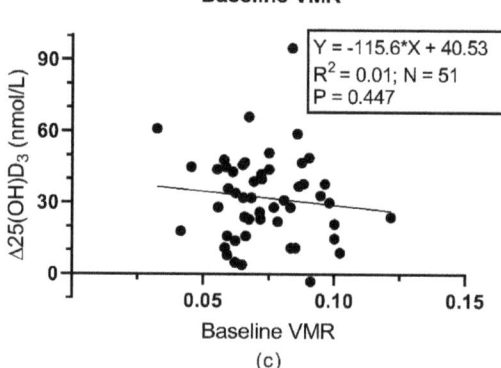

Figure 2. Univariate linear regression analysis for the change in 25(OH)D_3 concentration in the vitamin D intervention group and (**a**) baseline 25(OH)D_3, (**b**) baseline 24,25(OH)$_2$$D_3$ and (**c**) baseline VMR (Vitamin D Metabolite Ratio).

Table 3. Pearson correlations with unadjusted p-values and Bonferroni adjusted p-values of baseline vitamin-D-related parameters with the changes from baseline of 25(OH)D$_3$, 1,25(OH)$_2$D and 24,25(OH)$_2$D$_3$ after vitamin D supplementation.

Baseline Parameters		Δ25(OH)D$_3$	Δ1,25(OH)$_2$D	Δ24,25(OH)$_2$D$_3$
25(OH)D$_3$	r	−0.388	−0.142	−0.562
	p-value	0.005	0.322	<0.001
	Adjusted p-value	0.056	1.000	<0.001
1,25(OH)$_2$D	r	−0.287	−0.260	−0.272
	p-value	0.041	0.065	0.053
	Adjusted p-value	0.328	0.520	0.424
24,25(OH)$_2$D$_3$	r	−0.374	−0.122	−0.476
	p-value	0.007	0.392	<0.001
	Adjusted p-value	0.056	1.000	0.003
VMR	r	−0.109	−0.027	−0.015
	p-value	0.448	0.850	0.916
	Adjusted p-value	1.000	1.000	1.000
Calculated free 25(OH)D$_3$ *	r	−0.373	−0.281	−0.382
	p-value	0.007	0.046	0.006
	Adjusted p-value	0.056	0.368	0.048
Calculated bioavailable 25(OH)D$_3$ *	r	−0.375	−0.280	−0.393
	p-value	0.007	0.047	0.004
	Adjusted p-value	0.056	0.376	0.032
1,25(OH)$_2$D/25(OH)D$_3$ *	r	−0.004	−0.058	0.176
	p-value	0.980	0.687	0.216
	Adjusted p-value	1.000	1.000	1.000
1,25(OH)$_2$D /24,25(OH)$_2$D$_3$ *	r	0.053	−0.028	0.181
	p-value	0.711	0.843	0.204
	Adjusted p-value	1.000	1.000	1.000

* Log-transformed parameters.

4. Discussion

The goal of our study was to assess whether vitamin D metabolites can predict the increase of 25(OH)D after vitamin D supplementation. As elaborated above, CYP24A1 activity (24-hydroxylase) is reflected by the ratio of 24,25(OH)$_2$D over 25(OH)D, i.e. the VMR. In addition, the ratio between 1,25(OH)$_2$D and 24,25(OH)$_2$D$_3$ was recently proposed as part of a three-dimensional model for assessing vitamin D metabolic pathways [16]. It was previously suggested that vitamin D metabolites and their ratios could provide additional information for predicting vitamin D treatment response [8,9]. The findings in this vitamin D RC.T. in patients with 25(OH)D levels <75 nmol/L and hypertension do not support this hypothesis.

In our study, the VMR did not predict Δ25(OH)D$_3$ in the treatment arm of the RC.T.. In a regression model, baseline 24,25(OH)$_2$D$_3$ and baseline 25(OH)D$_3$ did, with comparable strength and magnitude, predict the increase in 25(OH)D$_3$ upon treatment. When adjusting for multiple testing in correlation analyses, no correlations of any of the included parameters with Δ25(OH)D$_3$ retained significance. Yet, we did observe trends for Δ25(OH)D$_3$ with baseline 25(OH)D$_3$, 24,25(OH)$_2$D$_3$, free 25(OH)D$_3$ and bioavailable 25(OH)D$_3$. Notwithstanding their borderline significance, the strength of the correlations is highly similar between these parameters and they do not seem to be superior to baseline 25(OH)D. According to these data, we can infer that CYP24A1 activity, measured by the VMR, does not predict the individual differences in the increase in 25(OH)D after vitamin D supplementation.

Concerning the VMR, the results of this study are in accordance with several other published reports. Saleh et al. performed an RC.T. of 4 weeks with 107 participants receiving a single 100,000 IU dose of vitamin D or placebo [11]. The VMR could not predict the increase of 25(OH)D after 4 weeks, whereas 25(OH)D did predict this increase with a similar R^2-value to our data. However, their data indicated that 24,25(OH)$_2$D$_3$ could not predict the Δ25(OH)D$_3$, whereas in our study it did. Aloia et al.

reported on the predictive properties of the VMR in four different small samples (between 14 and 16 participants per group) of placebo or 800, 2000 or 4000 IU vitamin D daily for 10 weeks [6]. They did not show an advantage of the VMR as a predictor, compared to baseline 25(OH)D, 24,25(OH)$_2$D$_3$ or free 25(OH)D. Binkley et al. investigated the effect of 1800IU of vitamin D in 62 postmenopausal women after 4 months and measured vitamin D metabolites [10]. They observed that neither VMR, 25(OH)D, 24,25(OH)$_2$D$_3$ nor free 25(OH)D was related to the observed increase in 25(OH)D.

On the contrary, other published studies did suggest a predictive role for the VMR. The study by Wagner et al. included young adults with a mean age of around 27 years that received 28,000 IU (equivalent to 4000 IU per day) of vitamin D once per week for 8 weeks in the form of a supplement or fortified cheese. Wagner et al. showed that the VMR predicted the increase in vitamin-D-receiving subjects ($R^2 = -0.38$, $p = 0.004$, $n = 60$) [8]. Also, Cashman et al. reported a significant correlation between the VMR and the change after vitamin D supplementation ($R^2 = 0.15$, $p < 0.01$) in a study including subjects above 50 years of age that were treated for 15 weeks by 20 µg vitamin D (800 IU) per day [9]. Of note, both studies did not report the R^2-value of baseline 25(OH)D with its increase after supplementation. Therefore, it is not possible to conclude whether the VMR was superior to 25(OH)D in this aspect.

Changes in other vitamin-D-related parameters after vitamin D treatment were also studied. To that end, we assessed if Δ1,25(OH)$_2$D and Δ24,25(OH)$_2$D$_3$ could be predicted by baseline parameters included in the study. We found no correlation between any tested baseline parameter and Δ1,25(OH)$_2$D. 1,25(OH)$_2$D levels are mainly regulated by calcium levels, which could explain this observation [12]. On the other hand, baseline 25(OH)D$_3$, 24,25(OH)$_2$D$_3$, calculated free 25(OH)D$_3$ and calculated bioavailable 25(OH)D$_3$ all showed a significant correlation with Δ24,25(OH)$_2$D$_3$. The clinical relevance of this observation is, in our opinion, unclear and should be further studied.

In our study, we observed an increase in the VMR upon vitamin D treatment. This suggests an increase in CYP24A1 activity and catabolism of 25(OH)D upon supplementation. A concurrent decrease in the 1,25(OH)$_2$D/25(OH)D$_3$ ratio implies a reduced conversion of 25(OH)D to 1,25(OH)$_2$D. Indeed, this suggests the physiological shift from anabolic to catabolic pathways when an excess of vitamin D exists. This is also supported by the significant decrease in the 1,25(OH)$_2$D/24,25(OH)$_2$D$_3$ ratio. In the present study, and all aforementioned studies, the correlation coefficients between baseline 25(OH)D and Δ25(OH)D$_3$ after supplementation were negative, which implies that the change in 25(OH)D$_3$ after vitamin D treatment is smaller in individuals with higher baseline 25(OH)D$_3$ levels [8–10].

We acknowledge that this study has several limitations. First, the results are derived from post-hoc analyses. Second, the study population consisted of hypertensive subjects with 25(OH)D levels <75 nmol/L; therefore, the findings might not be readily extrapolated to the general population. Furthermore, for the vitamin D level inclusion criterion, the 25(OH)D concentrations were measured at study baseline using a chemiluminescence assay, while mass-spectrometry-based methods are currently the gold standard [2]. However, for the current study, 25(OH)D and 24,25(OH)$_2$D were re-measured using a dedicated LC-MS/MS method. In addition, the intervention period of 8 weeks was relatively short and only a small number of subjects were severely vitamin D deficient. Vitamin D deficiency was defined as a 25(OH)D of <75 nmol/L in the original study by Pilz et al. [13]. There is still an ongoing debate as to whether the cut-off levels should be set at <50 nmol/L or <75 nmol/L [17,18]. In addition, vitamin D sufficiency was defined by measurements of baseline 25(OH)D$_3$, which is currently the critical measurement for defining vitamin D status [19]. Some studies suggest that free 25(OH)D$_3$ could be a better marker for assessing vitamin D status [20]. In our study, calculated free 25(OH)D$_3$ did not predict Δ25(OH)D$_3$ after supplementation better than baseline 25(OH)D$_3$. The RC.T. design and the successful vitamin D intervention are strengths of this study. Also, a high number of parameters were measured with gold-standard methods. In contrast to the majority of exploratory studies on the VMR, p-values of the correlations were adjusted for multiple testing.

In summary, we show that 25(OH)D$_3$, 24,25(OH)$_2$D$_3$ and the VMR increase after vitamin D treatment. However, 24,25(OH)$_2$D$_3$ and the VMR could not predict 25(OH)D$_3$ levels after vitamin

D treatment in this cohort better than baseline 25(OH)D$_3$. As this has been corroborated by other studies, it implicates the routine measurement of 24,25(OH)$_2$D$_3$ will probably be of no added value when personalizing the treatment dosage of vitamin D.

Author Contributions: Conceptualization, V.F., S.R.U., B.O.P., A.C.H.; methodology, N.F.D.; software, V.F., S.R.U., S.P., A.C.H., B.O.P., W.M., A.T.; validation, A.C.H., B.O.P.; formal analysis, V.F. and S.R.U..; investigation, M.H.K., V.T., C.T., M.P., V.B., M.R.G., N.D.V.; resources, S.P., A.C.H., B.O.P.; data curation, S.P., A.C.H., B.O.P.; writing—original draft preparation, V.F., S.R.U..; writing—review and editing, V.F., S.R.U., S.P., B.O.P., A.C.H., N.F.D.; visualization, V.F., S.R.U.; supervision, S.P., B.O.P., A.C.H.; project administration, S.P., A.C.H., B.O.P.; funding acquisition, n.a.

Funding: The Styrian Vitamin D Hypertension Trial was supported by funding from the Austrian National Bank (Jubilaeumsfond: project no.: 13878 and 13905).

Acknowledgments: The authors thank all study participants and also Fresenius Kabi for providing the study medication.

Conflicts of Interest: The authors declare no conflict of interest.

Appendix A

Table A1. Pearson correlations of baseline vitamin-D-related parameters adjusted for gender, age, BMI, PTH, eGFR, serum phosphate and serum calcium, with the changes from baseline of 25(OH)D, 1,25(OH)$_2$D and 24,25(OH)$_2$D after vitamin D supplementation. *p*-values without and with Bonferroni adjustment are shown.

Baseline Parameters		Δ25(OH)D$_3$	Δ1,25(OH)$_2$D	Δ24,25(OH)$_2$D$_3$
25(OH)D$_3$	r	−0.508	−0.277	−0.657
	p-value	0.013	0.201	0.001
	Adjusted *p*-value	0.104	1.000	0.008
1,25(OH)$_2$D	r	−0.350	−0.171	−0.430
	p-value	0.102	0.435	0.040
	Adjusted *p*-value	0.816	1.000	0.320
24,25(OH)$_2$D$_3$	r	−0.490	−0.129	−0.597
	p-value	0.018	0.559	0.003
	Adjusted *p*-value	0.440	1.000	0.096
VMR	r	−0.064	0.137	−0.516
	p-value	0.773	0.534	0.012
	Adjusted *p*-value	1.000	1.000	0.096
Calculated free 25(OH)D$_3$ *	r	−0.451	−0.363	−0.399
	p-value	0.031	0.089	0.059
	Adjusted *p*-value	0.248	0.712	0.472
Calculated bioavailable 25(OH)D$_3$ *	r	−0.451	−0.363	−0.404
	p-value	0.031	0.089	0.056
	Adjusted *p*-value	0.248	0.712	0.448
1,25(OH)$_2$D/25(OH)D$_3$ *	r	0.122	0.272	0.218
	p-value	0.578	0.209	0.318
	Adjusted *p*-value	1.000	1.000	1.000
1,25(OH)$_2$D /24,25(OH)$_2$D$_3$ *	r	0.126	0.136	0.211
	p-value	0.565	0.536	0.333
	Adjusted *p*-value	1.000	1.000	1.000

* Log-transformed parameters.

References

1. Bergwitz, C.; Jüppner, H. Regulation of Phosphate Homeostasis by PTH, Vitamin D, and FGF23. *Annu. Rev. Med.* **2010**, *61*, 91–104. [CrossRef] [PubMed]
2. Tuckey, R.C.; Cheng, C.Y.S.; Slominski, A.T. The Serum Vitamin D Metabolome: What We Know and What is Still to Discover. *J. Steroid Biochem. Mol. Biol.* **2019**, *186*, 4–21. [CrossRef] [PubMed]
3. Prietl, B.; Treiber, G.; Pieber, T.R.; Amrein, K. Vitamin D and immune function. *Nutrients* **2013**, *5*, 2502–2521. [CrossRef] [PubMed]

4. Jones, G.; Strugnell, S.A.; DeLuca, H.F. Current Understanding of the Molecular Actions of Vitamin D. *Physiol. Rev.* **1998**, *78*, 1193–1231. [CrossRef] [PubMed]
5. Dirks, N.; Ackermans, M.; Lips, P.; de Jongh, R.; Vervloet, M.; de Jonge, R.; Heijboer, A. The When, What & How of Measuring Vitamin D Metabolism in Clinical Medicine. *Nutrients* **2018**, *10*, 482.
6. Aloia, J.; Fazzari, M.; Shieh, A.; Dhaliwal, R.; Mikhail, M.; Hoofnagle, A.N.; Ragolia, L. The vitamin D metabolite ratio (VMR) as a predictor of functional biomarkers of bone health. *Clin. Endocrinol. (Oxf.)* **2017**, *86*, 674–679. [CrossRef] [PubMed]
7. Ginsberg, C.; Katz, R.; de Boer, I.H.; Kestenbaum, B.R.; Chonchol, M.; Shlipak, M.G.; Sarnak, M.J.; Hoofnagle, A.N.; Rifkin, D.E.; Garimella, P.S.; et al. The 24,25 to 25-hydroxyvitamin D Ratio and Fracture Risk in Older Adults: The Cardiovascular Health Study. *Bone* **2018**, *107*, 124–130. [CrossRef] [PubMed]
8. Wagner, D.; Hanwell, H.E.; Schnabl, K.; Yazdanpanah, M.; Kimball, S.; Fu, L.; Sidhom, G.; Rousseau, D.; Cole, D.E.C.; Vieth, R. The Ratio of Serum 24,25-dihydroxyvitamin D3 to 25-hydroxyvitamin D3 is Predictive of 25-hydroxyvitamin D3 Response to Vitamin D3 Supplementation. *J. Steroid Biochem. Mol. Biol.* **2011**, *126*, 72–77. [CrossRef] [PubMed]
9. Cashman, K.D.; Hayes, A.; Galvin, K.; Merkel, J.; Jones, G.; Kaufmann, M.; Hoofnagle, A.N.; Carter, G.D.; Durazo-Arvizu, R.A.; Sempos, C.T. Significance of Serum 24,25-Dihydroxyvitamin D in the Assessment of Vitamin D Status: A Double-edged Sword? *Clin. Chem.* **2015**, *61*, 636–645. [CrossRef] [PubMed]
10. Binkley, N.; Borchardt, G.; Siglinsky, E.; Krueger, D. Does Vitamin D Metabolite Measurement Help Predict 25(OH)D Change Following Vitamin D Supplementation? *Endocr. Pract.* **2017**, *23*, 432–441. [CrossRef] [PubMed]
11. Saleh, L.; Tang, J.; Gawinecka, J.; Boesch, L.; Fraser, W.D.; von Eckardstein, A.; Nowak, A. Impact of a Single Oral Dose of 100,000 IU Vitamin D3 on Profiles of Serum 25(OH)D3 and its Metabolites 24,25(OH)2D3, 3-epi-25(OH)D3, and 1,25(OH)2D3 in Adults with Vitamin D Insufficiency. *Clin. Chem. Lab. Med.* **2017**, *55*, 1912–1921. [CrossRef] [PubMed]
12. Mazahery, H.; von Hurst, P. Factors Affecting 25-Hydroxyvitamin D Concentration in Response to Vitamin D Supplementation. *Nutrients* **2015**, *7*, 5111–5142. [CrossRef] [PubMed]
13. Pilz, S.; Gaksch, M.; Kienreich, K.; Grübler, M.; Verheyen, N.; Fahrleitner-Pammer, A.; Treiber, G.; Drechsler, C.; Hartaigh, B.Ó.; Obermayer-Pietsch, B.; et al. Effects of Vitamin D on Blood Pressure and Cardiovascular Risk Factors. *Hypertension* **2015**, *65*, 1195–1201. [CrossRef] [PubMed]
14. Dirks, N.F.; Ackermans, M.T.; de Jonge, R.; Heijboer, A.C. Reference Values for 24,25-dihydroxyvitamin D and the 25-hydroxyvitamin D/24,25-dihydroxyvitamin D Ratio. *Clin. Chem. Lab. Med.* **2019**, *25*, 24–26. [CrossRef] [PubMed]
15. Powe, C.E.; Ricciardi, C.; Berg, A.H.; Erdenesanaa, D.; Collerone, G.; Ankers, E.; Wenger, J.; Karumanchi, S.A.; Thadhani, R.; Bhan, I. Vitamin D-binding protein modifies the vitamin D-bone mineral density relationship. *J. Bone Miner. Res.* **2011**, *26*, 1609–1616. [CrossRef] [PubMed]
16. Tang, J.C.Y.; Jackson, S.; Walsh, N.P.; Greeves, J.; Fraser, W.D. Bioanalytical Facility team The Dynamic Relationships Between the Active and Catabolic Vitamin D Metabolites, their ratios, and Associations with PTH. *Sci. Rep.* **2019**, *9*, 6974. [CrossRef] [PubMed]
17. Pilz, S.; Zittermann, A.; Trummer, C.; Theiler-Schwetz, V.; Lerchbaum, E.; Keppel, M.H.; Grübler, M.R.; März, W.; Pandis, M. Vitamin D testing and treatment: A narrative review of current evidence. *Endocr. Connect.* **2019**, *8*, R27–R43. [CrossRef] [PubMed]
18. Holick, M.F. Vitamin D Deficiency. *N. Engl. J. Med.* **2007**, *357*, 266–281. [CrossRef] [PubMed]
19. Sempos, C.T.; Heijboer, A.C.; Bikle, D.D.; Bollerslev, J.; Bouillon, R.; Brannon, P.M.; DeLuca, H.F.; Jones, G.; Munns, C.F.; Bilezikian, J.P.; et al. Vitamin D assays and the definition of hypovitaminosis D: Results from the First International Conference on Controversies in Vitamin D. *Br. J. Clin. Pharmacol.* **2018**, *84*, 2194–2207. [CrossRef] [PubMed]
20. Tsuprykov, O.; Chen, X.; Hocher, C.-F.; Skoblo, R.; Yin, L.; Hocher, B. Why should we measure free 25(OH) vitamin D? *J. Steroid Biochem. Mol. Biol.* **2018**, *180*, 87–104. [CrossRef] [PubMed]

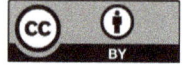

© 2019 by the authors. Licensee MDPI, Basel, Switzerland. This article is an open access article distributed under the terms and conditions of the Creative Commons Attribution (CC BY) license (http://creativecommons.org/licenses/by/4.0/).

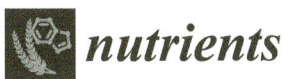

Article

Hypovitaminosis D in Postherpetic Neuralgia—High Prevalence and Inverse Association with Pain: A Retrospective Study

Jen-Yin Chen [1,2,*], Yao-Tsung Lin [1], Li-Kai Wang [1], Kuo-Chuan Hung [1], Kuo-Mao Lan [1], Chung-Han Ho [3] and Chia-Yu Chang [4,5]

1. Department of Anesthesiology, Chi Mei Medical Center, Tainan 71004, Taiwan; anekevin@hotmail.com (Y.-T.L); anesth@gmail.com (L.-K.W.); ed102605@gmail.com (K.-C.H.); albklan@gmail.com (K.-M.L.)
2. Department of the Senior Citizen Service Management, Chia Nan University of Pharmacy and Science, Tainan 71004, Taiwan
3. Department of Medical Research, Chi Mei Medical Center, Tainan 71004, Taiwan; ho.c.hank@gmail.com
4. Department of neurology, Chi Mei Medical Center, Tainan 71004, Taiwan; chiayu.chang7@msa.hinet.net
5. The center for General Education, Southern Taiwan University of Science and Technology, Tainan 71004, Taiwan
* Correspondence: chenjenyin@gmail.com; Tel.: +886-62812811

Received: 23 October 2019; Accepted: 13 November 2019; Published: 15 November 2019

Abstract: Hypovitaminosis D (25-hydroxyvitamin D (25(OH)D) <75 nmol/L) is associated with neuropathic pain and varicella-zoster virus (VZV) immunity. A two-part retrospective hospital-based study was conducted. Part I (a case-control study): To investigate the prevalence and risk of hypovitaminosis D in postherpetic neuralgia (PHN) patients compared to those in gender/index-month/age-auto matched controls who underwent health examinations. Patients aged ≥50 years were automatically selected by ICD-9 codes for shingle/PHN. Charts were reviewed. Part II (a cross-sectional study): To determine associations between 25(OH)D, VZV IgG/M, pain and items in the DN4 questionnaire at the first pain clinic visit of patients. Independent predictors of PHN were presented as adjusted odds ratios(AOR) and 95% confidence intervals (CI). Prevalence (73.9%) of hypovitaminosis D in 88 patients was high. In conditional logistic regressions, independent predictors for PHN were hypovitaminosis D (AOR3.12, 95% CI1.73–5.61), malignancy (AOR3.21, 95% CI 1.38–7.48) and *Helicobacter pylori*-related peptic ulcer disease (AOR3.47, 95% CI 1.71–7.03). 25(OH)D was inversely correlated to spontaneous/brush-evoked pain. Spontaneous pain was positively correlated to VZV IgM. Based on the receiver operator characteristic curve, cutoffs for 25(OH)D to predict spontaneous and brush-evoked pain were 67.0 and 169.0 nmol/L, respectively. A prospective, longitudinal study is needed to elucidate the findings.

Keywords: hypovitaminosis D; 25-hydroxyvitamin D; postherpetic neuralgia; spontaneous pain; brush-evoked pain; varicella-zoster virus immunoglobulin; DN4questionnaire

---

1. Introduction

Vitamin D is essential for musculoskeletal health in humans. The major circulating form of vitamin D is serum 25-hydroxyvitamin D (25(OH)D)—the main storage form. Currently, serum total 25(OH)D is considered to be the best marker of vitamin D status among the possible markers [1]. However, the definition of hypovitaminosis D is a central controversy in vitamin D research [1]. In the present study, sufficiency of vitamin D is defined as 25(OH)D ≥ 75 nmol/L (30 ng/mL) as defined by the Endocrine Society Clinical Practice Guideline [2]. Low vitamin D (hypovitaminosis D) includes insufficiency (50–75 nmol/L) and deficiency (< 50 nmol/L, 20 ng/mL) [2,3]. This cut-off is based on studies showing an increased intestinal calcium absorption and a decreased level of circulating parathyroid hormone when 25(OH)D levels were >75 nmol/L [2]. Notably, extra-skeletal functions of vitamin D are increasingly recognized. Vitamin D possesses anti-viral effects through vitamin D-induced peptides [4,5]. Vitamin D can inhibit neuroinflammation by downregulation of proinflammatory cytokines and upregulation of anti-inflammatory cytokines [6,7]. Vitamin D has concentration-dependent anti-inflammatory effects on glia and astrocytes through inhibiting the production of nitric oxide (NO) [8,9]. Importantly, NO increases phosphorylated N-methyl-D-aspartate (NMDA) receptors in spinal dorsal horn neurons which have been shown to be essential for the initiation of central sensitization and the development of mechanical allodynia [10]. In animal neuropathic pain models, vitamin D deficiency increases the production of reactive oxygen species (ROS) [11] which result in cold pain via the activation of transient receptor potential ankyrin 1 (TRPA1) [12,13] and contribute to mechanical hyperalgesia via the enhancement of NMDA receptor activation [14,15]. Vitamin D deficiency induces a marked dysbiosis and alters nociception possibly via molecular mechanisms involving the endocannabinoid and related mediator signaling system [16]. Vitamin D supplementation reduces mechanical hyperalgesia and cold allodynia [17]. Hypovitaminosis D has been demonstrated to increase neuropathic pain in patients with diabetic and rheumatoid arthritis [18–20]. Overall, vitamin D deficiency is associated with increased neuropathic pain.

Herpes zoster (shingles) is a common infectious disease resulting from reactivation of latent varicella-zoster virus (VZV). Patients with shingles suffer from herpetic pain which generally subsides within four weeks. Approximately 8%–24% of all zoster patients develop chronic herpetic pain known as postherpetic neuralgia (PHN) which lasts longer than 90 days after rash onset [21–23]. Although shingles vaccines are effective for preventing shingles and PHN, one-third of vaccinated persons aged ≥60 still develop PHN [24]. Besides, some PHN patients show inadequate responses to current therapies [25]. Thus far, PHN treatment remains challenging. Chronic pain in older patients may impair their ability to perform activities of daily living [26], leading to the development of vitamin D deficiency. Serum 25(OH)D status is positively associated with zoster immunity in dialysis patients [27]. We, therefore, conducted a two-part retrospective hospital-based study. In Part (a case-control study), we investigated the prevalence and the risk of hypovitaminosis D in PHN patients compared to those in controls receiving health examinations.

PHN is a peripheral neuropathy PHN patients experience various spontaneous and/or brush-evoked pain (allodynia) [28]. The Douleur Neuropathique 4 (DN4) questionnaire, which consists of seven symptoms (burning, painful cold, electric shocks, tingling, pins and needles, numbness, itching) and three items of physical examination (hypoesthesia to touch and pinprick as well as brush-evoked pain), is a popular tool for assessing the probability of neuropathic pain [29]. Following the protocol of our previous studies and that of others [28,30–33], zoster patients in the current study routinely received nutrient survey (e.g., serum 25(OH)D) and completed questionnaires including the DN4 questionnaire and those on pain intensity during their first visits to our pain clinic (Supplementary S1). Subsequently, the patients recruited for case-control study (i.e., Part I) were enrolled in Part II study (i.e., a cross-sectional study) that assessed the associations among vitamin D status, zoster immunity (VZV immunoglobulins), spontaneous/brush-evoked pain, and 10 items in the DN4 questionnaire [27,30,34,35] in PHN patients.

2. Materials and Methods

The study was conducted in accordance with the Declaration of Helsinki. This retrospective study was approved by the Institutional Review Board of the Chi Mei Medical Center in Tainan, Taiwan (IRB-10606-002). Patients' data in this study were drawn from the electronic medical database of Chi Mei Medical Center which is a 1200-bed tertiary referral center in Tainan, Taiwan.

During their first pain clinic visit, zoster patients routinely completed the DN4 questionnaires (seven questions and three clinical examinations) and received evaluation of their average daily spontaneous pain severity and the worst spontaneous pain on an 11-point numeric rating pain scale

(NRS, 0: no pain; 10: worst pain imaginable) [28] (Supplementary S1). Brush-evoked pain (mechanical allodynia) was assessed by using a manual handheld cotton swab swept three times approximately 3–5 cm in length over the skin, with a speed of 1 cm/s. A positive test of brush-evoked pain was defined as pain sensation elicited by at least two out of three strokes. The intensity of brush-evoked pain was graded on the 11-point NRS (0–10). Fasting blood samples were collected in the morning after the patients' pain clinic visits for 25(OH)D and VZV IgG/IgM antibody tests. In our pain clinic, a serum 25(OH)D survey has been performed routinely in zoster patients since 2011 [28,30,31,36]. Additionally, serological tests for VZV IgG/IgM have been a routine for the differential diagnosis of shingles from other skin diseases in zoster patients since mid-2012 [27,30,31,34,35]. Patients' information and data were collected and recorded in the electronic medical database.

2.1. Autosearch and Chart Review Criteria for Postherpetic Neuralgia

In this retrospective study, zoster/PHN patients aged ≥ 50 [37] receiving serum 25(OH)D and VZV IgG/IgM survey were selected by auto matched search from the computerized database (June 1, 2012–Dec. 31, 2016). Inclusion criteria for PHN were (1) International Classification of Diseases, Ninth Revision, Clinical Modification codes (ICD-9) 053 herpes zoster/053.X combined with new prescriptions of an analgesic, an anticonvulsant or an antidepressant for at least 90 days; (2) ICD-9 053.1X (herpes zoster with nervous system complications) [37,38]; and (3) patients with pain clinic visits ≥ 2 times during the study period [37,38]. Exclusion criteria were as follows: (1) patients diagnosed with herpes zoster ICD-9 053 in the preceding years; (2) patients who had diagnostic codes of human immunodeficiency virus infection (ICD-9 042, 043, 044) and organ transplants (ICD-9 3751, 1160, 1164, 1169, 5059, 5280, 5283, 5569, 3350–3352), which are potential confounders of shingles/PHN [21,38] and hypovitaminosis D [39,40]; and (3) patients whose medical records showed no evidence of serum 25(OH)D and VZV IgG/IgM survey during the study period.

Physicians (JYC and YTL) signed a patient confidentiality agreement before chart reviews. Each chart was reviewed for the inclusion and exclusion criteria. We included PHN patients who received a prescribed analgesic, anticonvulsant, or antidepressant or treatments by physicians for persisting pain ≥ 3 months and shorter than two years after zoster rash onset [28] as well as having a worst pain score ≥ 4 on the 11-point NRS [25]. In addition, no other cause for pain was considered more likely than PHN.

Age, gender and index-month are common confounders of vitamin D status [41]. Conditional logistic regression models were used by matching gender, index month, and age (i.e., ≤ 2 years between the two groups). The auto matched controls were individuals who received a health examination survey during the same period when the study patients visited the pain clinic. The ratio of controls to patients was 3 to 1 (Figure 1). The health survey package of our hospital included routine gastroduodenoscopy and 25(OH)D quantification [42].

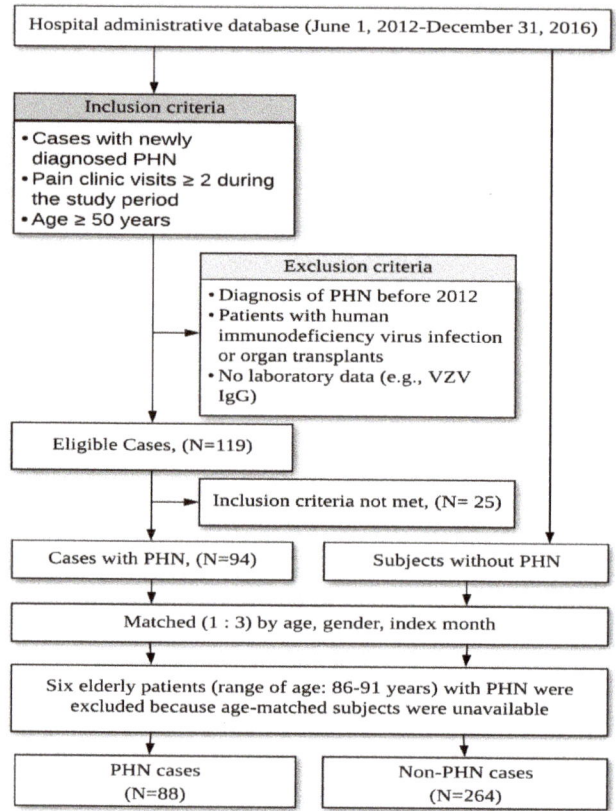

Figure 1. Flowchart of participant recruitment and case–control selection in Part I study.

The present study was a two-part retrospective hospital-based study including Part I (a case-control study) and Part II (a cross-sectional study). Using data from the electronic medical database of our hospital, we included automatically selected PHN patients and the gender/index-month/age-auto matched controls (non-PHN cases) in the case-control study. In the cross-sectional analysis, we included participants who were PHN patients of the case-control study.

2.2. Comorbidities

Hypertension/diabetes mellitus diagnosis was defined as patients who had ICD-9 codes for hypertension (ICD-9 401-405)/diabetes mellitus (ICD-9 250) and received a prescribed medication for hypertension/diabetes mellitus. Malignancy, autoimmune diseases, and chronic liver disease diagnosis were defined as patients who had ICD-9 code (malignancy 140-239; autoimmune diseases 710, 714, 725, 555, 556, 696, 340, 245.2; chronic liver disease 571) and received treatments by physicians for the diseases. Patients with chronic kidney disease were those who had ICD-9 585 and received dialysis regularly. *Helicobacter pylori*-related peptic ulcer disease was identified by ICD-9 530–534 and confirmed by positive findings on either hospital gastroduodenoscopy records or a self-reported gastroduodenoscopy history with prescriptions for the disease within one year prior to shingles outbreak [38].

2.3. Specimen Collection, Handling, and Biochemical Determination

2.3.1. Determination of 25(OH)D

Automated immunoassays are currently popular methods for measuring the circulating level of 25(OH)D. At our institute, a fasting blood sample was drawn in the morning from the testing subjects. Once the serum was separated, it was kept frozen at a temperature of −70°C until analysis. Serum 25(OH)D concentrations were measured by ARCHITECTi2000 (Abbott, Chicago, IL, USA) (Chemiluminescent Microparticle Immuno Assay) [43] every weekday.

2.3.2. Zoster Immunity—VZV IgG/IgM Detected by ELISA

Serum samples of PHN patients were routinely obtained for the VZV IgG and IgM antibody tests using enzyme-linked immunosorbent assay (ELISA) kits manufactured by Euroimmun (Lübeck, Germany) [44] and TECAN washer. The absorbance [44] was measured using ELISA reader Multiskan FC Thermo Scientific (Waltham, MA, USA). The result for VZV IgG was determined to be positive with the cut-off $\geq$ 110 mIU/mL. A positive result of VZV IgG was considered good immunity against VZV [44]. Positivity for VZV IgM was defined as an antibody index $\geq$ 1.0 [45]. A positive IgM result indicates recent or current VZV infection [27,34]. All assays were performed at the Chi Mei Medical Center Laboratory according to the instructions of the manufacturer.

2.4. Sample Size

In this study, the estimated rate of hypovitaminosis D in patients versus the controls was 70% versus 50% [3]. Therefore, a minimum sample size of patients (84 in each group) was determined to ensure a high power with a 5% significance level for an analysis of the difference between PHN patients and the controls.

2.5. Statistical Analysis

Data processing and statistical analysis were performed using SAS statistical software (Version 9.4; SAS Institute, Cary, NC, USA). The significance of difference among continuous data between the two groups was determined by student's t-test. Chi-square test or Fisher exact test was used to test the differences in categorical variables between the two groups. The risk of PHN was presented as an odds ratio (OR) and 95% confidence intervals (CI). Patients were divided into two groups according to age: patients aged 60years or older ($n = 64$) and patients aged 50–59 years ($n = 24$). Univariate logistic regression analysis was used to examine the associations between all selected predictors and PHN development in this study. A univariate association ($p < 0.10$) with PHN was included in the conditional multiple logistic regression model. Independent predictors for PHN were identified in the conditional multiple logistic regression model by gender, index month, and age (i.e., ≤ 2 years between two groups) match. Furthermore, patients were divided into two groups according to 25(OH)D levels: hypovitaminosis D (25(OH)D < 75 nmol/L) and sufficiency of vitamin D (25(OH)D $\geq$ 75 nmol/L). All of the demographic and clinical variables were compared between patients with sufficient-vitamin D and those with hypovitaminosis D.

The normality of variables was examined with the Kolmogorov–Smirnov test. Pearson's or Spearman's correlation was performed to test the significance of the association between clinical variables (e.g., 25(OH)D, VZV Ig) and severity of pain where appropriate. The correlation between clinical variables and severity of pain was considered to be clinically significant if the rho>0.3 [28]. According to pain severity, PHN patients were dichotomized into two pain groups: patients with mild pain (NRS $\leq$ 5) and those with moderate to severe pain (NRS 6–10). For identifying the optimal cutoff point for these clinical variables (e.g., 25(OH)D, VZV Ig) in predicting moderate to severe pain (i.e., NRS 6–10), a receiver operating characteristic (ROC) curve was plotted. The optimal cutoff value was determined with the Youden's index via maximizing the point on the ROC curve furthest from the line of equality. The area under the ROC curve (AUC) was used to measure the diagnostic ability of a variable (e.g., 25(OH)D, VZV Ig). Furthermore, the proportions of items in the DN4 questionnaire between patients with 25(OH)D /VZV IgM ≤ the cutoff point and those with levels > the cutoff point were compared to identify the associations between 25(OH)D /VZV IgM and symptoms/physical findings. A p value of <0.05 was considered statistically significant.

3. Results

A total of 119 PHN medical records were selected for review. Three patients were considered to experience other causes of chronic pain, while 19 patients were determined to suffer from zoster-associated pain which was defined as herpetic pain beyond 30 days but less than 90 days. Three patients were excluded due to incomplete records. In total, 25 patients were excluded after medical record review. Additionally, six elderly patients were excluded because of no age-matched controls (Figure 1).

3.1. Part I Study

Conditional Logistic Analysis for the Predictors of Postherpetic Neuralgia

The demographic characteristics of 88 patients and 264 controls are shown in Table 1. Comparisons between patients and the controls showed that PHN patients had significantly lower serum 25(OH)D (68.96 nmol/L, SD 18.72 nmol/L) and higher prevalence of hypovitaminosis D (73.9%) than those (75.13 nmol/L, SD17.47nmol/L; 47.0%) in the controls (p = 0.005; <0.001). Furthermore, PHN patients had higher prevalence of diabetes mellitus (29.5% vs. 15.9%, p = 0.005), malignancy (17.0% vs. 6.8%, p = 0.007) and *Helicobacter pylori*-related peptic ulcer disease (26.1% vs. 9.5%, p < 0.001) compared to that in the controls. There were no significant differences inbody mass index and the prevalence of hypertension, autoimmune diseases, chronic liver and kidney disease between the two groups.

Table 1. Conditional logistic regression analysis of potential predictors for PHN.

Predictors	PHN (n = 88)	Controls (n = 264)	Univariate OR (95% CI)	p	Adjusted OR (95% CI)	p
Age, years, mean (SD)	65.3 (9.4)	65.3 (9.0)		0.997		
Age groups						
≥60 years	64 (72.7%)	192 (72.7%)				
50–59 years	24 (27.3%)	72 (27.3%)				
Gender						
Male, n (%)	47 (53.4%)	141 (53.4%)				
Body mass index, mean (SD)	23.68 (3.26)	23.99 (3.07)		0.426		
Body mass index (kg/m²)			1.29 (0.54-3.06)	0.563	1.01 (0.36-2.79)	0.990
<18.5 or ≥30	8 (9.1%)	19 (7.2%)				
18.5–30	80 (90.0%)	245 (92.8%)				
25(OH)D (nmol/L), mean (SD)	68.96(18.72)	75.13 (17.47)		0.005		
Vitamin D status			3.31 (1.92-5.72)	<0.001	3.12 (1.73-5.61)	<0.001 *
Sufficiency, n (%)	23 (26.1%)	140 (51.9%)				
Hypovitaminosis D, n (%)	65 (73.9%)	124 (47.0%)				
Comorbidities						
Hypertension	33 (37.5%)	84 (31.8%)	1.35 (0.78-2.37)	0.279	1.14 (0.59-2.17)	0.702
Diabetes mellitus	26 (29.5%)	42 (15.9%)	2.22 (1.26-3.90)	0.005	1.97 (0.96-4.06)	0.065
Malignancy	15 (17.0%)	18 (6.8%)	2.71 (1.31-5.59)	0.007	3.21 (1.38-7.48)	0.007 *
Chronic liver disease	10 (11.4%)	28 (10.6%)	1.08 (0.51-2.28)	0.846	1.24 (0.52-2.93)	0.630
Chronic kidney disease	2 (2.3%)	6 (2.3%)	1.00 (0.20-4.95)	1.000	0.75 (0.13-4.48)	0.757
Autoimmune diseases	8 (9.1%)	10 (3.8%)	2.40 (0.95-6.08)	0.065	2.85 (0.98-8.27)	0.055
H. pylori-related PUD	23 (26.1%)	25 (9.5%)	3.15 (1.70-5.84)	<0.001	3.47 (1.71-7.03)	0.001 *
Antiviral therapy	38 (43.2%)	-				
Average spontaneous pain, mean (SD) (NRS 0–10)	5.84 (1.46)	-				
Brush-evoked pain, mean (SD) (NRS 0–10)	3.14 (3.10)	-				

n: number; SD: standard deviation; PHN: postherpetic neuralgia; 25(OH)D: serum 25-hydroxyvitamin D; PUD: peptic ulcer disease; NRS: numeric rating pain scale. T-test was used for continuous data. Chi Square or Fisher exact test was used for categorical data. Adjusted OR was determined using the conditional multiple logistic regression model by gender, age and index season match. * A p-value <0.05 was considered significant. Chronic liver disease: Patients had chronic hepatitis B and/or C or liver cirrhosis. Chronic kidney disease: Patients had hemodialysis. *Helicobacter pylori*-related PUD was defined as either positive findings on hospital gastroduodenoscopy records or a self-reported gastroduodenoscopy history with prescriptions for peptic ulcers/gastritis within one year prior to a shingles outbreak. -: The controls did not receive any antiviral therapy for VZV or pain measurement.

Although four risk factors for PHN were identified in univariate conditional logistic analysis, only three risk factors remained after conditional multivariate logistic analysis, including hypovitaminosis D (adjusted OR: 3.12, 95% confidence interval (CI) 1.73–5.61, $p < 0.001$), malignancy (adjusted OR: 3.21, 95% CI 1.38–7.48, $p = 0.007$) and *Helicobacter pylori*-related peptic ulcer disease (adjusted OR: 3.47, 95% CI 1.71–7.03, $p = 0.001$).

3.2. Part II Study

3.2.1. Comparison of Demographic and Clinical Characteristics Between Vitamin D-Deficient Patients and Vitamin D-Sufficient Patients

Patients with hypovitaminosis D had higher VZV IgM titers (0.63, SD 0.45), a lower vitamin D supplementation rate (1.5%) and greater spontaneous/brush-evoked pain intensity (6.1, SD 2.1; 4.3, SD 6.8), compared to those in patients with sufficient vitamin D (0.40, SD 0.25; 17.4%; 5.3, SD 1.8; 2.5, SD 8.3) ($p = 0.016$; 0.005; 0.021; 0.007) (Table 2).

Table 2. Demographic and clinical characteristics of patients with hypovitaminosis D vs. sufficiency of vitamin D.

	Hypovitaminosis D ($n = 65$)	Sufficiency of vitamin D ($n = 23$)	p
Age group			0.075
≥60 years, n (%)	44 (67.7)	20 (87.0)	
Gender			0.071
Male, n (%)	31 (47.7)	16 (69.6)	
Body mass index (kg/m^2)			0.357
<18.5 or ≥30, n (%)	7 (10.8)	1 (4.3)	
VZV-IgG (mIU/mL), mean (SD)	4239 (1382)	4281 (1066)	0.955
VZV-IgG, positive, n (%)	65 (100)	23 (100)	1.0
VZV-IgM, mean (SD)	0.63 (0.45)	0.40 (0.25)	0.016 *
VZV-IgM, positive, n (%)	8 (12.3)	1 (4.3)	0.279
Comorbidities, n (%)			
Hypertension	25 (38.5)	8 (34.8)	0.754
Diabetes mellitus	21 (32.3)	5 (21.7)	0.340
Malignancy	12 (18.5)	3 (13.0)	0.553
Chronic liver disease	8 (12.3)	2 (8.7)	0.639
Chronic kidney disease	2 (3.1)	0 (0.0)	0.416
Autoimmune diseases	6 (9.2)	2 (8.7)	0.939
Helicobacter pylori-related PUD	19 (29.2)	4 (17.4)	0.267
Vitamin D supplements★, n (%)	1 (1.5)	4 (17.4)	0.005 *
Average spontaneous pain, mean (SD) (NRS 0–10)	6.1 (2.1)	5.3 (1.8)	0.021 *
Brush-evoked pain, mean (SD) (NRS 0–10)	4.3 (6.8)	2.5 (8.3)	0.007 *

n: number; VZV: varicella-zoster virus; PUD: peptic ulcer disease; NRS: numeric rating pain scale. VZV-IgG, positive: >110 mIU/mL; VZV-IgM, positive: ≥1.0. T-test was used for continuous data. Chi Square or Fisher exact test was used for categorical data. ★ All of the five patients irregularly received a self-prescribed supplement of vitamin D (400 or 800 IU/day). * A p-value <0.05 was considered significant.

3.2.2. Correlations Between Pain and Serum 25(OH)D/VZV Igs in PHN

In Table 3, spontaneous pain was correlated to serum concentrations of 25(OH)D (Spearman correlation coefficient: −0.329, $p = 0.002$) and VZV IgM (Spearman correlation coefficient: 0.363, $p = 0.001$). Brush-evoked pain was correlated to the serum level of 25(OH)D (Spearman correlation coefficient: −0.311, $p = 0.003$). The other Spearman correlation coefficients were ≤ 0.3 indicating no clinical significance (Data not shown).

Table 3. Correlations between NRS of pain and serum concentrations of 25(OH)D/VZV Igs in PHN.

Correlation	Spearman's Correlation Coefficient	p
Spontaneous pain (NRS 0-10) vs.		
brush-evoked pain (NRS 0–10)	0.196	0.067
25(OH)D (nmol/L)	−0.329 *	0.002
VZV IgG(mIU/ml)	0.249	0.019
VZV IgM	0.363 *	0.001
Brush-evoked pain (NRS 0-10) vs.		
25(OH)D (nmol/L)	−0.311 *	0.003
VZV IgG(mIU/ml)	−0.181	0.092
VZV IgM	−0.183	0.088

Ig: Immunoglobulin; NRS: 11-point numeric rating pain scale (0–10); 25(OH)D: 25-hydroxyvitamin D; VZV: varicella-zoster virus; PHN: postherpetic neuralgia. * Spearman correlation coefficients indicate clinical significance if the value is greater than 0.3.

The cutoffs for serum 25(OH)D concentration to predict spontaneous pain and brush-evoked pain were 67.0 nmol/L (26.8 ng/mL) (sensitivity 71.4%; specificity 65.2%) and 169.0 nmol/L (67.6 ng/mL) (sensitivity 79.2%; specificity 59.4%), respectively. The cutoff for IgM titer to predict spontaneous pain was 0.60 with a sensitivity of 58.7% and a specificity of 76.2%. Based on the AUC values, we found that serum 25(OH)D status (0.704; 0.721) and IgM titers (0.689) were good predictors for pain in PHN (Figure 2a–c).

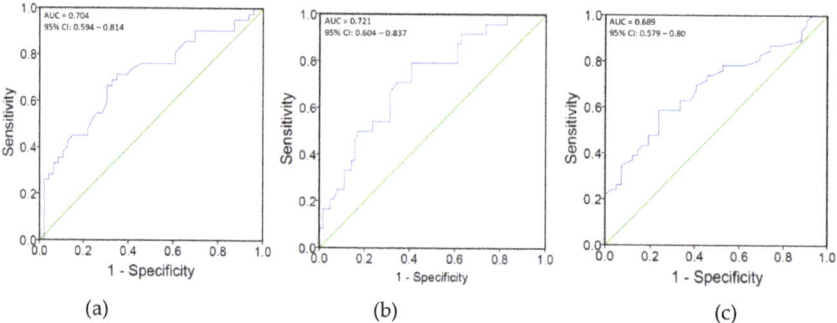

Figure 2. (a) area under the receiver operating characteristic curve for 25(OH)D concentration in spontaneous pain; (b) the area under the receiver operating characteristic curve for 25(OH)D status in brush-evoked pain; (c) the area under the receiver operating characteristic curve for IgM titer in spontaneous pain.

3.2.3. Proportions of 10 Items in the DN4 Questionnaire in Patients with Different Serum 25(OH)D/VZV Igs

In 88 PHN patients, 74 patients (84.1%) had a score greater or equal to 4 in the DN4 questionnaire. In 10 items of the DN4 questionnaire, patients with vitamin D ≤ 67.0 nmol/L had greater proportions of painful cold and brush-evoked pain compared to those in patients with vitamin D > 67.0 nmol/L ($p < 0.001$; $p = 0.002$). Although vitamin D-deficient patients (< 50.0 nmol/L) had greater proportions of painful cold and brush-evoked pain compared to those in vitamin D-insufficient patients ($p = 0.005$; $p = 0.225$), no statistically significant difference in brush-evoked pain was found between the two groups. Possibly, it was due to the small case number in the group with deficiency. (Table 4)

Table 4. Proportions of items in the DN4 questionnaire between patients with serum 25(OH)D concentration >the cutoff value vs.≤ the cutoff value.

Cutoff	25(OH)D			Insufficiency Deficiency		
	>67.0 nmol/L (n = 46)	≤ 67.0nmol/L (n = 42)	p	50–75nmol/L (n = 55)	<50.0 nmol/L (n = 10)	p
Burning pain, n (%)	28 (56.0)	22 (44.0)	0.422	14 (25.5)	2 (20.0)	0.713
Painful cold, n (%)	2 (11.8)	15 (88.2)	<0.001 *	10 (18.2)	6 (60.0)	0.005 *
Electric sharp pain, n (%)	35 (53.8)	30 (46.2)	0.619	9 (16.4)	2 (20.0)	0.778
Tingling, n (%)	35 (47.9)	38 (52.1)	0.073	33 (60.0)	7 (70.0)	0.550
Pins and needles, n (%)	36 (49.3)	37 (50.7)	0.220	31 (56.4)	6 (60.0)	0.831
Numbness, n (%)	19 (54.3)	16 (45.7)	0.759	17 (30.9)	4 (40.0)	0.572
Itching, n (%)	15 (32.6)	13 (31.0)	0.868	17 (30.9)	2 (20.0)	0.485
Hypoesthesia to touch, n (%)	17 (50.0)	17 (50.0)	0.735	21 (38.2)	4 (40.0)	0.913
Hypoesthesia to pinprick, n (%)	13 (46.4)	15 (53.6)	0.453	19 (34.5)	3 (30.0)	0.780
Brush-evoked pain, n (%)	27 (42.2)	37 (57.8)	0.002 *	43 (78.2)	10 (100.0)	0.225
DN4 ≥4, n (%)	39 (84.8)	35 (83.3)	0.853	45 (81.8)	9 (90.0)	0.526

n: number; VZV: varicella-zoster virus; DN4: the Douleur Neuropathique 4 questionnaire. * A p-value <0.05 was considered significant.

For the 10 items in the DN4 questionnaire, no significant finding was noted in patients with IgM ≤ 0.6 compared to those with IgM > 0.6. (Table 5).

Table 5. Proportions of items in the DN4 questionnaire between patients with VZV IgM titer ≥the cutoff value vs. < the cutoff value.

Cutoff	VZV IgM		p
	≥0.6 (n = 37)	<0.6 (n = 51)	
Burning pain, n (%)	19 (38.0)	31 (62.0)	0.378
Painful cold, n (%)	7 (41.2)	10 (58.8)	0.936
Electric sharp pain, n (%)	27 (41.5)	38 (58.5)	0.871
Tingling, n (%)	30 (41.1)	43 (58.9)	0.691
Pins and needles, n (%)	32 (43.8)	41 (56.2)	0.453
Numbness, n (%)	14 (40.0)	21 (60.0)	0.752
Itching, n (%)	12 (32.4)	16 (31.4)	0.916
Hypoesthesia to touch, n (%)	13 (38.2)	21 (61.8)	0.566
Hypoesthesia to pinprick, n (%)	12 (42.9)	16 (57.1)	0.916
Brush-evoked pain, n (%)	28 (43.8)	36 (56.3)	0.597
DN4 ≥4, n (%)	30 (81.1)	44 (86.3)	0.511

n: number; VZV: varicella-zoster virus; DN 4: the Douleur Neuropathique 4 questionnaire.

4. Discussion

The current study demonstrated a significantly higher prevalence of hypovitaminosis D in PHN patients than that in the controls. The rate in the controls was similar to that (44.1%) in subjects living on similar latitudes in our country located in the subtropical region [3]. The present study also showed that, compared to vitamin D-sufficient subjects, PHN patients with hypovitaminosis D had a lower vitamin D supplementation rate, greater pain intensity, and higher VZV IgM titers. There were several possible explanations for the high prevalence of hypovitaminosis D among PHN patients. First, compared to the healthy controls, PHN patients had a higher prevalence of diabetes mellitus [18], malignancy [46] and Helicobacter pylori-related peptic ulcer disease [42], all of which have been linked to hypovitaminosis D. Second, because low vitamin D intake is a known independent predictor of hypovitaminosis D [3], lack of vitamin D supplementation in the majority (94.3%) of patients may contribute to this condition. Third, previous studies have reported elevated titers of VZV

IgM titers in patients with hypovitaminosis D [27,45], indicating a current virus infection. Because vitamin D could enhance antimicrobial peptide expression [4,5], hypovitaminosis D may suppress antimicrobial peptide production and facilitate chronic infection. Moreover, higher VZV IgM titers in patients with hypovitaminosis D imply persistent VZV infection that may contribute to chronic pain and its severity. Chronic pain of high severity, in turn, could cause impaired activities of daily living in patients [26], leading to vitamin D deficiency. Interestingly, a previous report showed a high prevalence of hypovitaminosis D in hospitalized patients with shingles [47]. It raised a question of whether hypovitaminosis D in PHN was pre-existing at the onset of shingles or it was the consequence of depletion from PHN-related pain or chronic viral infection [27,30,35,47]. Instead of identifying causality, a retrospective case-control study could only establish an association. Longitudinal and experimental research is needed to further elucidate the findings.

In Part I study, hypovitaminosis D, malignancy and *Helicobacter pylori*-related peptic ulcer disease independently predicted PHN in conditional multiple logistic analysis. Because the pathogenesis of PHN includes neuronal excitability and persistent viral infection-induced neuroinflammation [48,49], there are probable molecular associations between hypovitaminosis D and PHN. First, activated microglia and astrocytes have been found to cause neuronal excitability, leading to neuropathic pain [49]. On the other hand, vitamin D can inhibit the activation of microglia [50] and astrocytes [51]. Second, vitamin D inhibits neuroinflammation by suppressing the production of pro-inflammatory cytokines and increasing that of anti-inflammatory cytokines [7,52]. Third, vitamin D possesses a direct anti-viral effect by enhancing the expression of antimicrobial peptides to suppress VZV replication in keratinocytes and B cells [4,5]. Taken together, hypovitaminosis D may induce PHN as a result of hyper-excitability of neurons, neuroinflammation and persistent viral replication.

PHN patients experience various spontaneous pain and brush-evoked pain (allodynia) [28]. Significant inverse associations were found between serum 25(OH)D level and the presence of spontaneous/brush-evoked pain in PHN patients. Spontaneous pain is related to the neuroinflammation-induced spontaneous firing of intact C-fiber nociceptors [53]. In a PHN rat model, inducible nitric oxide synthase (iNOS) in astrocytes, which produce large amounts of NO, is induced in response to VZV infection [54]. NO activates NMDA receptors in spinal dorsal horn neurons through phosphorylation, resulting in mechanical allodynia [10]. Therefore, the experimental model demonstrated VZV-NO-astrocyte-induced allodynia. Besides, vitamin D is anti-neuroinflammatory [6,7,52]. During inflammation, activated glia and astrocytes may synthesize 1,25(OH)D which inhibits iNOS expression and reduces the production of NO [8,9]. In mice, vitamin D deficiency generates reduced mechanical threshold without altering the thermal nociceptive threshold [16]. Vitamin D deficiency also induces a significant increase in the spontaneous activity and activation frequency of spinal nociceptive specific neurons as well as the duration of the evoked activity of spinal nociceptive specific neurons [16]. Accordingly, symptoms and signs in PHN patients may be augmented by hypovitaminosis D, perpetuating a vicious cycle involving spontaneous pain/allodynia and hypovitaminosis D at the molecular level. As for malignancy [55] and *Helicobacter pylori*-related peptic ulcer disease [38], both have been identified as the risk factors of PHN based on previous reports.

In Part II study, hypovitaminosis D was found to be associated with increased neuropathic pain in PHN patients. Vitamin D is a neuroactive steroid that may mediate pain processes by modulating several signal transduction systems. Patients with statin-induced musculoskeletal pain often have low vitamin D levels [56]. Statins decrease cholesterol synthesis through the reversible block of the hydroxy-3-methylglutaryl-coenzyme A reductase. As a result, statins may reduce the production of 7-dehydrocholesterol which can be photochemically converted to pre-vitamin D in the skin. Subsequently, pre-vitamin D is metabolized into 25(OH)D in the liver and is then converted into $1,25(OH)_2D$ in the kidney. Vitamin D is essential for the maintenance of musculoskeletal health; thus, its deficiency may produce muscular weakness and pain. A recent study showed a significant negative correlation between vitamin D levels and the severity of pain in patients with lower back pain [57]. Seemingly, patients suffering from chronic pain often have hypovitaminosis D. Recently, Guida et al. [16] demonstrated that spared nerve injury in normal or vitamin D deficient mice does not induce changes in gut microbiota. Nonetheless, vitamin D deficiency induces a marked dysbiosis (i.e., a lower microbial diversity characterized by an increase in Firmicutes and a decrease in Verrucomicrobia and Bacteroidetes). In addition, vitamin D deficiency alters the endocannabinoid system through reducing the expression of spinal cannabinoid receptor type 1, increasing levels of spinal cannabinoid receptor type 2 as well as changing endocannabinoid and endocannabinoid-like mediator levels in the gut. Concurrently, vitamin D deficiency causes tactile allodynia associated with spinal neuronal sensitization. Vitamin D deficiency affects nociception possibly via molecular mechanisms involving the endocannabinoid and related mediator signaling systems. Based on the findings of our studies and those of others, screening for hypovitaminosis D is suggested in the management of PHN.

In the current study, the cutoffs for 25(OH)D level to predict spontaneous pain and allodyniawere67.0 and 169.0 nmol/L, respectively. The difference in thresholds is consistent with the finding of a previous experimental study showing different thresholds for eliciting pain, allodynia, and hyperalgesia in rats [58]. In 88 PHN patients, 74 (84.1%) had a score greater or equal to 4 in the DN4 questionnaire. Our results suggest that a physical examination by the physician is still necessary [29]. Compared to patients with vitamin D >67.0 nmol/L, those with vitamin D ≤ 67.0 nmol/L had significantly greater proportions of painful cold among the seven symptoms in the DN4 questionnaire. The results support those of previous reports showing that lower 25(OH)D levels were correlated to lower cold detection thresholds in patients with painful diabetic peripheral neuropathy [19]. However, our findings demonstrated no association between 25(OH)D level and burning pain or other symptoms in PHN. In mice, vitamin D deficiency increases the production of ROS [11] which activates TRPA1 [12] and TRPV1 [59]. Sensitization of TRPA1 via ROS signaling causes noxious cold pain [13]. On the other hand, vitamin D inhibits TRPV1 channels which are involved in thermal hyperalgesia only in the acute phase of neuropathic pain [59]. The results of animal models support our clinical findings. Importantly, vitamin D supplementation has been demonstrated to reduce neuropathic pain in vitamin D-insufficient diabetic patients [18,60]. Optimization of vitamin D status may potentially prevent and treat PHN as an alternative therapy for spontaneous pain (painful cold) and allodynia.

The positive rate of VZV IgM in shingles ranges from 10% to 70% [45]. The positive rate of VZV IgM in our PHN patients was 11.4%. The current study is the first to report the positive rate of VZV IgM in patients with PHN. Our results showed that VZV IgM titer was positively correlated to spontaneous pain. Our findings support that some PHN is associated with VZV ganglionitis caused by persistent viral infection [48] and that high VZV IgM titers in zoster patients imply a high risk for PHN [61,62]. The cutoff for IgM to predict spontaneous pain was 0.60, indicating that antiviral therapy may decrease pain for patients with IgM ≥ 0.60. However, the analgesic efficacy of antiviral therapy for PHN remains conflicting [48,63,64]. This may be attributed to the lack of information on the concentrations of VZV immunoglobulins in those clinical trials. Further studies are needed to elucidate whether antiviral therapy is more effective in patients with high IgM titers than those with low titers as well as to assess the impact of hypovitaminosis D on the efficacy of antiviral therapy for PHN [35,65].

In terms of limitations, we did not assess sun exposure time, sunscreen use, daily activity, and vitamin D-rich food consumption [3], although the effects of these factors on our findings are likely to be limited. Second, patients aged >85 years were not included due to a lack of age-matched controls. Third, although race is a risk factor of hypovitaminosiss D [66], only Taiwanese were enrolled in this study. Further studies on other ethnic groups are warranted to generalize the results. Fourth, because of a small patient number and the retrospective nature of the present study, it is impossible to draw conclusions about causality. This demonstrates the need for large-scale prospective cohort studies to identify the causes and underlying mechanisms of hypovitaminosis D in PHN.

5. Conclusions

PHN patients aged 50–85 had a high prevalence of hypovitaminosis D which was associated with increased spontaneous and brush-evoked pain. PHN patients with hypovitaminosis D had greater pain, higher VZV IgM titers, and a lower vitamin D supplementation rate than those in subjects without the condition. The cutoffs for 25(OH)D to predict spontaneous pain and brush-evoked pain were 67.0 and 169.0 nmol/L, respectively. Patients with vitamin D ≤ 67.0 nmol/L had significantly greater proportions of painful cold. Spontaneous pain was also correlated to VZV Ig Mtiters. The cut-off for IgM to predict spontaneous pain was 0.60. Further prospective, longitudinal studies are warranted to confirm these findings.

Supplementary Materials: The following are available online at http://www.mdpi.com/2072-6643/11/11/2787/s1, Supplementary S1. First-visit questionnaire to the pain clinic at Chi Mei Medical Center.

Author Contributions: Conceptualization, J.-Y.C., Y.-T.L., L.-K.W., K.-C.H., K.-M.L., C.-H.H. and C.-Y.C.; methodology, J.-Y.C., Y.-T.L, L.-K.W., K.-C.H., K.-M.L., C.-H.H. and C.-Y.C.; software, K.-C.H., C.-H.H.; validation, J.-Y.C., Y.-T.L., L.-K.W. and K.-C.H.; formal analysis, C.-H.H.; investigation, J.-Y.C., Y.-T.L.; resources, J.-Y.C.; data curation, J.-Y.C.; writing—original draft preparation, J.-Y.C., Y.-T.L., L.-K.W.; writing—review and editing, J.-Y.C., Y.-T.L., L.-K.W., K.-C.H., K.-M.L., C.-H.H. and C.-Y.C.; visualization, C.-H.H.; supervision, J.-Y.C.; project administration, J.-Y.C.; funding acquisition, J.-Y.C.

Funding: MOST 107-2635-B-384-001(Ministry of Science and Technology, Taiwan), CMMOST 10717 (Chi Mei Medical Center, Tainan, Taiwan). The funders had no role in study design, data collection and analysis, decision to publish, or preparation of the manuscript.

Acknowledgments: We thank our pain assistant (Sherry Chen) for helping patients to complete the questionnaires at the first pain clinic visit.

Conflicts of Interest: The authors declare no conflict of interest.

Data Availability: Anonymized data not published within this article will be made available and shared by request from any qualified investigator.

Abbreviations

25(OH)D	25-hydroxyvitamin D
AUC	area under the ROC curve
DN4	Douleur Neuropathique 4
ELISA	Enzyme Linked Immunosorbent Assay
ICD-9	International Classification of Diseases, Ninth Revision, Clinical Modification
iNOS	inducible nitric oxide synthase
NMDA	N-methyl-D-aspartate
NO	nitric oxide
NRS	numeric rating pain scale
PHN	postherpetic neuralgia
ROC curve	receiver operating characteristic curve
ROS	reactive oxygen species
TLR	toll-like receptor
TRPA1	transient receptor potential ankyrin 1
VZV	varicella-zoster virus

References

1. Sempos, C.T.; Heijboer, A.C.; Bikle, D.D.; Bollerslev, J.; Bouillon, R.; Brannon, P.M.; DeLuca, H.F.; Jones, G.; Munns, C.F.; Bilezikian, J.P.; et al. Vitamin D assays and the definition of hypovitaminosis D: Results from the First International Conference on Controversies in Vitamin D. *Br. J. Clin. Pharmacol.* **2018**, *84*, 2194–2207. [CrossRef] [PubMed]
2. Holick, M.F.; Binkley, N.C.; Bischoff-Ferrari, H.A.; Gordon, C.M.; Hanley, D.A.; Heaney, R.P.; Murad, M.H.; Weaver, C.M. Evaluation, treatment, and prevention of vitamin D deficiency: An Endocrine Society clinical practice guideline. *J. Clin. Endocrinol. Metab.* **2011**, *96*, 1911–1930. [CrossRef] [PubMed]

3. Huang, C.H.; Huang, Y.A.; Lai, Y.C.; Sun, C.K. Prevalence and predictors of hypovitaminosis D among the elderly in subtropical region. *PLoS ONE* **2017**, *12*, e0181063. [CrossRef] [PubMed]
4. Crack, L.R.; Jones, L.; Malavige, G.N.; Patel, V.; Ogg, G.S. Human antimicrobial peptides LL-37 and human beta-defensin-2 reduce viral replication in keratinocytes infected with varicella zoster virus. *Clin. Exp. Dermatol.* **2012**, *37*, 534–543. [CrossRef]
5. Wang, T.T.; Nestel, F.P.; Bourdeau, V.; Nagai, Y.; Wang, Q.; Liao, J.; Tavera-Mendoza, L.; Lin, R.; Hanrahan, J.W.; Mader, S.; et al. Cutting edge: 1,25-dihydroxyvitamin D3 is a direct inducer of antimicrobial peptide gene expression. *J. Immunol.* **2004**, *173*, 2909–2912. [CrossRef]
6. Griffin, M.D.; Lutz, W.; Phan, V.A.; Bachman, L.A.; McKean, D.J.; Kumar, R. Dendritic cell modulation by 1alpha,25 dihydroxyvitamin D3 and its analogs: A vitamin D receptor-dependent pathway that promotes a persistent state of immaturity in vitro and in vivo. *Proc. Natl. Acad. Sci. USA* **2001**, *98*, 6800–6805. [CrossRef]
7. Piemonti, L.; Monti, P.; Sironi, M.; Fraticelli, P.; Leone, B.E.; Dal Cin, E.; Allavena, P.; Di Carlo, V. Vitamin D3 affects differentiation, maturation, and function of human monocyte-derived dendritic cells. *J. Immunol.* **2000**, *164*, 4443–4451. [CrossRef]
8. Lefebvre d'Hellencourt, C.; Montero-Menei, C.N.; Bernard, R.; Couez, D. Vitamin D3 inhibits proinflammatory cytokines and nitric oxide production by the EOC13 microglial cell line. *J. Neurosci. Res.* **2003**, *71*, 575–582. [CrossRef]
9. Garcion, E.; Nataf, S.; Berod, A.; Darcy, F.; Brachet, P. 1,25-Dihydroxyvitamin D3 inhibits the expression of inducible nitric oxide synthase in rat central nervous system during experimental allergic encephalomyelitis. *Brain Res. Mol. Brain Res.* **1997**, *45*, 255–267. [CrossRef]
10. Choi, S.R.; Roh, D.H.; Yoon, S.Y.; Choi, H.S.; Kang, S.Y.; Han, H.J.; Beitz, A.J.; Lee, J.H. Astrocyte D-serine modulates the activation of neuronal NOS leading to the development of mechanical allodynia in peripheral neuropathy. *Mol. Pain* **2019**, *15*, 1744806919843046. [CrossRef]
11. Liu, Y.; Chen, L.; Zhi, C.; Shen, M.; Sun, W.; Miao, D.; Yuan, X. 1,25(OH)2D3 Deficiency Induces Colon Inflammation via Secretion of Senescence-Associated Inflammatory Cytokines. *PLoS ONE* **2016**, *11*, e0146426. [CrossRef] [PubMed]
12. Arenas, O.M.; Zaharieva, E.E.; Para, A.; Vasquez-Doorman, C.; Petersen, C.P.; Gallio, M. Activation of planarian TRPA1 by reactive oxygen species reveals a conserved mechanism for animal nociception. *Nat. Neurosci.* **2017**, *20*, 1686–1693. [CrossRef] [PubMed]
13. Miyake, T.; Nakamura, S.; Zhao, M.; So, K.; Inoue, K.; Numata, T.; Takahashi, N.; Shirakawa, H.; Mori, Y.; Nakagawa, T.; et al. Cold sensitivity of TRPA1 is unveiled by the prolyl hydroxylation blockade-induced sensitization to ROS. *Nat. Commun.* **2016**, *7*, 12840. [CrossRef] [PubMed]
14. Lee, I.; Kim, H.K.; Kim, J.H.; Chung, K.; Chung, J.M. The role of reactive oxygen species in capsaicin-induced mechanical hyperalgesia and in the activities of dorsal horn neurons. *Pain* **2007**, *133*, 9–17. [CrossRef] [PubMed]
15. Gao, X.; Kim, H.K.; Chung, J.M.; Chung, K. Reactive oxygen species (ROS) are involved in enhancement of NMDA-receptor phosphorylation in animal models of pain. *Pain* **2007**, *131*, 262–271. [CrossRef]
16. Guida, F.; Boccella, S.; Belardo, C.; Iannotta, M.; Piscitelli, F.; De Filippis, F.; Paino, S.; Ricciardi, F.; Siniscalco, D.; Marabese, I.; et al. Altered gut microbiota and endocannabinoid system tone in vitamin D deficiency-mediated chronic pain. *Brain Behav. Immun.* **2019**, in press. [CrossRef]
17. Poisbeau, P.; Aouad, M.; Gazzo, G.; Lacaud, A.; Kemmel, V.; Landel, V.; Lelievre, V.; Feron, F. Cholecalciferol (Vitamin D3) Reduces Rat Neuropathic Pain by Modulating Opioid Signaling. *Mol. Neurobiol.* **2019**, *56*, 7208–7221. [CrossRef]
18. Soderstrom, L.H.; Johnson, S.P.; Diaz, V.A.; Mainous, A.G. Association between vitamin D and diabetic neuropathy in a nationally representative sample: Results from 2001–2004 NHANES. *Diabet. Med.* **2012**, *29*, 50–55. [CrossRef]
19. Shillo, P.; Selvarajah, D.; Greig, M.; Gandhi, R.; Rao, G.; Wilkinson, I.D.; Anand, P.; Tesfaye, S. Reduced vitamin D levels in painful diabetic peripheral neuropathy. *Diabet. Med.* **2019**, *36*, 44–51. [CrossRef]
20. Yesil, H.; Sungur, U.; Akdeniz, S.; Gurer, G.; Yalcin, B.; Dundar, U. Association between serum vitamin D levels and neuropathic pain in rheumatoid arthritis patients: A cross-sectional study. *Int. J.Rheum. Dis.* **2018**, *21*, 431–439. [CrossRef]

21. Yawn, B.P.; Itzler, R.F.; Wollan, P.C.; Pellissier, J.M.; Sy, L.S.; Saddier, P. Health care utilization and cost burden of herpes zoster in a community population. In *Mayo Clinic Proceedings*; Elsevier: Amsterdam, The Netherlands, 2009; Volume 84, pp. 787–794.
22. Massengill, J.S.; Kittredge, J.L. Practical considerations in the pharmacological treatment of postherpetic neuralgia for the primary care provider. *J. Pain Res.* **2014**, *7*, 125–132. [CrossRef] [PubMed]
23. Drolet, M.; Brisson, M.; Schmader, K.E.; Levin, M.J.; Johnson, R.; Oxman, M.N.; Patrick, D.; Blanchette, C.; Mansi, J.A. The impact of herpes zoster and postherpetic neuralgia on health-related quality of life: A prospective study. *CMAJ* **2010**, *182*, 1731–1736. [CrossRef] [PubMed]
24. Marin, M.; Yawn, B.P.; Hales, C.M.; Wollan, P.C.; Bialek, S.R.; Zhang, J.; Kurland, M.J.; Harpaz, R. Herpes zoster vaccine effectiveness and manifestations of herpes zoster and associated pain by vaccination status. *Hum. Vaccines Immunother.* **2015**, *11*, 1157–1164. [CrossRef] [PubMed]
25. van Seventer, R.; Bach, F.W.; Toth, C.C.; Serpell, M.; Temple, J.; Murphy, T.K.; Nimour, M. Pregabalin in the treatment of post-traumatic peripheral neuropathic pain: A randomized double-blind trial. *Eur. J. Neurol.* **2010**, *17*, 1082–1089. [CrossRef]
26. Stamm, T.A.; Pieber, K.; Crevenna, R.; Dorner, T.E. Impairment in the activities of daily living in older adults with and without osteoporosis, osteoarthritis and chronic back pain: A secondary analysis of population-based health survey data. *BMC Musculoskelet. Disord.* **2016**, *17*, 139. [CrossRef]
27. Chao, C.T.; Lee, S.Y.; Yang, W.S.; Yen, C.J.; Chiang, C.K.; Huang, J.W.; Hung, K.Y. Serum vitamin D levels are positively associated with varicella zoster immunity in chronic dialysis patients. *Sci. Rep.* **2014**, *4*, 7371. [CrossRef]
28. Chen, J.Y.; Chang, C.Y.; Feng, P.H.; Chu, C.C.; So, E.C.; Hu, M.L. Plasma vitamin C is lower in postherpetic neuralgia patients and administration of vitamin C reduces spontaneous pain but not brush-evoked pain. *Clin. J. Pain* **2009**, *25*, 562–569. [CrossRef]
29. Timmerman, H.; Steegers, M.A.H.; Huygen, F.; Goeman, J.J.; van Dasselaar, N.T.; Schenkels, M.J.; Wilder-Smith, O.H.G.; Wolff, A.P.; Vissers, K.C.P. Investigating the validity of the DN4 in a consecutive population of patients with chronic pain. *PLoS ONE* **2017**, *12*, e0187961. [CrossRef]
30. Bartley, J. Post herpetic neuralgia, schwann cell activation and vitamin D. *Med. Hypotheses* **2009**, *73*, 927–929. [CrossRef]
31. Chen, J.Y.; Chu, C.C.; Lin, Y.S.; So, E.C.; Shieh, J.P.; Hu, M.L. Nutrient deficiencies as a risk factor in Taiwanese patients with postherpetic neuralgia. *Br. J. Nutr.* **2011**, *106*, 700–707. [CrossRef]
32. Chen, J.Y.; Chu, C.C.; So, E.C.; Hsing, C.H.; Hu, M.L. Treatment of postherpetic neuralgia with intravenous administration of vitamin C. *Anesth. Analg.* **2006**, *103*, 1616–1617. [CrossRef] [PubMed]
33. Lin, Y.T.; Lan, K.M.; Wang, L.K.; Chen, J.Y. Treatment of Postherpetic Neuralgia with Intravenous Administration of Zinc Sulfate: A Case Report. *A A Pract.* **2018**, *11*, 8–10. [CrossRef] [PubMed]
34. Mathiesen, T.; Linde, A.; Olding-Stenkvist, E.; Wahren, B. Antiviral IgM and IgG subclasses in varicella zoster associated neurological syndromes. *J. Neurol. Neurosurg. Psychiatry* **1989**, *52*, 578–582. [CrossRef] [PubMed]
35. Chao, C.T.; Chiang, C.K.; Huang, J.W.; Hung, K.Y. Vitamin D is closely linked to the clinical courses of herpes zoster: From pathogenesis to complications. *Med. Hypotheses* **2015**, *85*, 452–457. [CrossRef]
36. Chen, J.Y.; Chang, C.Y.; Lin, Y.S.; Hu, M.L. Nutritional factors in herpes zoster, postherpetic neuralgia, and zoster vaccination. *Popul. Health Manag.* **2012**, *15*, 391–397. [CrossRef]
37. Yawn, B.P.; Saddier, P.; Wollan, P.C.; St Sauver, J.L.; Kurland, M.J.; Sy, L.S. A population-based study of the incidence and complication rates of herpes zoster before zoster vaccine introduction. In *Mayo Clinic Proceedings*; Elsevier: Amsterdam, The Netherlands, 2007; Volume 82, pp. 1341–1349.
38. Chen, J.Y.; Lan, K.M.; Sheu, M.J.; Tseng, S.F.; Weng, S.F.; Hu, M.L. Peptic ulcer as a risk factor for postherpetic neuralgia in adult patients with herpes zoster. *J. Med. Virol.* **2015**, *87*, 222–229. [CrossRef]
39. Mansueto, P.; Seidita, A.; Vitale, G.; Gangemi, S.; Iaria, C.; Cascio, A. Vitamin D Deficiency in HIV Infection: Not Only a Bone Disorder. *BioMed Res. Int.* **2015**, *2015*, 735615. [CrossRef]
40. Stein, E.M.; Shane, E. Vitamin D in organ transplantation. *Osteoporos. Int.* **2011**, *22*, 2107–2118. [CrossRef]
41. Levis, S.; Gomez, A.; Jimenez, C.; Veras, L.; Ma, F.; Lai, S.; Hollis, B.; Roos, B.A. Vitamin d deficiency and seasonal variation in an adult South Florida population. *J. Clin. Endocrinol. Metab.* **2005**, *90*, 1557–1562. [CrossRef]

42. Mut Surmeli, D.; Surmeli, Z.G.; Bahsi, R.; Turgut, T.; Selvi Oztorun, H.; Atmis, V.; Varli, M.; Aras, S. Vitamin D deficiency and risk of Helicobacter pylori infection in older adults: A cross-sectional study. *Aging Clin. Exp. Res.* **2018**, *31*, 985–991. [CrossRef]
43. Koivula, M.K.; Matinlassi, N.; Laitinen, P.; Risteli, J. Four automated 25-OH total vitamin D immunoassays and commercial liquid chromatography tandem-mass spectrometry in Finnish population. *Clin. Lab.* **2013**, *59*, 397–405. [CrossRef] [PubMed]
44. van Rijckevorsel, G.G.; Bovee, L.P.; Damen, M.; Sonder, G.J.; Schim van der Loeff, M.F.; van den Hoek, A. Increased seroprevalence of IgG-class antibodies against cytomegalovirus, parvovirus B19, and varicella-zoster virus in women working in child day care. *BMC Public Health* **2012**, *12*, 475. [CrossRef] [PubMed]
45. Min, S.W.; Kim, Y.S.; Nahm, F.S.; Yoo da, H.; Choi, E.; Lee, P.B.; Choo, H.; Park, Z.Y.; Yang, C.S. The positive duration of varicella zoster immunoglobulin M antibody test in herpes zoster. *Medicine* **2016**, *95*, e4616. [CrossRef] [PubMed]
46. Grant, W.B. A Review of the Evidence Supporting the Vitamin D-Cancer Prevention Hypothesis in 2017. *Anticancer Res.* **2018**, *38*, 1121–1136. [PubMed]
47. Han, G.Y.; Choi, Y.A.; Lee, K.Y.; Park, Y.O.; Cho, S.U.; Shim, M.; Kim, B.; Kim, S.O. The Comparison of the Blood Level of 25-Hydroxyvitamin D3 in Healthy Adult and Patients with Herpes Zoster. *Korean J. Fam. Pract.* **2016**, *6*, 288–292. [CrossRef]
48. Gilden, D.H.; Cohrs, R.J.; Mahalingam, R. VZV vasculopathy and postherpetic neuralgia: Progress and perspective on antiviral therapy. *Neurology* **2005**, *64*, 21–25. [CrossRef]
49. Ellis, A.; Bennett, D.L. Neuroinflammation and the generation of neuropathic pain. *Br. J. Anaesth.* **2013**, *111*, 26–37. [CrossRef]
50. Boontanrart, M.; Hall, S.D.; Spanier, J.A.; Hayes, C.E.; Olson, J.K. Vitamin D3 alters microglia immune activation by an IL-10 dependent SOCS3 mechanism. *J. Neuroimmunol.* **2016**, *292*, 126–136. [CrossRef]
51. Jiao, K.P.; Li, S.M.; Lv, W.Y.; Jv, M.L.; He, H.Y. Vitamin D3 repressed astrocyte activation following lipopolysaccharide stimulation in vitro and in neonatal rats. *Neuroreport* **2017**, *28*, 492–497. [CrossRef]
52. White, J.H. Vitamin D metabolism and signaling in the immune system. *Rev. Endocr. Metab. Disord.* **2012**, *13*, 21–29. [CrossRef]
53. Djouhri, L.; Koutsikou, S.; Fang, X.; McMullan, S.; Lawson, S.N. Spontaneous pain, both neuropathic and inflammatory, is related to frequency of spontaneous firing in intact C-fiber nociceptors. *J. Neurosci.* **2006**, *26*, 1281–1292. [CrossRef] [PubMed]
54. Zhang, G.H.; Lv, M.M.; Wang, S.; Chen, L.; Qian, N.S.; Tang, Y.; Zhang, X.D.; Ren, P.C.; Gao, C.J.; Sun, X.D.; et al. Spinal astrocytic activation is involved in a virally-induced rat model of neuropathic pain. *PLoS ONE* **2011**, *6*, e23059. [CrossRef] [PubMed]
55. Forbes, H.J.; Bhaskaran, K.; Thomas, S.L.; Smeeth, L.; Clayton, T.; Mansfield, K.; Minassian, C.; Langan, S.M. Quantification of risk factors for postherpetic neuralgia in herpes zoster patients: A cohort study. *Neurology* **2016**, *87*, 94–102. [CrossRef] [PubMed]
56. Pennisi, M.; Di Bartolo, G.; Malaguarnera, G.; Bella, R.; Lanza, G.; Malaguarnera, M. Vitamin D Serum Levels in Patients with Statin-Induced Musculoskeletal Pain. *Dis. Mark.* **2019**, *2019*, 3549402. [CrossRef]
57. Gokcek, E.; Kaydu, A. Assessment of Relationship between Vitamin D Deficiency and Pain Severity in Patients with Low Back Pain: A Retrospective, Observational Study. *Anesth. Essays Res.* **2018**, *12*, 680–684. [CrossRef]
58. Allchorne, A.J.; Broom, D.C.; Woolf, C.J. Detection of cold pain, cold allodynia and cold hyperalgesia in freely behaving rats. *Mol. Pain* **2005**, *1*, 36. [CrossRef]
59. Caterina, M.J.; Julius, D. The vanilloid receptor: A molecular gateway to the pain pathway. *Annu. Rev. Neurosci.* **2001**, *24*, 487–517. [CrossRef]
60. Lee, P.; Chen, R. Vitamin D as an analgesic for patients with type 2 diabetes and neuropathic pain. *Arch. Intern. Med.* **2008**, *168*, 771–772. [CrossRef]
61. Kim, Y.G.; Paek, J.O.; Kim, J.S.; Yu, H.J. Clinical significance of serum varicella zoster virus immunoglobulin M and G in varicella and herpes zoster. *Korean J. Dermatol.* **2015**, *53*, 441–448.
62. Higa, K.; Dan, K.; Manabe, H.; Noda, B. Factors influencing the duration of treatment of acute herpetic pain with sympathetic nerve block: Importance of severity of herpes zoster assessed by the maximum antibody titers to varicella-zoster virus in otherwise healthy patients. *Pain* **1988**, *32*, 147–157. [CrossRef]

63. Acosta, E.P.; Balfour, H.H., Jr. Acyclovir for treatment of postherpetic neuralgia: Efficacy and pharmacokinetics. *Antimicrob. Agents Chemother.* **2001**, *45*, 2771–2774. [CrossRef] [PubMed]
64. Quan, D.; Hammack, B.N.; Kittelson, J.; Gilden, D.H. Improvement of postherpetic neuralgia after treatment with intravenous acyclovir followed by oral valacyclovir. *Arch. Neurol.* **2006**, *63*, 940–942. [CrossRef] [PubMed]
65. Lin, Y.T.; Wang, L.K.; Hung, K.C.; Wu, Z.F.; Chang, C.Y.; Chen, J.Y. Patient characteristics and analgesic efficacy of antiviral therapy in postherpetic neuralgia. *Med. Hypotheses* **2019**, *131*, 109323. [CrossRef] [PubMed]
66. Holick, M.F. Vitamin D deficiency. *N. Engl. J. Med.* **2007**, *357*, 266–281. [CrossRef] [PubMed]

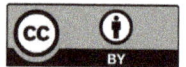

© 2019 by the authors. Licensee MDPI, Basel, Switzerland. This article is an open access article distributed under the terms and conditions of the Creative Commons Attribution (CC BY) license (http://creativecommons.org/licenses/by/4.0/).

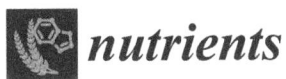

Article

Factors Predicting the Response to a Vitamin D-Fortified Milk in Healthy Postmenopausal Women

Rebeca Reyes-Garcia [1,2], Antonia Garcia-Martin [1,3], Santiago Palacios [4], Nancy Salas [4], Nicolas Mendoza [5], Miguel Quesada-Charneco [3], Juristo Fonolla [6], Federico Lara-Villoslada [7] and Manuel Muñoz-Torres [1,3,8,9,*]

1. Centro de Investigación Biomédica en Red sobre Fragilidad y Envejecimiento Saludable (CIBERFES), Instituto de Salud Carlos III, 28029 Madrid, Spain; rebeca.reyes.garcia@gmail.com (R.R.-G.); garciamartin_t@hmail.com (A.G.-M.)
2. Unidad de Endocrinología y Nutrición. Hospital Universitario Torrecárdenas, 04009 Almería, Spain
3. Unidad de Gestión Clínica Endocrinología y Nutrición, Hospital Universitario San Cecilio de Granada, Avenida de la Innovacion, 18016 Granada, Spain; charneco@me.com
4. Palacios Institute of Women's Health, 28029 Madrid, Spain; santiago.palacios@institutopalacios.com (S.P.); nancy.salas@institutopalacios.com (N.S.)
5. Department of Obstetrics and Gynecology, University of Granada, 18016 Granada, Spain; NICOMENDOZA@telefonica.net
6. Nutrition Department, Biosearch S.A, 18016 Granada, Spain; juristo.fonollajoya@biosearchlife.com
7. Research and Development Department of Lactalis Puleva, Nutrition Department, Biosearch S.A, 18004 Granada, Spain; federico.laravilloslada@puleva.es
8. Department of Medicine, University of Granada, 18016 Granada, Spain
9. Instituto de Investigación Biosanitaria (Ibs.GRANADA), 18106 Granada, Spain
* Correspondence: mmt@mamuto.es; Tel.: +34-950023000

Received: 14 September 2019; Accepted: 25 October 2019; Published: 4 November 2019

Abstract: Background: Milk products fortified with vitamin D may constitute an alternative to pharmacological supplements for reaching the optimal levels of serum 25-hydroxyvitamin D [25(OH)D]. Our aim was to analyze the response of serum 25(OH)D and its predictive factors in postmenopausal healthy women after a dietary intervention with a milk fortified with vitamin D and calcium. Methods: We designed a prospective study including 305 healthy postmenopausal women who consumed a fortified milk with calcium (900 mg/500 mL) and vitamin D3 (600 IU/500 mL) daily for 24 months. Results: The 25(OH)D concentrations at 24 months were correlated to weight, to body mass index, to the percentage of fat, triglycerides and to baseline 25(OH)D levels. We found significant differences in the levels of 25(OH)D at 24 months according to baseline 25(OH)D levels ($p < 0.001$) and body mass index ($p = 0.019$) expressed at quartiles. Multivariate analysis showed an association between levels of 25(OH)D after the intervention and at baseline 25(OH)D (Beta = 0.47, $p < 0.001$) and percentage of body fat (Beta = −0.227, $p = 0.049$), regardless of the body mass index. Conclusions: In healthy postmenopausal women, the improvement in 25(OH)D after an intervention with a fortified milk for 24 months depends mainly on the baseline levels of serum 25(OH)D and on the percentage of body fat.

Keywords: Vitamin D; postmenopausal women; obesity; fat mass

1. Introduction

The Institute of Medicine (IOM) states that the Recommended Dietary Allowance (RDA) of vitamin D is 15 µg (600 IU, international units) for 97.5% of the population aged 1–70, and 20 µg (800 IU) for 97.5% of the population >70 years. These are the recommendations for achieving the circulating levels of 25-hydroxyvitamin D (25(OH)D) ≥ 20 ng/mL needed to maintain bone health [1].

However, other guidelines recommend serum levels of at least 20–30 ng/mL [2,3], and according to these recommendations, many people are vitamin D deficient and will need vitamin D supplementation [4]. However, there is an important controversy about the target serum levels of 25(OH)D that must be reached to achieve the maximum health benefits and how to supplement 25(OH)D in cases where it is indicated [5].

The consumption of foods fortified with vitamin D is an alternative to treatment with pharmacological supplements to reach the optimal serum levels of 25(OH)D. Factors influencing the response to this strategy constitute an interesting area of research to optimize the nutritional recommendations about fortified foods. Although there is no consensus, several clinical factors have been reported to influence the dose–response relationships between vitamin D supplementation and serum 25(OH)D [6,7], such as body weight, percentage of fat, age, baseline 25(OH)D levels, and type and the duration of the intervention. In addition, genetic factors like single nucleotide polymorphisms in the vitamin D-binding protein gene can also be significant [8].

Obesity is one of the main factors related to a lower response after vitamin D supplementation [7]. Different causes have been proposed to explain this finding, one of them is a decreased bioavailability of vitamin D_3 from skin and from dietary source due to its deposition in body fat compartments. Also, an increased distribution volume for vitamin D has been proposed. Vitamin D deficiency is related to obesity regardless of age and the latitude, and it is also independent of the cut-offs to define vitamin D deficiency [9]. In the context of the increasing prevalence of obesity in the worldwide population, a better knowledge of the relationship between obesity and vitamin D after nutritional interventions is of interest.

Therefore, the aim of our study was to evaluate the changes occurring in serum 25(OH)D levels and their predictive factors in postmenopausal Spanish women after a nutritional intervention with a dairy product fortified with vitamin D.

2. Materials and Methods

2.1. Study Design

The findings presented in this study are a post-hoc analysis of data from a previously published clinical trial [10]. Here we analyze the predictive factors of response of vitamin D after 24 months of a nutritional intervention with a fortified milk with calcium (900 mg/500 mL) and vitamin D3 (600 IU/500 mL) on serum 25(OH)D. For this analysis, we selected 305 postmenopausal healthy women (mean age 59 ± 6 years) who completed 24 months of follow up. Inclusion and exclusion criteria of the study have been previously published [10].

Women consumed the dairy drinks for 24 months (500 mL/day, two intakes per day of 250 mL each), in the context of their usual diet. Counselling about Mediterranean diet and physical activity were provided to all women. The adherence to the intervention was evaluated every three months by telephone calls and empty dairy containers were collected. Compliance with the intervention was above 90%. The dairy drinks were produced in white 1 L Tetra Bricks by Lactalis Puleva (Granada, Spain).

The study was approved by the Ethics Committee of Hospital Universitario San Cecilio of Granada. All the volunteers provided informed written consent. The study was conducted in accordance with the ethical principles of the Declaration of Helsinki, following the EEC Good Clinical Practice guidelines (July 1996).

2.2. Anthropometric Measurements

In the first visit anthropometric measurements were obtained, and also after 24 months of intervention. We measured body weight (kg) using a standard balance beam scale (Seca), and body height (cm) using a precision stadiometer (Seca), attached to the balance beam scale. Obesity was defined as body mass index >30 kg/m^2.

2.3. Body Composition Measurements

Skeletal muscle mass was estimated from bioelectrical impedance analysis (Tanita BC418) at baseline and at 24 months after the onset of the intervention. This device calculates the percentage of body fat, fat mass, fat-free mass, and the predicted muscle mass, based on the data obtained by Dual-Energy X-ray Absorptiometry (DXA), using Bioelectrical Impedance Analysis with an operating frequency of 50 kHz at 500 lA. Obesity was defined as percentage of fat mass above 35% [11].

2.4. Biochemical Parameters

Blood samples were obtained at 0 and at 24 months after a 12 hour overnight fast. The blood was collected in a SST-Vacutainer (BD) and serum was separated by centrifugation at 3000 rpm for 15 min at 22–24 °C, then it was divided into aliquots and frozen and stored at −80 °C until analysis. Serum total cholesterol, high-density lipoprotein cholesterol (HDL-c), triglycerides (TGs), glucose levels, HbA_{1c}, and apo B were determined by standard automated procedures (Biosystems, Barcelona, Spain). LDL-c was calculated using the Friedewald formula. Serum 25(OH)D levels were measured by chemiluminescence immunoassay from Diasorin (LIAISON® 25 OH Vitamin D TOTAL Assay).

2.5. Statistical Analyses

Data were evaluated for normality and homogeneity of variance, and they are expressed as mean standard ± deviation. The relationship between serum vitamin D and biochemical and clinical factors were assessed by univariate analysis. A logistic regression and multiple regression analysis were performed to analyze the association between vitamin D levels at baseline and the levels found after 24 months of intervention. The variables related to vitamin D after 24 months of intervention (percentage of fat mass, weight, BMI, triglycerides and baseline 25 OH vitamin D) were included as covariates. SPSS software (version 17.0, IBM, Armonk, NY, USA) was used for doing statistical analysis. We considered p values < 0.05 as significant.

3. Results

Baseline clinical characteristics are shown in Table 1. Mean age was 59.3 ± 5.9 years.

Table 1. Characteristics of study subjects at baseline and after 24 months of intervention.

	Baseline	24 months	p
Weight (kg)	70 ± 11	70 ± 11	0.5
Body mass index (kg/m^2)	28 ± 4	28 ± 4	0.084
Obesity (%)	28	32	
Overweight (%)	47	48	
Percentage of fat mass	37 ± 5	37 ± 5	0.047
Serum calcium (mg/dL)	9.7 ± 0.6	9.8 ± 0.6	<0.001
Parathyroid hormone (pg/mL)	57 ± 21	58 ± 20	0.102
25(OH)D (ng/mL)	22 ± 8	25± 6	<0.001
Total cholesterol (mg/dL)	214 ± 33	208 ± 32	<0.001
HDL colesterol (mg/dL)	55 ± 15	55 ± 14	0.62
LDL colesterol (mg/dL)	141 ± 32	135 ± 32	<0.001
Triglycerides (mg/dL)	87 ± 44	88 ± 46	0.6

3.1. Changes in Biochemical Parameters

Serum 25(OH)D concentrations increased significantly at 24 months compared to the baseline values (25.4 ± 6.3 ng/dL vs. 21.7 ± 8.3 ng/dL, respectively, $p < 0.001$). At baseline, 51.3% of the women had 25(OH)D concentrations > 20 ng/mL, and 14.1% > 30 ng/mL. After 24 months of intervention, we observed a significant increase in the percentage of women with 25(OH)D levels > 20 ng/mL (78.5%) and > 30 ng/mL (18.8%) compared to baseline, $p < 0.001$ for both.

3.2. Factors Related to 25(OH)D Levels after the Intervention

Serum 25(OH)D levels at 24 months were correlated to weight ($r = -0.243$, $p < 0.001$), BMI ($r = -0.177$, $p = 0.006$), percentage of fat mass ($r = -0.32$, $p < 0.001$), triglycerides ($r = -0.301$, $p < 0.001$) and baseline 25(OH)D levels ($r = 0.5$, $p < 0.001$). (Figure 1). We found statistically significant differences in the levels of 25(OH)D at 24 months according to baseline 25(OH)D ($p < 0.001$) and BMI ($p = 0.019$) distributed by quartiles (Figure 2).

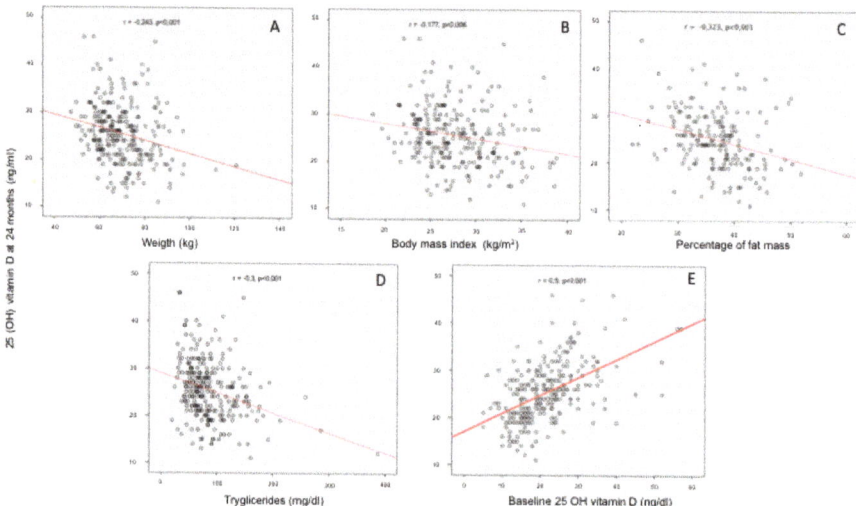

Figure 1. Correlations between serum 25(OH)D levels at 24 months and weight (**A**), body mass index (**B**), percentage of fat mass (**C**), triglycerides (**D**) and baseline 25(OH)D levels (**E**).

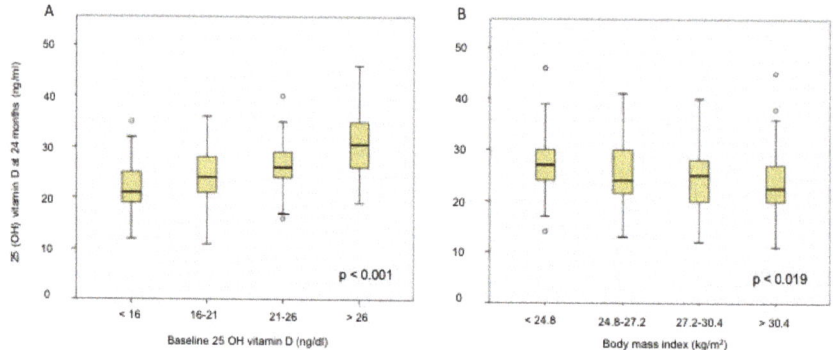

Figure 2. The 25(OH) D levels at 24 months according to quartiles of baseline 25(OH) vitamin D (**A**) and quartiles of body mass index (**B**).

We did not find differences in baseline 25(OH)D according to BMI: (<30 kg/m^2) 21.9 ± 8 vs. (>30 kg/m^2) 21.3 ± 8.5, $p > 0.05$. However, lower 25(OH)D levels were observed in women with BMI > 30 kg/m^2 (24.1 ± 6.5 ng/mL) vs. those women with a BMI < 30 kg/m^2 (26.2 ± 6 ng/mL) at 24 months ($p = 0.026$).

In women with obesity, defined by percentage of fat mass, baseline levels of 25(OH)D were lower (21.2 ± 8.1 ng/mL) compared to women with percentage of fat mass below 35%: (24.6 ± 9 ng/mL), $p < 0.01$. Women with obesity, defined by percentage of fat mass, also reached lower 25(OH)D levels after 24 months of intervention: 23.7 ± 5.9 ng/mL vs. 27.4 ± 5.9 ng/mL, $p < 0.001$, compared to women with percentage of fat mass below 35%.

3.3. Multivariate Analysis

When we analyzed the probability of reaching adequate vitamin D levels after 24 months of intervention, women with obesity (defined as BMI > 30 kg/m^2 or percentage of fat mass above 35%) have a higher risk of 25(OH)D < 20 ng/mL at 24 months: odds ratio (OR) 2.3, confidence interval, CI, 95%: 1.2–4.4, $p = 0.013$ for BMI > 30 and OR 5, CI 95% 2–12.6, $p < 0.001$, for percentage of fat mass. The influence of adiposity, defined as percentage of fat mass, in 25(OH)D levels after 24 months persisted after adjusting for BMI: 25(OH)D < 20 ng/mL OR 4.5 CI 95% 1.6–12.3, $p = 0.003$, 25(OH)D < 30 ng/mL OR 3.2 CI 95% 1.2–8.9, $p = 0.02$.

In women with percentage of fat mass above 35%, there was a 3.2 times higher probability of reaching 25(OH)D levels < 30 ng/dL at 24 months, regardless of the BMI. However, when we adjusted by baseline 25(OH)D levels, only the relationship with 25(OH)D < 20 ng/dL persisted (OR 3.6, CI 1.3–10.1, $p = 0.007$).

In the multivariate analysis, we observed an association between serum 25(OH)D after 24 months of intervention, baseline 25(OH)D levels (Beta = 0.47, $p < 0.001$) and percentage of fat mass (Beta = −0.227, $p = 0.049$), regardless of weight, BMI and triglycerides.

4. Discussion

The daily consumption of a dairy product providing 600 IU of vitamin D3 for 24 months is effective to improve serum concentrations of 25(OH)D in healthy postmenopausal women. The nutritional intervention described in our study allows that 78.5% of women reach 25(OH)D levels > 20 ng/mL, and 18.8% of women reach 25(OH)D > 30 ng/mL. Baseline 25(OH)D levels and the percentage of body fat mass are the main factors explaining the responsiveness. The risk of having 25(OH)D below 20 ng/mL after 24 months of intervention was 3.6 times higher in the women with fat mass above 35%, regardless of BMI and baseline 25(OH)D levels.

This study shows that a simple nutritional intervention with a vitamin D3-enriched milk that supplies 600 IU/day is effective in increasing 25(OH)D levels and helps to reach adequate 25(OH)D levels in a high percentage of women. These results are comparable to those described when pharmacological supplements of vitamin D were used, which often are not well tolerated by patients, especially if combined with calcium [12]. Although there is not a total consistency regarding the adequate 25(OH)D levels in healthy subjects [1–3,13], the most accepted serum values are 20 ng/mL, which will be reached for most of the women after this intervention.

Basel concentrations of 25(OH)D influence the achievement of adequate 25(OH)D levels after 24 months, regardless of other factors. This fact reinforces previous data found in older [14,15] and younger adults [16], and confirms the importance of considering baseline vitamin D in postmenopausal healthy women who receive a nutritional intervention with vitamin D.

Another independent predictor of the response of 25(OH)D levels after 24 months of intervention was body fat. Although weight, triglycerides and BMI showed and association with 25(OH)D levels at 24 months, only the percentage of fat mass persisted in multivariate analysis. BMI is a simple and worldwide measurement of obesity. However, its validity has been discussed in recent years [17], and other measures of fat may provide a better estimation of obesity, as percentage of fat mass. In the present study, only the percentage of fat mass remained as an independent factor influencing the response of vitamin D after the nutritional intervention, and not BMI. In older healthy women, fat mass was negatively related to 25(OH)D in a cross-sectional study [18]. Our data showing an independent association between the fat mass percentage and the evolution of 25(OH) D after 24 months confirms this relationship, and reinforces the utility of this measurement when addressing the response to an intervention with vitamin D. Other authors [16] found that body fat mass and BMI were not related the 25(OH)D response, speculating that total body mass instead than fat mass may determine the 25(OH)D response. The disparity in the results may be explained by the duration of the intervention and also by the mean BMI of the subjects included in the study.

There is no agreement regarding why obesity would affect serum 25(OH)D levels. This influence could be explained by a reduced intake of vitamin D, a reduced sun exposure, an increased storage and/or sequestration of vitamin D in the adipose tissue. A volumetric dilution due to the distribution of 25(OH)D in larger fat volumes [6,7,19,20]. In addition, vitamin D stored in the adipose tissue may be less available for hydroxylation [14,16]. Therefore, if the increased prevalence of obesity worldwide is the explanation for the high rates of hypovitaminosis D reported is a matter that should be investigated. However, our study could not demonstrate a favorable effect of the consumption of a dairy product supplemented with vitamin D on the loss of body weight or fat mass. This finding is consistent with previously described findings [21].

Although BMI is the most widely used method to evaluate the presence of overweight and obesity, it has been criticized because BMI does not always reflect true body fatness, that may be better evaluated by the assessment of body fat and fat-free mass [22]. Bioelectrical impedance analysis is considered as the simplest, most reproducible and least expensive method for the evaluation of body composition in clinical practice. It has shown a high accuracy and an excellent correlation with DXA when assessing the percentage of body fat [23]. Therefore, bioelectrical impedance is cost-effective and feasible, and may replace DXA in assessing the body composition. Our results highlight the usefulness of bioelectrical impedance analysis in the evaluation of healthy postmenopausal women. This analysis may be useful in the selection of women at higher risk of vitamin D deficiency or in the selection of women who need a higher supplementation of a more frequent evaluation of vitamin D levels.

Our results show that, in healthy postmenopausal women, baseline 25(OH)D levels and obesity, defined as the percentage of fat mass, are independent determinants of 25(OH)D levels after 24 months of a nutritional intervention, and they are of clinical relevance. These findings may allow a better personalization of the supplementation with vitamin D for reaching adequate levels after the intervention. Moreover, it has been described that the response to vitamin D may differ according to the dose of vitamin D and the duration of the intervention [24]. Furthermore, the factors influencing this response may differ between pharmacological and nutritional supplementation, and this potential difference must be addressed. Considering our findings, the recommended vitamin D dose may be adapted to baseline vitamin D levels. In addition, the estimation of the percentage of fat mass may be better for predicting the response to nutritional interventions with vitamin D.

Our study has several strengths, as the long follow-up for a nutritional intervention, and the exhaustive evaluation of compliance with the intervention. Limitations of the study are the absence of a comprehensive assessment of dietary intake of vitamin D, which may influence the results. However, women were advised not to change their lifestyle habits, and exercise was evaluated semi-quantitatively and showed no changes during the intervention, as an example of no changes. In addition, we evaluated Caucasian healthy women, and the generalization of this finding to males or to other ethnic groups must be confirmed. Moreover, we only measured total 25(OH)D, and we did not evaluate other metabolites.

5. Conclusions

In summary, the response of serum 25(OH)D levels to the supplementation with a fortified milk consumed for 24 months depend on baseline levels of serum 25(OH)D and on the percentage of body fat, regardless of BMI, in healthy postmenopausal women. In these women, the determination of the percentage of fat mass by bioelectrical impedance may allow a better prediction of the response to vitamin D after a nutritional intervention.

Author Contributions: Designed research: M.M.-T., N.M., S.P., J.F. and F.L.-V.; conducted research: N.M., S.P., N.S., M.Q.-C., M.M.T., R.R.-G., J.F. and F.L.-V.; analyzed data: R.R.-G. and A.G.-M.; wrote the manuscript: R.R.-G. and M.M.-T.; and had the primary responsibility for final content: R.R.-G. and M.M.-T. All authors have approved the final version of the article.

Funding: This research received no external funding.

Acknowledgments: This study has been financed by Lactalis Puleva. We thank Nutraceutical Translations for English language editing of this manuscript.

Conflicts of Interest: J.F. is an employee at Nutrition Department of Biosearch Life, F.L.-V. is an employee at Research and Development Department of Lactalis Puleva. The rest of the authors have no conflict of interest.

References

1. Heaney, R.P. Health is better at serum 25(OH)D above 30ng/mL. *J. Steroid Biochem. Mol. Biol.* **2013**, *136*, 224–228. [CrossRef] [PubMed]
2. Holick, M.F.; Binkley, N.C.; Bischoff-Ferrari, H.A.; Gordon, C.M.; Hanley, D.A.; Heaney, R.P.; Murad, M.H.; Weaver, C.M. Guidelines for preventing and treating vitamin D deficiency and insufficiency revisited. *J. Clin. Endocrinol. Metab.* **2012**, *97*, 1153–1158. [CrossRef] [PubMed]
3. Rosen, C.J.; Abrams, S.A.; Aloia, J.F.; Brannon, P.M.; Clinton, S.K.; Durazo-Arvizu, R.A.; Gallagher, J.C.; Gallo, R.L.; Jones, G.; Kovacs, C.S.; et al. IOM committee members respond to Endocrine Society vitamin D guideline. *J. Clin. Endocrinol. Metab.* **2012**, *97*, 1146–1152. [CrossRef] [PubMed]
4. Roth, D.E.; Abrams, S.A.; Aloia, J.; Bergeron, G.; Bourassa, M.W.; Brown, K.H.; Calvo, M.S.; Cashman, K.D.; Combs, G.; De-Regil, L.M.; et al. Global prevalence and disease burden of vitamin D deficiency: A roadmap for action in low- and middle-income countries. *Ann N. Y. Acad. Sci.* **2018**, *430*, 44–79. [CrossRef]
5. Giustina, A.; Adler, R.A.; Binkley, N.; Bouillon, R.; Ebeling, P.R.; Lazaretti-Castro, M.; Marcocci, C.; Rizzoli, R.; Sempos, C.T.; Bilezikian, J.P. Controversies in Vitamin D: Summary Statement From an International Conference. *J. Clin. Endocrinol. Metab.* **2019**, *104*, 234–240. [CrossRef]
6. Drincic, A.T.; Armas, L.A.G.; Van Diest, E.E.; Heaney, R.P. Volumetric dilution, rather than sequestration best explains the low vitamin D status of obesity. *Obes. Silver Spring Md* **2012**, *20*, 1444–1448. [CrossRef]
7. Wortsman, J.; Matsuoka, L.Y.; Chen, T.C.; Lu, Z.; Holick, M.F. Decreased bioavailability of vitamin D in obesity. *Am. J. Clin. Nutr.* **2000**, *72*, 690–693. [CrossRef]
8. Didriksen, A.; Grimnes, G.; Hutchinson, M.S.; Kjærgaard, M.; Svartberg, J.; Joakimsen, R.M.; Jorde, R. The serum 25-hydroxyvitamin D response to vitamin D supplementation is related to genetic factors, BMI, and baseline levels. *Eur. J. Endocrinol.* **2013**, *169*, 559–567. [CrossRef]
9. Pereira-Santos, M.; Costa, P.R.F.; Assis, A.M.O.; Santos, C.A.S.T.; Santos, D.B. Obesity and vitamin D deficiency: A systematic review and meta-analysis. *Obes. Rev. Off. J. Int. Assoc. Study Obes.* **2015**, *16*, 341–349. [CrossRef] [PubMed]
10. Reyes-Garcia, R.; Mendoza, N.; Palacios, S.; Salas, N.; Quesada-Charneco, M.; Garcia-Martin, A.; Fonolla, J.; Lara-Villoslada, F.; Muñoz-Torres, M. Effects of Daily Intake of Calcium and Vitamin D-Enriched Milk in Healthy Postmenopausal Women: A Randomized, Controlled, Double-Blind Nutritional Study. *J. Womens Health 2002* **2018**, *27*, 561–568. [CrossRef]
11. De Lorenzo, A.; Deurenberg, P.; Pietrantuono, M.; Di Daniele, N.; Cervelli, V.; Andreoli, A. How fat is obese? *Acta Diabetol.* **2003**, *40* (Suppl. 1), S254–S257. [CrossRef] [PubMed]
12. Sanfelix-Genovés, J.; Gil-Guillén, V.F.; Orozco-Beltran, D.; Giner-Ruiz, V.; Pertusa-Martínez, S.; Reig-Moya, B.; Carratalá, C. Determinant factors of osteoporosis patients' reported therapeutic adherence to calcium and/or vitamin D supplements: A cross-sectional, observational study of postmenopausal women. *Drugs Aging* **2009**, *26*, 861–869. [CrossRef] [PubMed]
13. Ross, A.C.; Manson, J.E.; Abrams, S.A.; Aloia, J.F.; Brannon, P.M.; Clinton, S.K.; Durazo-Arvizu, R.A.; Gallagher, J.C.; Gallo, R.L.; Jones, G.; et al. The 2011 report on dietary reference intakes for calcium and vitamin D from the Institute of Medicine: What clinicians need to know. *J. Clin. Endocrinol. Metab.* **2011**, *96*, 53–58. [CrossRef] [PubMed]
14. Blum, M.; Dallal, G.E.; Dawson-Hughes, B. Body size and serum 25 hydroxy vitamin D response to oral supplements in healthy older adults. *J. Am. Coll. Nutr.* **2008**, *27*, 274–279. [CrossRef]
15. Waterhouse, M.; Tran, B.; Armstrong, B.K.; Baxter, C.; Ebeling, P.R.; English, D.R.; Gebski, V.; Hill, C.; Kimlin, M.G.; Lucas, R.M.; et al. Environmental, personal, and genetic determinants of response to vitamin D supplementation in older adults. *J. Clin. Endocrinol. Metab.* **2014**, *99*, E1332–E1340. [CrossRef]

16. Lehmann, U.; Riedel, A.; Hirche, F.; Brandsch, C.; Girndt, M.; Ulrich, C.; Seibert, E.; Henning, C.; Glomb, M.A.; Dierkes, J.; et al. Vitamin D3 supplementation: Response and predictors of vitamin D3 metabolites—A randomized controlled trial. *Clin. Nutr. Edinb. Scotl.* **2016**, *35*, 351–358. [CrossRef]
17. Adab, P.; Pallan, M.; Whincup, P.H. Is BMI the best measure of obesity? *BMJ* **2018**, *360*, k1274. [CrossRef]
18. Trevisan, C.; Veronese, N.; Berton, L.; Carraro, S.; Bolzetta, F.; De Rui, M.; Miotto, F.; Inelmen, E.M.; Coin, A.; Perissinotto, E.; et al. Factors Influencing Serum-Hydroxivitamin D Levels and Other Bone Metabolism Parameters in Healthy Older Women. *J. Nutr. Health Aging* **2017**, *21*, 131–135. [CrossRef]
19. Jorde, R.; Sneve, M.; Emaus, N.; Figenschau, Y.; Grimnes, G. Cross-sectional and longitudinal relation between serum 25-hydroxyvitamin D and body mass index: The Tromsø study. *Eur. J. Nutr.* **2010**, *49*, 401–407. [CrossRef]
20. Carrelli, A.; Bucovsky, M.; Horst, R.; Cremers, S.; Zhang, C.; Bessler, M.; Schrope, B.; Evanko, J.; Blanco, J.; Silverberg, S.J.; et al. Vitamin D Storage in Adipose Tissue of Obese and Normal Weight Women. *J. Bone Miner. Res. Off. J. Am. Soc. Bone Miner. Res.* **2017**, *32*, 237–242. [CrossRef]
21. Golzarand, M.; Hollis, B.W.; Mirmiran, P.; Wagner, C.L.; Shab-Bidar, S. Vitamin D supplementation and body fat mass: A systematic review and meta-analysis. *Eur. J. Clin. Nutr.* **2018**, *72*, 1345–1357. [CrossRef] [PubMed]
22. Liu, P.; Ma, F.; Lou, H.; Liu, Y. The utility of fat mass index vs. body mass index and percentage of body fat in the screening of metabolic syndrome. *BMC Public Health* **2013**, *13*, 629. [CrossRef] [PubMed]
23. Bolanowski, M.; Nilsson, B.E. Assessment of human body composition using dual-energy x-ray absorptiometry and bioelectrical impedance analysis. *Med. Sci. Monit. Int. Med. J. Exp. Clin. Res.* **2001**, *7*, 1029–1033.
24. Gallagher, J.C.; Sai, A.; Templin, T.; Smith, L. Dose response to vitamin D supplementation in postmenopausal women: A randomized trial. *Ann. Intern. Med.* **2012**, *156*, 425–437. [CrossRef] [PubMed]

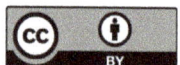

© 2019 by the authors. Licensee MDPI, Basel, Switzerland. This article is an open access article distributed under the terms and conditions of the Creative Commons Attribution (CC BY) license (http://creativecommons.org/licenses/by/4.0/).

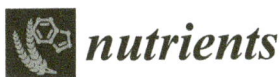

Article

Association between Dietary Calcium Intake and Adiposity in Male Adolescents

Jaak Jürimäe [1],*, Evelin Mäestu [1], Eva Mengel [2], Liina Remmel [1], Priit Purge [1] and Vallo Tillmann [2,3]

[1] Institute of Sport Sciences and Physiotherapy, University of Tartu, 51007 Tartu, Estonia
[2] Children's Clinic of Tartu University Hospital, 50406 Tartu, Estonia
[3] Institute of Clinical Medicine, University of Tartu, 50406 Tartu, Estonia
* Correspondence: jaak.jurimae@ut.ee; Tel.: +372-7376276

Received: 4 June 2019; Accepted: 25 June 2019; Published: 27 June 2019

Abstract: The aim was to investigate the possible association of dietary calcium intake with adiposity, insulin resistance, and adipocytokine values in adolescent boys. In this cross-sectional study, participants were 123 adolescent boys aged 13–15 years, who were divided into tertiles according to their dietary calcium intake. Dietary calcium intake was assessed using three 24 h dietary recalls. In addition, energy intake, body composition, physical activity (PA), and blood biochemical values were also measured. Mean body fat%, fat mass (FM), trunk FM, trunk fat%, and leptin differed between high and low tertiles of calcium intake after adjustment for age, pubertal stage, and PA. For the entire cohort, mean calcium intake was 786 ± 380 mg/day and was related to body mass index (BMI), FM, and trunk fat% but not to insulin resistance or adipocytokine values after adjusting for possible confounders. In addition, only 15.4% of the participants obtained or exceeded their mean dietary calcium intake requirements. These subjects who met their dietary calcium intake had significantly lower body fat% in comparison with subjects not meeting their dietary calcium intake. Odds ratio of being in the highest tertile of FM, trunk FM, and trunk fat% was 3.2–4.4 (95% confidence interval 1.19–12.47; $p < 0.05$) times higher for boys in low calcium intake tertile, compared to those boys in high calcium intake tertile. In conclusion, dietary calcium intake is inversely associated with total body and abdominal adiposity values in a specific group of healthy male adolescents with different body mass values.

Keywords: dietary calcium intake; adolescent boys; adiposity; percentage of body fat; insulin resistance; adipocytokines

1. Introduction

Obesity during childhood has become a major health issue that can lead to several chronic diseases and health problems later in life [1]. While some plateauing or decline in the prevalence of obesity has been observed in younger children [2], it is not the case in adolescents [1]. Childhood obesity appears to be the most common cause of insulin resistance in children and adolescents [3], and has been associated with type 2 diabetes mellitus, dyslipidemia, atherosclerosis, and coronary artery diseases [4] as well as with increased morbidity and mortality in later adulthood [5]. Adolescence is recognized as a critical period for the development of obesity [6]. Accordingly, it is important to identify modifiable risk factors during adolescence to prevent lifelong diseases related to obesity.

These modifiable risk factors include dietary habits, as dietary intervention is an important aspect in the treatment of obesity [7]. While it is commonly accepted that various combinations of macronutrients are able to regulate body mass, there is a need to further explore the effects of different micronutrients on body adiposity values [3,7,8]. Among different micronutrients, calcium and vitamin D intake may influence obesity and other health characteristics [9]. Studies with adults have reported inverse associations of calcium intake with body mass index (BMI) [10], body fat% [9], body fat mass (FM) [11], waist circumference [12], insulin resistance [13], and systemic inflammation [14] values. However, only few investigations have examined the association between dietary calcium intake and body adiposity values in children and adolescents with conflicting results [7]. There are studies to suggest that daily calcium intake may play a role in the modulation of body fat during growth and maturation [15,16], while other investigations have not found a relationship between daily calcium intake and body adiposity values in children and adolescents [17,18].

The association between dietary calcium intake with adiposity, insulin resistance, and adipocytokine values during growth and maturation has not yet been clarified. Accordingly, the aim of the present study was to investigate the possible association of daily calcium intake with adiposity, insulin resistance, and adipocytokine values in a specific group of healthy adolescent boys with a wide range of BMI values. It was hypothesized that adolescent boys with higher calcium intake would have lower body fat, insulin resistance, and adipocytokine values compared with adolescent boys with lower calcium intake values.

2. Material and Methods

2.1. Participants

The participants of the study were 123 pubertal boys aged between 13 and 15 years from different schools in Tartu, Estonia. The inclusion criteria for current study were that a boy had to be healthy and took part in obligatory physical education lessons at school. Participants were recruited as a part of larger longitudinal study. Boys using calcium supplementation were not included, nor were those taking any medications or having a clinical history of endocrine or metabolic problems, or cardiovascular, respiratory, or musculoskeletal diseases. All participants had their ordinary everyday diet. All procedures were approved by the Medical Ethics Committee of the University of Tartu, Estonia (Consent No 179/T-4, issue date 16.02.2009), and were explained to the boys and their parents who signed a consent form. Boys were divided in tertiles (low, medium, high) according to energy-adjusted calcium intake [16]. According to the previous study [19], where participants in the low calcium intake group ($n = 26$) compared with those in the high calcium intake group ($n = 31$) exhibited significantly higher values for BMI after adjustments for confounders, we should have had 50 participants per group to have a 0.80 chance (80% power) to detect the difference at 0.05 level of significance between the groups. In our study with 41 boys per group, we had 72% power to detect the difference of similar significance between the low calcium intake goup and high calcium intake group.

2.2. Maturity Assessment

Pubertal development was assessed by self-report using an illustrated questionnaire on pubertal stages according to Tanner [20]. Each boy was given line drawings, pictures, and descriptions representing genitalia and pubic hair development stages. The pubertal stage assessment according to the Tanner method, which uses the self-assessment of genitalia and pubic hair stage, has been previously validated [21] and used in our laboratory with previous studies with boys [22–25].

2.3. Anthropometry and Body Composition

Body mass and height were measured using calibrated medical digital scales (A&D Instruments, Abington, UK) and portable stadiometer (GMP anthropological instruments, Zurich, Switzerland) to the nearest 0.05 kg and 0.1 cm, respectively, with the participant wearing light clothing without shoes. Body mass index (BMI; kg/m^2) was calculated as body mass in kg divided by squared height in meters. Whole body fat percentage, fat mass (FM), fat free mass (FFM), trunk FM, and trunk fat percentage were measured by dual-energy X-ray absorptiometry (DXA) using the DPX-IQ densitometer (Lunar Corporation, Madison, WI, USA) equipped with proprietary software, version 3.6. During DXA measurements, subjects were scanned in a light clothing while lying flat on their backs with arms on their sides. The medium scan mode and the standard subject positioning was used for whole body measurements, which were analyzed using the extended analysis option. The DXA measurements and results were evaluated by the same examiner. The precision of measurement expressed as coefficient of variation (CV) was less than 2% for all measurements [25].

2.4. Dietary Intake

Dietary intake was assessed using the average of three 24-h dietary recalls, including two weekdays (i.e., Thursday and Friday) and one weekend day (Saturday). Participants were asked to record everything they ate and drank for these days, and cup and bowl sizes were provided to help estimate portion sizes. The same dietitian interviewed all participants face-to-face and asked probing questions about their diet recalls. The nutrition data were entered into Nutridata System for Research (National Institute for Health Development, Tallinn, Estonia) and were analyzed for total daily energy (kcal/day), calcium (mg/day), and vitamin D (μg/day) intakes [22]. To estimate the prevalence of nutrient intake below or above the recommendations, the intakes of calcium and vitamin D were compared with their estimated average requirement (EAR), which are 1100 mg/day and 10 μg/day, respectively, according to the Institute of Medicine [26]. Finally, to control for confounding and mitigate for extraneous variation, calcium intake was adjusted for energy intake and expressed as mg per 1000 kcal consumed (i.e., energy-adjusted calcium intake) as suggested previously [27].

2.5. Physical Activity

The Actigraph uniaxial physical activity monitor (model GT1M; ActiGraph, Pensacola, CA), USA) was used to measure physical activity (PA) level and pattern for seven consecutive days. Epoch length was set at 15 s, and data were expressed as counts per min [23,28]. All participants were asked to wear accelerometer on the right hip, allowing removal for sleeping, bathing, and swimming. Physical activity was included for further analyses, if the participant had accumulated a minimum of 10 h of activity data for at least two weekdays and one weekend day [23,28].

2.6. Blood Analysis

After an overnight fast, between 08:00 and 09:00, a 10 mL blood sample was collected from the antecubital vein with the participant in an upright position. Blood serum was separated and then frozen at −80 °C for further analysis. Leptin was determined by radioimmunoassay (RIA) (Mediagnost Reutlingen, Germany) with intra- and inter-assay CVs <5%, and the least detection limit was 0.01 ng/mL. Adiponectin was also determined with a commercially available RIA kit (Linco Research, St. Charles, MO; USA). The intra- and inter-assay CVs were <7%, and the least detection limit was 1 μg/mL. Insulin was analyzed using Immulite 2000 (DPC, Los Angeles, USA). The intra- and inter-assay CVs for insulin were 4.5% and 12.2% at an insulin concentration of 6.6 μIU/mL, respectively. Glucose was measured with a commercial kit (Boehringer, Mannheim, Germany). Insulin resistance index was calculated using homeostasis model assessment (HOMA-IR): Fasting insulin (μIU/mL) × fasting glucose (mmol/L)/22.5 [29].

2.7. Statistical Analysis

Data analysis was performed using SPSS 25.0 for Windows (Chicago, IL, USA). Descriptive data are presented as means and standard deviations (SD). Boys were divided in tertiles according to energy-adjusted calcium intake [16]. Differences between tertiles (Low, Medium, High) groups were assessed by ANOVA using Bonferroni method. In addition, differences between tertiles were assessed after adjustment for age, pubertal stage, and total PA using univariate analysis of covariance (ANCOVA). Spearman correlation and partial correlation (controlling for age, pubertal stage, and total PA) coefficients were conducted to describe relationships of energy-adjusted calcium intake with body composition, insulin resistance, and adipocytokine values. Differences between EAR of calcium and vitamin D intake were assessed by ANOVA. Regression analyses were used to examine the relationships between energy-adjusted calcium intake and body fatness components through two separate models, where body fatness components were inserted as dependent variables and energy-adjusted calcium intake as independent variable. Model 1 was unadjusted model, while Model 2 was adjusted for age, pubertal stage, and total PA to determine the independent association with energy-adjusted calcium intake. Logistic regression analysis was also used to describe the odds ratio (OR) (95% confidence interval (CI)) of being at the highest tertile of each body fatness components according to the energy-adjusted calcium intake tertiles. Significance was set at $p < 0.05$.

3. Results

The study population included 123 adolescent boys, including 4 boys at pubertal stage 2, 30 boys at pubertal stage 3, 55 boys at pubertal stage 4, and 34 boys at pubertal stage 5, with the mean age of 13.9 ± 0.6 years. The mean BMI was 21.6 ± 5.4 kg/m^2, with a range from 13.8 to 45.5 kg/m^2 including 71% normal weight and 29% overweight/obese boys. Participants presented mean energy intake of 1798 ± 535 kcal/day, and the range was 622 to 3300 kcal/day. The mean calcium intake for all adolescent boys ($n = 123$) was 786 ± 380 mg/day, with a large range from 123 to 2460 mg/day. Data indicated that only 15.4% ($n = 19$) of the participants obtained or exceeded their calcium intake EAR [26]. The mean vitamin D intake was 3.2 ± 4.3 µg/day and only 8.1% ($n = 10$) of the participants met the recommended vitamin D intake EAR [26]. Boys who met their calcium intake EAR ($n = 19$) had a mean vitamin D intake of 5.1 µg/day, energy intake was 2330 kcal/day, and body fat% was 18.1 ± 9.1%, while boys who did not meet their calcium intake EAR ($n = 104$) had a mean vitamin D intake of 2.8 µg/day, their energy intake was 1700 kcal/day, and body fat% was 24.0 ± 12.%. These values were significantly different ($p < 0.05$) from the corresponding values in those boys who met their calcium intake EAR.

Body composition, PA, dietary intake, and blood biochemical characteristics of the study population are presented in Table 1. When the study participants were grouped by energy-adjusted calcium intake tertiles, body mass, and body adiposity values were lower with increasing tertile of calcium intake. The participants in the high calcium intake tertile had significantly lower body mass, BMI, body fat%, FM, FFM, trunk FM, and trunk fat% than those in the low calcium intake group. In addition, body fat%, FM, FFM, trunk FM, and trunk fat% remained significantly different between the high and low calcium intake tertiles after adjustment for age, pubertal stage, and total PA. No significant differences between different calcium tertiles were seen in blood biochemical characteristics. However, after controlling for confounding factors, participants in the high calcium intake tertile had significantly lower leptin levels when compared with the boys at the low calcium intake tertile. In addition, no significant differences between the three studied groups were seen in energy intake and vitamin D intake values (Table 1).

Bivariate correlation analysis revealed that calcium intake was inversely related to BMI, FM, trunk FM, and trunk fat% values (Table 2). The correlations between calcium intake and BMI, FM, and trunk fat% remained significant after adjusting for age, pubertal stage, and total PA values. In addition, calcium intake was correlated with body mass and FFM values after controlling for these confounding factors. In contrast, calcium intake was not associated with leptin, adiponectin, or insulin resistance (glucose, insulin, HOMA-IR) values (Table 2). Linear regression analysis showed that in unadjusted model (Model 1), the energy-adjusted calcium intake was negatively associated with trunk FM ($\beta = -0.183$; $p = 0.043$) (Table 3). After adjustment for age, pubertal stage and total PA (Model 2), the association slightly increased ($\beta = -0.185$; $p = 0.042$). There were no associations between calcium intake and other body fatness parameters in Model 1 as well as in Model 2 ($p > 0.05$) (Table 3). In addition, the OR of being in the highest tertile of FM was 4.4 (95% CI 1.55–12.47; $p = 0.005$) times higher for participants with low calcium intake tertile compared to those with high calcium intake tertile (Table 4). Similarly, the OR of being highest tertile of trunk FM and trunk fat% was 3.2 (95% CI 1.19–8.35; $p = 0.021$) and 3.3 (95% CI 1.19–9.05; $p = 0.021$) times higher, respectively, in the participants with low calcium intake tertile, compared to those with high calcium intake tertile (Table 4).

Table 1. Mean (± SD) descriptive characteristics of the studied sample according to tertiles of energy-adjusted calcium intake.

Variable	Total (n = 123)	Low Ca Intake Tertile (n = 41)	Medium Ca Intake Tertile (n = 41)	High Ca Intake Tertile (n = 41)
Age (yrs)	13.9 ± 0.6	13.9 ± 0.6	13.8 ± 0.6	14.1 ± 0.6 [#]
Height (cm)	169.0 ± 8.6	170.7 ± 8.7	167.5 ± 8.4	168.9 ± 8.7
Body mass (kg)	62.5 ± 19.4	70.5 ± 24.1	58.7 ± 15.2 *	58.2 ± 15.4 *
BMI (kg/m^2)	21.6 ± 5.4	23.8 ± 6.5	20.7 ± 4.3 *	20.3 ± 4.4 *
Overweight/obese (n/%)	36/29.3	16/39.0	12/29.3	8/19.5
Body fat%	23.1 ± 11.7	26.6 ± 12.1	22.3 ± 11.4 [†]	20.3 ± 11.0 *[†]
FM (kg)	15.2 ± 12.3	19.8 ± 15.4	13.6 ± 9.4 *[†]	12.2 ± 10.0 *[†]
FFM (kg)	46.5 ± 10.0	49.8 ± 11.4	44.4 ± 8.6 *	45.3 ± 9.3 *[†]
Trunk FM (kg)	6.3 ± 5.6	8.5 ± 7.2	5.6 ± 4.3 *[†]	4.7 ± 4.4 *[†]
Trunk fat%	21.4 ± 12.1	25.3 ± 12.7	20.7 ± 11.7 [†]	18.1 ± 11.0 *[†]
Total PA (counts/min)	398 ± 161	397 ± 165	403 ± 145	393 ± 174
Energy intake (kcal/day)	1798 ± 535	1785 ± 543	1769 ± 561	1839 ± 512
Calcium intake (mg/day)	786 ± 380	515 ± 189	738 ± 240 *	1104 ± 408 *[#]
Calcium intake (mg/1000 kcal)	434 ± 146	287 ± 60	418 ± 40 *	597 ± 98 *[#]
Vitamin D intake (μg/day)	3.2 ± 4.3	2.7 ± 3.0	3.5 ± 5.4	3.5 ± 4.1
Leptin (ng/mL)	6.1 ± 8.6	8.1 ± 11.2	5.6 ± 7.5	4.6 ± 6.2 [†]
Adiponectin (μg/mL)	8.0 ± 4.4	7.5 ± 4.1	8.3 ± 4.3	8.3 ± 4.9
Glucose (mmol/L)	5.1 ± 0.4	5.1 ± 0.4	5.0 ± 0.4	5.1 ± 0.4
Insulin (μIU/mL)	14.2 ± 7.7	15.8 ± 8.5	12.7 ± 6.4	14.2 ± 7.9
HOMA-IR	3.2 ± 1.8	3.6 ± 1.9	2.9 ± 1.5	3.3 ± 1.9

* Significantly different from Low Ca intake tertile; $p < 0.05$; [#] Significantly different from Medium Ca intake tertile; $p < 0.05$; [†] Significantly different from Low Ca intake tertile after adjustment for age, pubertal stage, and total PA; $p < 0.05$.

Table 2. Correlation coefficients of energy-adjusted calcium intake with body composition and blood biochemical variables.

Variables	Bivariate Correlation	Partial Correlation Adjusted for Age, Pubertal Stage, and Total Physical Activity
Body mass (kg)	−0.157	−0.211 *
BMI (kg/m^2)	−0.192 *	−0.205 *
Body fat%	−0.167	−0.132
FM (kg)	−0.195 *	−0.190 *
FFM (kg)	−0.104	−0.194 *
Trunk FM (kg)	−0.188 *	−0.150
Trunk fat%	−0.189 *	−0.199 *
Leptin (ng/mL)	−0.111	−0.103
Adiponectin (μg/mL)	0.072	0.130
Glucose (mmol/L)	0.022	0.033
Insulin (μIU	−0.061	−0.059
HOMA-IR	−0.064	−0.053

* Statistically significant; $p < 0.05$.

Table 3. Linear regression coefficients examining the associations of energy-adjusted calcium intake with body fatness components.

	Calcium Intake				
	B ± SE	95% CI	R^2	β	p value
Model 1					
Body fat%	−0.01 ± 0.01	−0.03; 0.01	0.13	−0.128	0.157
FM	−14.60 ± 7.58	−29.61; 0.41	0.03	−0.172	0.056
Trunk FM	−7.10 ± 3.47	−13.97; −0.23	0.03	−0.183	0.043
Trunk fat%	−0.01 ± 0.01	−0.03; 0.003	0.02	−0.147	0.104
Model 2					
Body fat%	−0.01 ± 0.01	−0.03; 0.001	0.06	−0.125	0.168
FM	−14.70 ± 7.65	−29.84; 0.45	0.05	−0.174	0.057
Trunk FM	−7.20 ± 3.50	−14.13; −0.26	0.05	−0.185	0.042
Trunk fat%	−0.01 ± 0.01	−0.03; 0.003	0.05	−0.146	0.108

Model 1: Unadjusted model. Model 2: Adjusted for age, pubertal stage, and total PA. B—unstandardized coefficient. SE—standard error. CI—confidence interval. β—standardized coefficient.

Table 4. Odds ratios of highest tertile of body fat components versus other tertiles (medium+lower) of body fat components.

	Body Fat%			FM			Trunk FM			Trunk Fat%		
Ca tertiles	OR	95%CI	p value	OR	95%CI	p value	OR	95%CI	p value	OR	95%CI	p value
High	Ref			Ref			Ref			Ref		
Medium	0.92	0.36; 2.35	0.867	1.56	0.62; 3.93	0.342	1.97	0.78; 4.97	0.154	1.24	0.49; 3.12	1.24
Low	2.79	0.99; 7.83	0.051	4.39	1.55; 12.47	0.005	3.15	1.19; 8.35	0.021	3.29	1.19; 9.05	0.021

All models were adjusted for age, pubertal stage, and total PA.

4. Discussion

This study was aimed to investigate the possible associations between calcium intake with adiposity, insulin resistance, and adipocytokine values in a heterogeneous group of 123 male adolescents with different adiposity values. An independent inverse association of calcium intake with different adiposity, but not with insulin resistance and adipocytokine values was observed in adolescent boys. Individuals with higher calcium intake had lower body adiposity values. Furthermore, those boys who met their calcium intake EAR had lower body fat% in comparison with those who did not met their daily calcium intake EAR. Accordingly, it could be suggested that adequate calcium intake is needed to maintain lower body fat values in adolescent boys during pubertal growth and maturation.

Our results demonstrated that lower calcium intake was associated with higher total body adiposity values in adolescent boys in this important developmental age, which is a critical period for the development of obesity [6]. These results are in accordance with a recent study in a large European cohort of children and adolescents [16]. In that study, an inverse correlation of total calcium intake with different adiposity indices was consistently observed in boys but not in girls, and the prevalence of obesity decreased significantly across tertiles of calcium intake [16]. While relatively few investigations have studied the role of calcium intake in modulating adiposity in children and adolescents [16], most of them have supported a significant association between calcium intake and adiposity measures [3,15,16,30], similarly to our results. In contrast, other studies have not found this relationship in children and adolescents [17,18,31]. The relationship between calcium intake and body adiposity has also been evaluated longitudinally demonstrating that lower calcium intake at baseline was associated with an increase in adiposity indices over a six-year period in boys with a wide range of BMI values but not in girls [16]. Similarly, calcium intake was not related to two-year change in body fat in lean peripubertal girls [17]. In addition to possible gender differences, it has been suggested that a certain threshold for calcium intake and/or BMI may be needed to observe the relationship between calcium intake and total body adiposity values [13]. It has also been argued that the effects of calcium intake on body adiposity depend on higher percentage of body fat in children [7].

In accordance with this, the OR being in the highest tertile of FM in our study was more than four times higher for participants with low calcium intake compared to those with high calcium intake and more than three times higher being in the highest tertile of trunk FM or trunk fat%.

Inverse association of calcium intake with abdominal adiposity was also identified in the current investigation, which is in accordance with the results of other studies carried out with 8–9-year-old [32], 9–12-year-old [17], and 12–19-year-old [3] children with various BMI values as well as 7–18-year-old children and adolescents with obesity [33]. Interestingly, Barr [17] demonstrated that calcium intake below the median was independently associated with higher trunk fat% in 9–12-year-old girls. Similarly, calcium intake was negatively correlated with trunk fat% after controlling for potentially confounding variables in our study. It has been suggested that trunk fat may be preferentially affected by calcium intake [17,34], and abdominal adiposity is closely related to metabolic syndrome, type 2 diabetes mellitus, and cardiovascular diseases [3,4].

Another important finding of the present study was the inadequate calcium intake in majority of studied adolescents. It appeared that only 15.4% ($n = 19$) met their daily calcium intake EAR, similarly to the results of other studies in children and adolescents [3,32,35]. In fact, most studies have observed that more than 90% of studied children and adolescents do not meet the required daily calcium intake [3,32,35]. Therefore, calcium appears to be one of the micronutrients with the highest rate of inadequate consumption worldwide [36]. In our study, adolescent boys with adequate calcium intake had significantly lower body fat% in comparison with adolescents with inadequate daily calcium intake. The importance of adequate calcium intake in adolescent boys should be emphasized because about 45% of bone mineral accrual occurs during early adolescence [37]. This age and maturation period provides a limited window of opportunity for maximizing peak bone mass [38], which is a major determinant of fractures, a major public health problem in adults [6].

Different mechanisms have been proposed to explain the association between calcium intake and body adiposity. For example, it has been suggested that adequate calcium intake increases the oxidative capacity of adipose tissue [32]. Higher calcium intake is associated with reduced 1,25-vitamin D levels, which in turn induce intracellular calcium content to decrease in adipose tissue, stimulating lipolysis, and inhibiting lipogenesis in the adipocyte [39]. In contrast, low calcium intake is associated with high intracellular calcium concentrations, which may then increase the rate of lipogenesis and inhibit lipolysis, resulting in increased adiposity [39]. Furthermore, dietary calcium intake may influence fat metabolism by increased faecal fat excretion [40] and decreased hunger or increased satiety [41]. Anti-obesity mechanisms of vitamin D have also been suggested [16], with vitamin D interacting in a complex system of absorptive and endocrine functions [10]. However, it has to be considered that all these suggested mechanisms still lack confirmation in human longitudinal studies [16].

There was no association between daily calcium intake and measured adipocytokine values in adolescent boys with various adiposity values. Therefore, leptin is synthesized by adipocytes and is directly related to the amount of body fat [42]. While calcium intake was related to body FM in current study, it would have expected to also observe an association between calcium intake and leptin values, similarly to a study with premenopausal women [13]. The differences between the results of our study and that of da Silva Ferreira et al. [13] could be explained by different leptin levels in these studies, premenopausal women having considerably higher leptin and adiposity values compared to adolescent boys in the present study. However, leptin concentration was significantly lower in high calcium intake tertile compared with leptin value in low calcium intake tertile after controlling for energy intake, PA and maturation values in adolescent boys, which was also observed in premenopausal women [13]. Further studies are needed before any conclusion about possible association of daily calcium intake with leptin can be drawn.

The possible relationship of calcium intake and insulin resistance has not yet been fully clarified. Unlike previously reported investigations in adults [13,43,44] and adolescents [28], no association between calcium intake and HOMA-IR as an index of insulin resistance was seen in our specific group of adolescent boys with different adiposity values. While dos Santos et al. [30] found a significant inverse association between calcium intake and HOMA-IR among obese but not normal weight adolescents. In accordance with our results, a recent study reported no relationship between calcium intake and HOMA-IR in adult males, while calcium intake was related to HOMA-IR in adult females [43]. Accordingly, the reported association between calcium intake and insulin resistance that has been found in adults [13,43,44], should be further investigated in adolescents using a direct measure of insulin resistance.

There are some limitations in our study that should be considered. Firstly, this is a cross-sectional study, which limits our ability to make causal inferences. In addition, although the same dietitian interviewed all participants and reviewed their diet recalls with each participant, self-reported dietary intakes are subject to error as it depends on the memory of adolescents, and is susceptible to under- and over-reporting. Another potential limitation is that some significant associations would have not been detected due to slightly underpowered study, although the number of participants was similar to previous cross-sectional studies in this area [3,9,13,19]. The specific information about socioeconomic status and/or maternal/paternal overweight/obesity was also not collected. Finally, our findings are limited to a specific group of Caucasian male adolescents with specific age and maturation range, and wide range of total body adiposity values.

This study has also some strengths. Firstly, objective assessment of PA by accelerometry and body composition by DXA were used in this study. In addition, the present study is one of the few studies that has evaluated possible associations of calcium intake with adiposity, insulin resistance, and adipocytokines taking into account several confounders including pubertal maturation, energy intake, and PA. These findings help to understand the possible associations between calcium intake levels and adiposity values during growth and maturation.

5. Conclusions

Dietary calcium intake is inversely associated with total body and abdominal adiposity values in a specific group of healthy male adolescents with different body mass values. In contrast, no relationships of calcium intake with adipocytokine and insulin resistance values were observed. In addition, adolescents with adequate calcium intake had significantly lower body fat% in comparison with those adolescents with inadequate daily calcium intake. Odds ratio of being in the highest tertile of FM, trunk FM, or trunk fat% was more than three times higher for participants in low calcium intake tertile compared to those with high calcium intake tertile.

Author Contributions: Conceptualization, J.J., E.M. (Evelin Mäestu), E.M. (Eva Mengel), and V.T.; methodology, J.J. and V.T.; formal analysis, J.J. and E.M. (Evelin Mäestu); investigation E.M. (Evelin Mäestu), L.R., and P.P.; data curation, E.M. (Evelin Mäestu); writing—original draft preparation, J.J.; writing—review and editing, E.M. (Evelin Mäestu), E.M. (Eva Mengel), L.R., P.P., and V.T.; project administration, J.J.; funding acquisition, J.J. and V.T.

Funding: This research was funded by the Estonian Ministry of Education and Science Institutional Grant IUT 20-58 and Personal Grant PUT 1382.

Conflicts of Interest: The authors declare no conflict of interest.

Abbreviations

BMI, body mass index; EAR, estimated average requirement; DXA, dual- energy X-ray absorptiometry; FM, fat mass; FFM, fat free mass; HOMA-IR, homeostasis model assessment of insulin resistance; OR, odds ratio; PA, physical activity.

References

1. Olds, T.; Maher, C.; Zumin, S.; Peneau, S.; Lioret, S.; Castetbon, K.; Bellisle, K.; de Wilde, J.; Hohepa, M.; Maddison, R.; et al. Evidence that the prevalence of childhood overweight is plateauing: Data from nine countries. *Int. J. Pediatr. Obes.* **2011**, *6*, 342–360. [CrossRef]
2. Chung, A.; Backholer, K.; Wong, E.; Palermo, C.; Keating, C.; Peeters, A. Trends in child and adolescent obesity prevalence in economically advanced countries according to socioeconomic position: A systematic review. *Obes. Rev.* **2016**, *17*, 276–295. [CrossRef] [PubMed]
3. Castro Burbano, J.; Fajardo Venegas, P.; Robles Rodriguez, J.; Pazmino Estevez, K. Relationship between dietary calcium intake and adiposity in female adolescents. *Endocrinol. Nutr.* **2016**, *63*, 58–63. [CrossRef] [PubMed]
4. Gupta, N.; Goel, K.; Shah, P.; Misra, A. Childhood obesity in developing countries: Epidemiology, determinants, and prevention. *Endocr. Rev.* **2012**, *33*, 48–70. [CrossRef] [PubMed]
5. Reilly, J.J.; Kelly, J. Long-term impact of overweight and obesity in childhood and adolescence on morbidity and premature mortality in adulthood: Systematic review. *Int. J. Obes.* **2011**, *35*, 891–898. [CrossRef] [PubMed]
6. Lappe, J.M.; McMahon, D.J.; Laughlin, A.; Hanson, C.; Desmangles, J.C.; Begley, M.; Schwartz, M. The effect of increasing dairy calcium intake of adolescent girls on changes in body fat and weight. *Am. J. Clin. Nutr.* **2017**, *105*, 1046–1053. [CrossRef]
7. da Cunha, K.A.; da Silva Magalhaes, E.I.; Rodrigues Loreiro, L.M.; da Rocha Sant'Ana, L.F.; Queiroz Ribeiro, A.; de Novaes, J.F. Calcium intake, serum vitamin D and obesity in children: Is there an association? *Rev. Paul. Pediatr.* **2015**, *33*, 222–229. [CrossRef]
8. Skrypnik, K.; Suliburska, J. Association between the gut microbiota and mineral metabolism. *J. Sci. Food Agric.* **2018**, *98*, 2449–2460. [CrossRef]
9. Tidwell, D.K.; Valliant, M.W. Higher amounts of body fat are associated with inadequate intakes of calcium and vitamin D in African American women. *Nutr. Res.* **2011**, *31*, 527–536. [CrossRef]
10. Eilat-Adar, S.; Xu, J.; Loria, C.; Mattil, C.; Goldbourt, U.; Howard, B.V.; Resnick, H.E. Dietary calcium is associated with body mass index and body fat in American Indians. *J. Nutr.* **2007**, *137*, 1955–1960. [CrossRef]
11. Jacqmain, M.; Doucet, E.; Despres, J.P.; Bouchard, C.; Tremblay, A. Calcium intake, body composition, and lipoprotein-lipid concentrations in adults. *Am. J. Clin. Nutr.* **2003**, *77*, 1448–1452. [CrossRef] [PubMed]
12. Sadeghi, O.; Keshteli, A.H.; Doostan, F.; Esmaillzadeh, A.; Adibi, P. Association between dairy consumption, dietary calcium intake and general and abdominal obesity among Iranian adults. *Diabetes Metab. Syndr. Clin. Res. Rev.* **2018**, *12*, 769–775. [CrossRef] [PubMed]
13. da Silva Ferreira, T.; Goncalves Torres, M.R.S.; Sanjuliani, A.F. Dietary calcium intake is associated with adiposity, metabolic profile, inflammatory state and blood pressure, but not with erythrocyte intracellular calcium and endothelial function in healthy pre-menopausal women. *Br. J. Nutr.* **2013**, *110*, 1079–1088. [CrossRef] [PubMed]
14. Zemel, M.B.; Sun, X. Dietary calcium and dairy products modulate oxidative and inflammatory stress in mice and humans. *J. Nutr.* **2008**, *138*, 1047–1052. [CrossRef] [PubMed]
15. Keast, D.R.; Hill Gallant, K.M.; Albertson, A.M.; Gugger, C.K.; Holschuh, N.M. Associations between yogurt, dairy, calcium, and vitamin D intake and obesity among U.S. children aged 8–18 years: NHANES, 2005–2008. *Nutrients* **2015**, *7*, 1577–1593. [CrossRef] [PubMed]
16. Nappo, A.; Sparano, S.; Intermann, T.; Kourides, Y.A.; Lissner, L.; Molnar, D.; Moreno, L.A.; Pala, V.; Sioen, I.; Veidebaum, T.; et al. Dietary calcium intake and adiposity in children and adolescents: Cross-sectional and longitudinal results from IDEFICS/I.Family cohort. *Nutr. Metab. Cardiovasc. Dis.* **2019**, *29*, 440–449. [CrossRef] [PubMed]
17. Barr, S.I. Calcium and body fat in peripubertal girls: Cross-sectional and longitudinal observations. *Obesity* **2007**, *15*, 1302–1310. [CrossRef]
18. Phillips, S.M.; Bandini, L.G.; Cyr, H.; Colclough-Douglas, S.; Naumova, E.; Must, A. Dairy food consumption and body weight and fatness studied longitudinally over the adolescent period. *Int. J. Obes. Relat. Metab. Disord.* **2003**, *27*, 1106–1113. [CrossRef]

19. Torres, M.R.S.G.; da Silva Ferreira, T.; Carvalho, D.C.; Sanjuliani, A.F. Dietary calcium intake and its relationship with adiposity and metabolic profile in hypertensive patients. *Nutrition* **2011**, *27*, 666–671. [CrossRef]
20. Tanner, J.M. *Growth at Adolescence*, 2nd ed.; Blackwell Scientific Publications: Oxford, UK, 1962.
21. Leone, M.; Comtois, A.S. Validity and reliability of self-assessment of sexual maturity in elite adolescent athletes. *J. Sports Med. Phys. Fit.* **2007**, *47*, 361–365.
22. Jürimäe, J.; Lätt, E.; Mäestu, J.; Saar, M.; Purge, P.; Maasalu, K.; Jürimäe, T. Osteocalcin is inversely associated with adiposity and leptin in adolescent boys. *J. Pediatr. Endocr. Metab.* **2015**, *28*, 571–577. [CrossRef] [PubMed]
23. Lätt, E.; Mäestu, J.; Ortega, F.B.; Rääsk, T.; Jürimäe, T.; Jürimäe, J. Vigorous physical activity rather than sedentary behaviour predicts overweight and obesity in pubertal boys: A 2-year follow-up study. *Scand. J. Public Health* **2015**, *43*, 276–282. [CrossRef] [PubMed]
24. Utsal, L.; Tillmann, V.; Zilmer, M.; Mäestu, J.; Purge, P.; Jürimäe, J.; Saar, M.; Lätt, E.; Maasalu, K.; Jürimäe, T. Elevated serum IL-6, IL-8, MCP-1, CRP, and IFN-γ levels in 10- to 11-year-old boys with increased BMI. *Horm. Res. Pediatr.* **2012**, *78*, 31–39. [CrossRef] [PubMed]
25. Vaitkeviciute, D.; Lätt, E.; Mäestu, J.; Jürimäe, T.; Saar, M.; Purge, P.; Maasalu, K.; Jürimäe, J. Physical activity and bone mineral accrual in boys with different body composition parameters during puberty: A longitudinal study. *PLoS ONE* **2014**, *9*, e107759. [CrossRef] [PubMed]
26. Institute of Medicine. *Dietary Reference Intakes for Calcium and Vitamin D*; The National Academies Press: Washington, WA, USA, 2011.
27. Willett, W.C.; Howe, G.R.; Kushi, L.H. Adjustment for total energy intake in epidemiologic studies. *Am. J. Clin. Nutr.* **1997**, *65*, 1220S–1228S. [CrossRef] [PubMed]
28. Ivuškāns, A.; Mäestu, J.; Jürimäe, T.; Lätt, E.; Purge, P.; Saar, M.; Maasalu, K.; Jürimäe, J. Sedentary time has a negative influence on bone mineral parameters in peripubertal boys: A 1-year prospective study. *J. Bone Miner. Metab.* **2015**, *33*, 85–92. [CrossRef] [PubMed]
29. Wallace, T.M.; Levy, J.C.; Matthews, D.R. Use and abuse of HOMA modelling. *Diabetes Care* **2004**, *27*, 1487–1495. [CrossRef] [PubMed]
30. dos Santos, L.C.; de Padua Cintra, I.; Fisberg, M.; Martini, L.A. Calcium intake and its relationship with adiposity and insulin resistance in post-pubertal adolescents. *J. Hum. Nutr. Diet.* **2008**, *21*, 109–116. [CrossRef] [PubMed]
31. Wiley, A.S. Dairy and milk consumption and child growth: Is BMI involved? An analysis of NHANES 1999–2004. *Am. J. Hum. Biol.* **2010**, *22*, 517–525. [CrossRef]
32. Gomes Suhett, L.; Souza Silveira, K.; De Santis Filgueiras, M.; do Carmo Gouveia Peluzio, M.; Hermsdorff, H.H.M.; Farias de Novaes, J. Inverse association of calcium intake with abdominal adiposity and C-reactive protein in Brazilian children. *Public Health Nutr.* **2018**, *21*, 1912–1920. [CrossRef]
33. Czerwonogradzka, A.; Pyzak, B.; Majcher, A.; Rumińska, M.; Rymkiewicz-Kluczyńska, B.; Jeznach-Steinhagen, A. Assessment of dietary calcium intake on metabolic syndrome frequency in obese children and adolescents. *Pediatr. Endocrinol. Diabetes Metab.* **2008**, *14*, 231–235.
34. Zemel, M.B.; Richards, J.; Mathis, S.; Milstead, A.; Gebhardt, L.; Silva, E. Dairy augmentation of total and central fat loss in obese subjects. *Int. J. Obes.* **2005**, *29*, 391–397. [CrossRef] [PubMed]
35. Magalhaes, E.I.; Pessoa, M.C.; Franceschini, S.D.; Novaes, J.F. Dietary calcium intake is inversely associated with blood pressure in Brazilian children. *Int. J. Food Sci. Nutr.* **2017**, *68*, 331–338. [CrossRef] [PubMed]
36. Beal, T.; Massiot, E.; Arsenault, J.E.; Smith, M.R.; Hijmans, R.J. Global trends in dietary micronutrient supplies and estimated prevalence of inadequate intakes. *PLoS ONE* **2017**, *12*, e0175554. [CrossRef] [PubMed]
37. Bailey, D.A.; Martin, A.; McKay, H.; Whiting, S.; Mirwald, R. Calcium accretion in girls and boys during puberty: A longitudinal analysis. *J. Bone Miner. Res.* **2000**, *15*, 2245–2250. [CrossRef] [PubMed]
38. Jürimäe, J.; Gruodyte-Raciene, R.; Baxter-Jones, A.D.G. Effects of gymnastics activities on bone accrual during growth: A systematic review. *J. Sports Sci. Med.* **2018**, *17*, 245–258.
39. Zemel, M.B.; Miller, S.L. Dietary calcium and dairy modulation of adiposity and obesity risk. *Nutr. Rev.* **2004**, *62*, 125–131. [CrossRef]
40. Bendsen, N.T.; Hother, A.L.; Jensen, S.K.; Lorenzen, J.K.; Astrup, A. Effect of dairy calcium on fecal fat excretion: A randomized crossover trial. *Int. J. Obes.* **2008**, *32*, 1816–1824. [CrossRef]

41. Gilbert, J.A.; Joanisse, D.R.; Chaput, J.P.; Miegueu, P.; Cianflone, K.; Almeras, N.; Tremblay, A. Milk supplementation facilitates appetite control in obese women during weight loss: A randomised, single-blind, placebo-controlled trial. *Br. J. Nutr.* **2011**, *105*, 133–143. [CrossRef]
42. Jürimäe, J. Adipocytokine and ghrelin responses to acute exercise and sport training in children during growth and maturation. *Pediatr. Exerc. Sci.* **2014**, *26*, 392–403. [CrossRef]
43. Kim, J.H.; Lee, S.H.; Park, S.J.; Yeum, K.J.; Choi, B.; Joo, N.S. Dietary calcium intake may contribute to the HOMA-IR score in Korean females with vitamin D deficiency (2008–2012 Korea National Health and Nutrition Examination Survey). *J. Obes. Metab. Syndr.* **2017**, *26*, 274–280. [CrossRef] [PubMed]
44. Tremblay, A.; Gilbert, J. Milk products, insulin resistance syndrome and type 2 diabetes. *J. Am. Coll. Nutr.* **2009**, *28*, 91S–102S. [CrossRef] [PubMed]

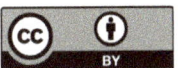

© 2019 by the authors. Licensee MDPI, Basel, Switzerland. This article is an open access article distributed under the terms and conditions of the Creative Commons Attribution (CC BY) license (http://creativecommons.org/licenses/by/4.0/).

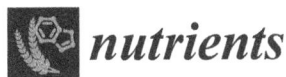

Review

Vitamin D Food Fortification and Nutritional Status in Children: A Systematic Review of Randomized Controlled Trials

Paula Nascimento Brandão-Lima [1], Beatriz da Cruz Santos [2], Concepción Maria Aguilera [3,4,5,*], Analícia Rocha Santos Freire [2], Paulo Ricardo Saquete Martins-Filho [1,6] and Liliane Viana Pires [2]

[1] Health Sciences Post-Graduation Program, Department of Medicine, Federal University of Sergipe, Rua Cláudio Batista, S/N, Cidade Nova, Aracaju, 49060-108 Sergipe, Brazil; paulanblima@gmail.com (P.N.B.-L.); saqmartins@hotmail.com (P.R.S.M.-F.)
[2] Nutrition Sciences Post-Graduation Program, Department of Nutrition, Federal University of Sergipe, Avenida Marechal Rondon, S/N, Jardim Rosa Elze, São Cristovão, 49100-000 Sergipe, Brazil; cruz14_bia@outlook.com (B.d.C.S.); alicia.nutri@gmail.com (A.R.S.F.); lvianapires@gmail.com (L.V.P.)
[3] Department of Biochemistry and Molecular Biology II, Institute of Nutrition and Food Technology, Center of Biomedical Research, University of Granada, Avda. del Conocimiento s/n. Armilla, 18100 Granada, Spain
[4] Instituto de Investigación Biosanitaria IBS.GRANADA, Complejo Hospitalario Universitario de Granada, 18014 Granada, Spain
[5] CIBEROBN (Physiopathology of Obesity and Nutrition Network CB12/03/30038), Institute of Health Carlos III (ISCIII), 28029 Madrid, Spain
[6] Investigative Pathology Laboratory, Federal University of Sergipe, Rua Cláudio Batista, S/N, Cidade Nova, Aracaju, 49060-108 Sergipe, Brazil
* Correspondence: caguiler@ugr.es; Tel.: +34-958-241-000 (ext. 20314)

Received: 27 September 2019; Accepted: 12 November 2019; Published: 14 November 2019

Abstract: Children are in the risk group for developing hypovitaminosis D. Several strategies are used to reduce this risk. Among these, fortification of foods with vitamin D (25(OH)D) has contributed to the achievement of nutritional needs. This systematic review aims to discuss food fortification as a strategy for maintenance or recovery of nutritional status related to vitamin D in children. The work was developed according to Preferred Reporting Items for Systematic Reviews and Meta-Analyses (PRISMA) and registered in the International prospective register of systematic reviews (PROSPERO) database (CRD42018052974). Randomized clinical trials with children up to 11 years old, who were offered vitamin D-fortified foods, and who presented 25(OH)D concentrations were used as eligibility criteria. After the selection stages, five studies were included, totaling 792 children of both sexes and aged between two and 11 years. Interventions offered 300–880 IU of vitamin D per day, for a period of 1.6–9 months, using fortified dairy products. In four of the five studies, there was an increase in the serum concentrations of 25(OH)D with the consumption of these foods; additionally, most children reached or maintained sufficiency status. Moreover, the consumption of vitamin D-fortified foods proved to be safe, with no concentrations of 25(OH)D > 250 nmol/L. Based on the above, the fortification of foods with vitamin D can help maintain or recover the nutritional status of this vitamin in children aged 2–11 years. However, it is necessary to perform additional randomized clinical trials in order to establish optimal doses of fortification, according to the peculiarities of each region.

Keywords: enriched food; child; cholecalciferol; ergocalciferols; dairy products

1. Introduction

Vitamin D (25(OH)D) is an important nutrient during childhood because of its involvement in bone formation, as well as in the immune system, which can result in higher body needs for this vitamin [1–3]. Thus, children are among the groups at risk of developing hypovitaminosis D [4].

Dietary intake is one of the ways to obtain this vitamin, but the food contribution is limited (10% to 20%) [4–6]. The main way of obtaining vitamin D is endogenously from sun exposure: ultraviolet B (UVB) rays are absorbed by 7-dehydrocholesterol, producing a thermally unstable compound that is converted in the liver to 25(OH)D, and subsequently converted to the active form 1,25-dihydroxycholecalciferol in the kidneys [3,6–9].

Even in sunny countries, vitamin D deficiency is observed in different population groups [10–13]. Considering the issue raised, the fortification of foods with vitamin D is an alternative for wide population coverage for reducing the risk of vitamin D deficiency, and its adoption is increasing worldwide [14,15]. In some countries with high prevalence of vitamin D deficiency and ineffective sun exposure, fortification of foods with vitamin D is compulsory or voluntary, with dairy products being the most frequently fortified foods [16–18].

There are few clinical trials evaluating food fortification as a strategy to improve or maintain vitamin D nutritional status in child population [14,16–19], as well as systematic reviews and meta-analysis have evaluated this outcome [20,21]. In this context, the fortification of ready-to-eat foods may contribute to the achievement of the nutritional needs of vitamin D in children, who commonly present a high inadequacy in vitamin D intake [15,22]. Although promising, vitamin D fortification is not yet widely explored by public health policies because more studies are needed to assess the contribution of fortified foods consumption to serum 25(OH)D levels in children and other risk groups of hypovitaminosis D, given the need to obtain information regarding dose, safety, and fortification food vehicle. The objective of this study is to evaluate the available evidence of dairy food fortification as a strategy for maintenance or recovery of nutritional status related to vitamin D in children.

2. Materials and Methods

This study was conducted following the Preferred Reporting Items for Systematic Reviews and Meta-Analyses statement (PRISMA) [23] (Supplementary 1) and supplemented by guidance from the Cochrane Collaboration Handbook for Systematic Reviews of Interventions [24]. Institutional review board approval and informed consent were not required for this systematic review. A study protocol was designed a priori and was registered in the International prospective register of systematic reviews PROSPERO database (registration number CRD42018052974).

2.1. Eligibility Criteria

For the construction of this review randomized clinical trials (RCTs) with children up to 11 years old, who presented data regarding serum or plasma vitamin D (25(OH)D) concentrations at baseline and after the intervention, were considered eligible. The comparators were foods fortified with cholecalciferol or ergocalciferol with non-fortified foods.

Animal or in vitro studies, manuscript published only in summary form, and review studies were excluded. In addition, studies including children diagnosed with diseases that compromised vitamin D metabolism were excluded. To avoid interference from other nutrients, studies who offered fortified foods with vitamin D in conjunction with other nutrients were not considered.

2.2. Search Strategy

Searches for RCTs were performed in PubMed, SCOPUS, Bireme, Lilacs, and the website ClinicalTrials.gov from inception to January 2019. A gray-literature search included Google Scholar and OpenThesis. The structured search strategy used the following terms: (child) AND ("vitamin d" OR cholecalciferol OR ergocalciferol OR "fortified food" OR "fortified foods") (Supplementary 2).

The search was limited to studies published in full-text versions, without language restriction. The reference lists of all eligible studies and reviews were scanned to identify additional studies for inclusion.

2.3. Study Selection and Data Extraction

Two evaluators (B.C.S and P.N.B-L) conducted all the selection stages of studies independently, first reading the Titles and Abstracts, and subsequently reading the full studies selected in the first stage. Any disagreement was resolved in conjunction by three evaluators (B.C.S, P.N.B-L, and L.V.P).

To evaluate the agreement between the evaluators in the selection stages of the studies, the kappa coefficient proposed by Landis and Koch [25] was used. The results were classified according to the interval <0 to 1, where <0 = no agreement, 0–0.19 = poor agreement, 0.20–0.39 = fair agreement, 0.40–0.59 = moderate agreement, 0.60–0.79 = substantial agreement, and 0.80–1= almost perfect agreement [25].

The following information was extracted from studies: characteristics of the participants; season of the year; dosage and food matrix used as the fortification vehicle; sun exposure; duration of intervention; and 25(OH)D status. The cut-off points proposed by the World Health Organization were adopted for the classification of BMI (Body Mass Index) for age, with z-score values ≥ -2 and $\leq +1$ considered normal weight [26].

In the included study that presented the serum 25(OH)D concentration as a graph [16], mean and standard deviation values were extracted using Web Plot Digitizer software version 4.1 (Ankit Rohatgi, Austin, Texas, USA). If the means and standard deviations were not directly reported in the publication, indirect methods of extracting estimates were used [27,28].

2.4. Assessment of Risk of Bias

The risk of bias in the studies was independently assessed by two reviewers using the Cochrane Collaboration's tool for assessing risk of bias in randomized trials [24]. The tool presents seven domains in which random sequence generation, allocation concealment, blinding of participants and professionals, blinding of outcome evaluators, incomplete outcomes, selective outcome reporting, and other sources of bias are evaluated. Other sources of bias were non-descriptions of skin color and frequency of sun exposure of children assessed in the studies. The items contained in this checklist were classified as low risk, high risk, or unclear risk of bias.

2.5. Data Synthesis

In order to assess the main outcome, vitamin D intake values were converted into international units per day ($\mu g \times 40 = IU$) [4] when not provided by the studies. Furthermore, serum concentrations of 25(OH)D were presented in nanomoles per liter (ng/mL $\times$ 2.5 = nmol/L) [4]. 25(OH)D levels were analyzed based on change-from-baseline measures [24]. However, due to the heterogeneity observed between the studies, the meta-analysis of the data was not performed. Thus, the results of the studies were reported individually and were not summarized.

The graphical representation of the bias risk analysis was elaborated with Review Manager software 5.3 (The Nordic Cochrane Centre, The Cochrane Collaboration, Copenhagen, Denmark, 2008).

3. Results

3.1. General Characteristics

The initial search identified 1778 studies, and, after all the selection stages, five studies met the inclusion criteria and were included in this review [14,16–19]. The kappa coefficient for two selection stages was, respectively, 0.664 and 0.683, which characterizes a substantial agreement between the evaluators in both stages. The selection stages of the studies are presented in Figure 1.

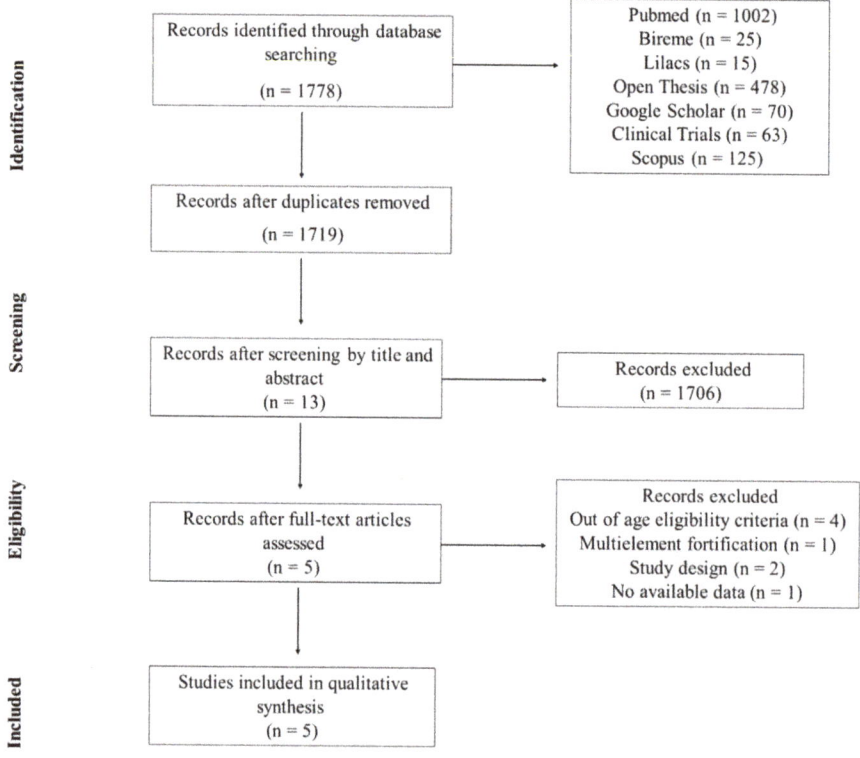

Figure 1. Flowchart of search and selection steps of the studies.

Of the included randomized clinical trials, four are double-blind type [14,16,17,19], and one is blind [18]. The studies were conducted in four different countries, two being conducted in Canada (latitude > 40° N) [16,17], and the others in Sweden (latitude 55° N e 63° N) [19], Germany (latitude > 50° N) [14], and Mongolia (latitude 48° N) [18].

3.2. Risk of Bias

Regarding the analysis of bias risk (Figure 2), among the five included studies, 100% were classified as low risk of selection bias (random sequence generation). This result was due to the studies using a table of random numbers [14,17] or a computer program [16,18,19] to generate the random sequence. In relation to selection bias (allocation concealment), 100% of the studies presented low risk, while 80% of the studies presented a low risk for the performance bias domain, with only one of the studies lacking sufficient information on the blinding process of participants and professionals [18].

The evaluation of detection, attrition, and reporting bias showed that 100% of the studies presented low risk of bias [14,16,17,19], considering the description of the blinding, the loss of data, and their respective reasons, together with the intention-to-treat analysis, as well as the proposed outcomes were reported, and no bias was observed in the observed effect size.

According to the analysis of other sources of bias (assessment of sun exposure and skin color), 60% of the studies presented low risk [16,17,19]. Only one study did not evaluate such information, being assigned a high risk of bias [18], and another did not clearly describe the method used to evaluate these aspects, being classified as an unclear risk of bias [14].

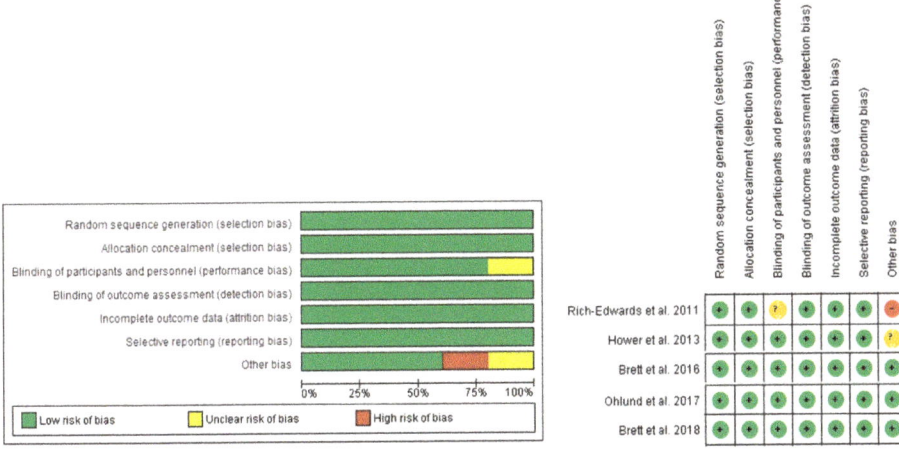

Figure 2. Authors' judgment about the risk of bias for each included study. Caption: (+) indicates low risk; (−) high risk; and (?) unclear risk.

3.3. Sample Characterization

The five studies selected present data on 792 children of both sexes and aged between two and 11 years, distributed in the intervention groups with vitamin D-fortified foods (n = 568) and control (n = 224). Regarding nutritional status, three studies were conducted with normal weight children according to BMI for age [16–18]. Two other studies included in the sample children with normal weight, thinness [14], overweight, and obesity [14,19]. In the studies, no differences were observed between the intervention and control groups in relation to age, sex, and BMI. The general characteristics of the study and the children at baseline are presented in Table 1.

Skin pigmentation was evaluated in four studies, and three of these studies [16,17,19] classified skin pigmentation according to Fitzpatrick's scale, which considers the existence of six phototypes according to the person's skin color and response to sun exposure (degree of burning and tanning).

Two studies used a spectrophotometer to measure the individual typological angle and found that more than 50% of the children evaluated had types I to III skin [16,17], whereas Ohlund et al. [19] evaluated the pigmentation of the skin through visual means, characterizing 52% of the children with skin types I to IV in the fair skin group. One of the studies observed that 98% of the children in the sample had a fair skin color, but the methodology used for this classification was not described by the authors [14]. Only the study by Rich-Edwards et al. [18] did not evaluate this information.

The incidence of UVB rays is also a variable that can influence the availability of vitamin D. Two studies were conducted exclusively during a period with no efficient sun exposure (autumn and winter) [18,19], and two other studies also included spring [16,17]; only the study by Hower et al. [14] covered all seasons.

Another relevant aspect to be evaluated is sun exposure. In two studies, no significant differences were observed regarding direct sun exposure among the evaluated children [16,17]. The other studies did not present this information clearly [14,19] or did not evaluate it [18]. Regarding the use of sunscreens, only three studies presented this information [16,17,19].

Table 1. General characteristics of the studies and the children at baseline.

Author	Country	Duration of Study/Season	Group	No. of Children	Age (Years)	Vitamin D Status (n) Deficiency and Insufficiency	Vitamin D Status (n) Sufficiency	BMI for Age Classification ‡	Skin Phototype (n) §
Rich-Edwards et al. [18]	Mongolia	January to March/Winter	Mongolian Milk UHT USA Milk Control	140 137 101	10.0 ± 1.0	NA	1 5 1	Normal weight	NA
Hower et al. [14]	Germany	November to July/Fall to Summer	Intervention Control	46 34	3.8 (2.0–6.8) 3.7 (2.0–6.2)	21 19	25 15	Thickness, normal weight, overweight and obesity	Light skin: 78 ¥ Dark skin: 2 ¥
Brett et al. [16]	Canada	January to April/Winter to mid-spring	EAR RDA Control	27 26 24	4.9 ± 2.1 5.3 ± 2.0 5.0 ± 1.8	7 4 7	20 22 17	Normal weight	Phototype I to III: 43 Phototype IV to VI: 34
Ohlund et al. [19]	Sweden	November to March/Fall to Winter	10 µg 25 µg Control	80 86 40	6.3 (6.2;6.7) 6.3 (6.2;6.4) 6.3 (6.1;6.5)	NA	47 54 20	Normal weight, overweight and obesity	Phototype I to IV: 108 Phototype V to VI: 98
Brett et al. [17]	Canada	October to March/Fall to Winter	Intervention Control	26 25	5.0 ± 1.8 5.4 ± 2.0	2 2	24 23	Normal weight	Phototype I to III: 34 Phototype IV to VI: 17

Data presented as mean ± standard deviation, median (minimum–maximum) or mean (95% confidence interval); ‡ Classification of BMI for age according to the World Health Organization [26]; § Skin phototypes classified by the authors of the studies using the Fitzpatrick scale or ¥ by method not informed. BMI: Body Mass Index; EAR: Estimated Average Requirement; RDA: Recommended Dietary Allowances; UHT: Ultra-High Temperature; USA: United States; NA: Data not available in the papers.

The children's vitamin D status at baseline was variable, with the presence of children at risk of deficiency (<30 nmol/L) and of insufficiency (30–49 nmol/L), and with status classified as sufficiency (≥50 nmol/L) of vitamin D (Table 1). However, the experimental design by Hower et al. [14] took into consideration the previous nutritional status as inclusion criterion for the study (>25 nmol/L). The study sample by Rich-Edwards et al. [18] was almost completely composed of children at risk for vitamin D insufficiency and deficiency.

3.4. Food Fortification and Intervention Outcomes

Corroborating aspects of vitamin D status, four studies also considered the usual intake of this vitamin. Different methods of assessing food intake were used; among them, semiquantitative food frequency questionnaire (FFQ) [14], short FFQ [19], and the combination of 24-h dietary recall (24HR) and 13-item semiquantitative FFQ [16,17]. The FFQs used were composed of food items with a known contribution to the daily intake of vitamin D (e.g., milk and dairy products, fish, mushrooms) in the study countries. The study by Rich-Edwards et al. [18] was the only one that did not assess the habitual vitamin D intake, only used 24HR to quantify the number of portions of Mongolia's dairy products consumed daily.

The results showed that at baseline, dietary vitamin D intake was lower than the adequacy recommendations adopted in each study. Dairy products used as vehicles for vitamin D fortification were cheddar cheese, yogurt [16,17], and milk [14,18,19], with concentrations ranging from 42 to 880 IU of vitamin D per serving. Thus, the results were discussed considering the exclusive intervention of the fortified foods offered [14,18,19] or in association with usual daily diet [16,17], for periods ranging from 1.6 to 9 months (Table 2).

By observing the effects of intake of fortified foods on serum vitamin D levels, in three studies, an increase of 25(OH)D levels after the intervention period was observed in all groups receiving fortified foods, whereas the respective control groups did not present alteration of this vitamin in the serum [16,17,19] (Table 3).

In the study by Hower et al. [14], the fortified milk intervention was evaluated during different climatic seasons, showing an increase in the serum 25(OH)D levels after winter in the intervention group that was statistically different from the control group, which presented a reduction in the concentrations of vitamin. In contrast, during the summer, the intervention and control groups remained similar.

Different behavior was observed in the study by Brett et al. [17], in which the fortified dairy products (yogurt and cheddar cheese) promoted maintenance of serum 25(OH)D concentrations during the first 3 months, but at the end of the study (6 months) those concentrations were reduced (Δ = −6.9 nmol/L). On the other hand, in the control group, serum 25(OH)D concentrations reduced at 3 months of the study and remained unchanged until the end of the study (6 months).

Differently, Ohlund et al. [19] observed differences in the 25(OH)D concentrations at baseline according to skin color (dark skin and fair skin) and, with this, the post-intervention data were compared using the analysis of covariance with study groups as a fixed factor and the skin type as a random factor.

The methods used to determine serum 25(OH)D concentrations were liquid chromatography coupled with tandem mass spectrometry (LC-MS/MS) [18,19], high performance liquid chromatography (HPLC) [17], and chemiluminescence immunoassays [14,16]. The quantified forms corresponded to total vitamin D [14,16], and the D2 [18,19] and D3 forms [17–19] (Table 3).

In none of the studies, serum 25(OH)D concentrations were above safety limits (>250 nmol/L) in the groups receiving fortified foods, even during the months with abundant sunshine.

Table 2. Characteristics of interventions and food fortification of the studies.

Author	Duration of Study (Months)	Group	Food/Portion Size	Vitamin D Content in Food	Total Vitamin D (IU/Day)
Rich-Edwards et al. [18]	1.6	Mongolian milk	Mongolian milk/710 mL	100 IU/236 mL	300
		UHT USA milk	UHT USA milk/710 mL	100 IU/236 mL	300
		Control	Non-fortified milk/710 mL	NA	NA
Hower et al. [14]	9	Intervention	fortified milk /350 mL	114 IU/100 mL	400
		Control	Non-fortified milk /350 mL	1.2 IU/100 mL	4.2
Brett et al. [16]	3	EAR	Yogurt/186 mL Cheddar cheese /21 g	42 IU/ 93 mL 200 IU/21 g	400 ¥
		RDA	Yogurt/186 mL Cheddar cheese/21 g	125 IU/93 mL 200 IU/21 g	600 ¥
		Control	Non-fortified yogurt/186 mL Non-fortified cheddar cheese/21 g	15 IU/93 mL NA	140–195 ¥
Ohlund et al. [19]	3	10 µg	UHT milk/200 mL	480 IU/200 g	480
		25 µg	UHT milk/ 200 mL	880 IU/200 g	880
		Control	Non-fortified UHT milk/200 mL	80 IU/200 mL	80
Brett et al. [17]	6	Intervention	Yogurt/186 mL Cheddar cheese/33g	Yogurt: 150 IU/93 mL Cheddar cheese: 300 IU/33 g	400 ¥
		Control	Non-fortified yogurt/186 mL Non-fortified cheddar cheese/33 g	NA	140–195 ¥

¥ Studies have counted the usual intake of 110–165 IU of vitamin D from foods routinely consumed in the total daily intake. EAR: Estimated Average Requirement; NA: Data not available in the papers; RDA: Recommended Dietary Allowances; UHT: Ultra-High Temperature; USA: United States.

Table 3. Effect of consumption of the vitamin D-fortified foods in children.

Author	Methods of Vitamin D Assessment	Group	25(OH)D (nmol/L)			Δ Change (nmol/L)	
			Baseline	End Point			
Rich-Edwards et al. [18]	LC-MS/MS	Mongolian milk UHT USA milk Control	20.0 ± 10.0 a 25.0 ± 12.5 a 20.0 ± 10.0 a	50.0 ± 15.0 b,# 72.4 ± 25.0 b,# 20.0 ± 10.0 a		30.0 ± 13.2 47.4 ± 21.7 0 ± 10.0	
Hower et al. [14]	CLIA	Intervention	53.7 ± 20.6 a	After winter 62.0 ± 25.8 b,#	Summer 69.0 ± 13.6 b	After winter 8.3 ± 23.6	Summer 15.3 ± 18.1
		Control	46.0 ± 21.2 a	After winter 34.0 ± 18.6 b	Summer 68.5 ± 13.0 c	After winter −12.0 ± 20.0	Summer 22.5 ± 18.5
Brett et al. [16]	CLIA	EAR RDA Control	59.7 ± 13.0 a 60.9 ± 10.1 a 58.6 ± 14.5 a	64.2 ± 9.7 b,# 64.1 ± 11.8 b,# 56.1 ± 11.9 a		4.5 ± 11.7 3.2 ± 11.0 −2.5 ± 13.4	
Ohlund et al. [19]	LC-MS/MS	10 μg 25 μg Control	56.0 ± 18.3 a 58.0 ± 21.3 a 49.0 ± 19.4 a	69.0 ± 9.1 b,# 82.0 ± 14.2 b,# 50.0 ± 14.5 a		13.0 ± 15.8 24.0 ± 18.8 1.0 ± 17.5	
Brett et al. [17]	HPLC	Intervention	65.3 ± 12.2 a	3 months 64.7 ± 12.2 a,#	6 months 58.4 ± 8.7 b	3 months −0.6 ± 12.2	6 months −6.9 ± 10.9
		Control	67.5 ± 15.1 a	3 months 58.3 ± 15.3 b	6 months 56.6 ± 13.9 b	3 months −9.2 ± 15.2	6 months −10.9 ± 14.5

Data presented as mean ± standard deviation; # denotes significant difference in relation to the control group; different superscript letters denote significant differences within the group over time. 25(OH)D: serum vitamin D concentration; CLIA: chemiluminescence immunoassay; EAR: Estimated Average Requirement; HPLC: High Performance Liquid Chromatography; LC-MS/MS: liquid chromatography coupled with tandem mass spectrometry; RDA: Recommended Dietary Allowances; UHT: Ultra-High Temperature; USA: United States.

4. Discussion

This study evaluated the available evidence regarding food fortification as a strategy for maintenance or recovery of vitamin D nutritional status in children. The results of the individual studies suggest that consumption of vitamin D-fortified foods seems to be an important strategy to reduce the prevalence of hypovitaminosis D in this age group, which present greater vulnerability to developing this deficiency. However, due to the clinical and methodological heterogeneity of these studies, a meta-analysis could not be performed.

Previous systematic reviews and meta-analysis sought to evaluate the effect of fortification of foods with vitamin D, demonstrating a significant increase in 25(OH)D concentrations from the consumption of these foods in different population groups [15,20,21,29]. However, when considering only the child group, only one systematic review and meta-analysis has been observed in the literature, with children aged 2–18 years [20].

The effects of fortification with vitamin D are reported to be dependent on increased intake of fortified foods, previous vitamin D status, age, body composition, skin pigmentation, sun exposure, geographic aspects, and food intake [14,18,30–32]. In addition, for food fortification there is also a need to evaluate the population's eating habits, especially in the children's group, so that the used vehicle is routinely present in the food in order to guarantee greater acceptance [14,16].

As noted in the included studies, the use of fortified foods to improve or maintain vitamin D status considered the consumption of milk and dairy products as part of the population's eating habits. Milk and its products are among the foods often fortified with vitamin D, as they are widely consumed by children, especially in developed countries, and have good bioavailability of the vitamin [33,34].

Dairy products naturally feature in their composition nutrients that act together with vitamin D, thus contributing to the metabolism of this vitamin, as well as in the physiological processes in which it is active [35].

Furthermore, vitamin D is directly related to the calcium present in these foods, in which the 1,25(OH)2D stimulates the intestinal absorption and renal reabsorption of this mineral, as well as acting in the processes of bone mineralization, due its participation in the synthesis of osteocalcin [34]. At the same time, calcium participates in the processes of biosynthesis and regulation of vitamin D, and the reduced content of dietary calcium stimulates the catabolism of 25(OH)D as a result of the elevation of parathormone and 1,25(OH)2D concentrations [34,36]. Despite its sensitivity to light, vitamin D is considered as good micronutrient for fortification [30].

In the countries of origin of the included clinical trials, in areas with restricted sun exposure, it is noted that, although increasing, food fortification is still not widely adopted. In Canada, where two of the five included studies were conducted [16,17], only liquid cow's milk (35–45 UI/100 mL), and margarine (530 UI/100 g) must be fortified in accordance with current legislation [4,31]. In Sweden, the Swedish National Food Agency has established recent changes in fortification policy by expanding the list of foods and the levels to be fortified [37]. However, in Germany and Mongolia there is no food fortification policy, although they are located in a region with a latitude greater than 45° N and have a high prevalence of vitamin D deficiency [14,18,38].

Different responses to food fortification at serum vitamin D concentrations can be observed depending on previous nutritional status [16,18]. Children with poor or insufficient vitamin D status had a significant increase in serum 25(OH)D concentrations after the intervention [14,16,18,19], which was not identified in children with sufficient status [17]. This is because the evidence of the relationship between vitamin D intake and serum concentrations is non-linear in nature; that is, the intake of vitamin D has less impact on their serum concentrations when they are at high or sufficient levels [4,39]. Considering this, Aloia et al. [39] showed that in order to alter serum vitamin D concentrations above 50 nmol/L, there would be a need for a higher intake of vitamin D when compared to the amount necessary to increase serum vitamin D levels under 50 nmol/L.

When circulating 25(OH)D concentrations are present in sufficiency, a portion of this vitamin can be transferred to body stores once saturation of the vitamin D 25-hydroxylase (CYP2R1)—the enzyme responsible for vitamin D hydroxylation in the liver—occurs [16,17]. The aspects related to the tissue distribution of vitamin D in children are not widely known; however, studies indicate that vitamin D intake is associated with an increase in lean mass and bone mineral density in healthy children [17,36].

The discussion of dose-response of fortification at 25(OH)D concentrations is little explored. Brett et al. [16] observed, by linear regression analysis, that each 100 IU per day increase in vitamin D intake by through fortified foods resulted in an increase in serum 25(OH)D concentrations of 0.6–10 nmol/L in the children. A similar result could be observed in the study by Rich-Edwards et al. [18] in which the increase in serum concentrations of 25(OH)D was 15 nmol/L per 100 IU of vitamin D intake. In the only systematic review and meta-analysis performed in children (2–18 years) to date, the authors sought to investigate the effect of vitamin D interventions (fortified foods, supplements, bolus injections) on vitamin D status. In this study, the authors observed greater results in the mean change in serum 25(OH)D per 100 IU vitamin D/d in trials only using fortified food ($n = 7$; 6.9 nmol/L; 95% CI: 3.7, 10.0 nmol/L; $I^2 = 99.9\%$) than trials that offered daily supplements ($n = 15$; 2.9 nmol/L; 95% CI: 2.4, 3.5 nmol/L; $I^2 = 56\%$) ($p = 0.001$), and bolus injections ($n = 2$; 2.3 nmol/L; 95% CI: 0.9, 3.9 nmol/L; $I^2 = 0\%$) ($p = 0.04$). The authors demonstrated that the serum 25(OH)D response to vitamin D intake differed on the basis of baseline status, intakes, and delivery mode, but not age, sex, or latitude [20]. However, the overall results should be used cautiously due to the high level of heterogeneity observed.

A meta-analysis published by Black et al. [15], performed with adults, showed similar results. The increase of 1.2 nmol/L (95% CI: 0.72, 1.68; $I^2 = 89\%$) was observed in the 25(OH)D concentrations for each 40 IU day of vitamin D ingested from fortified foods. In the paper by O'Donnell et al. [29], the combining results of four trials that offered vitamin D fortified-milk ($n = 466$ individuals; 138–800 IU vitamin D/day) also demonstrated an increase in the 25(OH)D concentrations in adults (15.63 (12.79, 18.48) nmol/L; $I^2 = 0.0\%$; $p = 0.77$).

From the evaluated results, it is not possible to determine the optimal fortification dose, since changes in 25(OH)D concentrations were observed in almost all trials in different populations. However, the dose range of vitamin D used in fortification of foods from included studies (300–800 IU/day) were effective in maintaining or recovering vitamin D status in children. Besides, the optimal dose could be dependent on the characteristics of the population targeted, including those with vitamin D deficiency.

The intervention period, another relevant aspect for the study outcome, varied among the studies. In some of the included studies, this variable was chosen because it corresponds to the length of the season of interest. Even so, all studies exceeded the considered half-life of 25(OH)D which is between 2 and 3 weeks [40]. Vitamin D3 obtained orally has a circulatory peak of 12 h, returning to basal concentrations within 7 days, even when given high doses [41]. Chronic vitamin D supplementation is shown to be the best alternative for promoting gradual increase and sustaining constant 25(OH)D concentrations [20,42], reaching a steady state in healthy adult subjects at 3 months, approximately [43,44]. More importantly, there is not enough evidence on vitamin D metabolism in children [45,46].

In children, deficient vitamin D status is the main cause of rickets, a disorder characterized by disturbances in bone growth and skeletal abnormalities, besides negatively influencing cognitive development, hormone formation, and immune function [32,47,48]. It is important to consider that the early years of childhood are characterized by high rates of growth velocity, requiring specific values of energy and micronutrients such as vitamin D [32,49].

In addition, other variables that may affect the vitamin D bioavailability should be considered. Body composition is an important aspect for understanding the metabolism of this vitamin because adiposity has been inversely associated with 25(OH)D concentrations by acting on vitamin D storage, increasing its clearance [4,17,50,51]. Thus, children with excess body fat may present an increased risk for the development of 25(OH)D deficiency, requiring two to three times higher concentrations of vitamin D to meet bodily needs [50].

Overall, studies have shown that fair-skinned individuals have higher levels of 25(OH)D compared to darker skinned individuals [6,52], a fact that could be observed in one of the included studies [19].

The variation in skin pigmentation depends on the type and amount of melanin generated, as well as on the activity of keratinocytes, which are responsible for the sequestration and degradation of melanin [53]. Thus, the greater the pigmentation of the skin, the lower the vitamin D production, since the melanin absorbs the UVB radiation that would act in the synthesis of this vitamin [36].

Geographical location and climatic characteristics also directly influence the synthesis of vitamin D in the skin, with low or absent synthesis observed during most of the winter in places with latitudes above 33° [50]. In this study, all studies included were performed in countries with a latitude greater than 35°, and the individuals studied presented mostly fair skin (Fitzpatrick classification I to III). Since during a part of the year the UVB radiation in these places is not sufficient to activate the endogenous synthesis and consequently maintain the status of this vitamin [50], food fortification takes on greater importance in the context of public policy.

It is known that diet has a lower participation in 25(OH)D concentrations [47]. This is because the reduced variety of vitamin D food sources means they cannot be part of the eating habits of individuals, especially children [14,18,33]. Among the available food sources, we can mention fatty fish, cod liver oil, mushrooms, egg yolk, and liver steak [4,29,33]. In addition, regular consumption of vitamin D-fortified foods can provide better results in maintaining sufficient vitamin D status compared to other strategies such as seasonal capsule supplementation or the supply of high-dose vitamin D acutely [14,16].

In addition, methods of serum 25(OH)D assessment have a strong influence on the diagnosis of vitamin D status. There is no consensus regarding the reference standard due to susceptibility to problems in the pre-analytical, analytical, and post-analytical phases. Immunoassays are dependent on the specificity of the antibodies used, not being able to identify the 3-epi-25(OH)D molecule. The HPLC method has been replaced by the LC-MS/MS method, currently considered the gold standard because of its higher sensitivity [4,54]. It should be noted the included studies showed clinical and methodological heterogeneity that could not be sufficiently explored in the subgroup analysis and could produce clinically inconsistent results. Thus, the food fortification strategy is promising, but there is a need to evaluate the dose-response of vitamin D-fortified foods in vitamin D status, considering all aspects involved in bioavailability, especially population-wide implementation.

This is the first systematic review that addresses the effects of vitamin D-fortified food intake by children aged 2–11 years, taking into account the other factors that influence vitamin D metabolism, such as latitude, sun exposure, skin color, use of sunscreen, and usual dietary intake. Furthermore, this review included studies that offered fortified foods exclusively with vitamin D in order to minimize additional factors that could interfere in the bioavailability of this vitamin.

Regarding limitations of the present study, it is possible to mention the low number of studies available in the literature that offered vitamin D-fortified foods for children. Thus, this study recommends further randomized clinical trials of this age group to increase evidence and identify the optimal dose for vitamin D food fortification. Moreover, it should be emphasized that the habitual consumption of the evaluated groups should be considered, even in the face of the limitations inherent in the methods used to evaluate habitual nutrient intake.

5. Conclusions

The results of the individual studies suggest that the fortification of foods with vitamin D can be used for maintaining or recovering the vitamin's nutritional status in children aged 2–11 years. In addition, the intake of 300–880 IU of vitamin D per day through the consumption of fortified foods appears to be safe under the conditions studied, with no increase in serum 25(OH)D concentrations above the tolerable limits. However, due to the insufficient number and heterogeneity between the studies, a meta-analysis evaluating the outcomes of interest was not performed, and a pragmatic recommendation on the fortification of foods with vitamin D is not possible. It is necessary to carry out additional randomized clinical trials in order to increase the strength of evidence, and to establish ideal doses of fortification at the population level.

Supplementary Materials: The following are available online at http://www.mdpi.com/2072-6643/11/11/2766/s1, Supplementary 1: PRISMA 2009 checklist; Supplementary 2: Structured search strategy used for systematic search on databases.

Author Contributions: Conceptualization, P.N.B.-L. and L.V.P.; investigation, B.d.C.S., P.N.B.-L. and L.V.P.; writing—original draft preparation, B.d.C.S., P.N.B.-L. and L.V.P.; writing—review and editing, B.d.C.S., P.N.B.-L., C.M.A., P.R.S.M.-F., A.R.S.F. and L.V.P.

Funding: This research was funded by the National Council for Scientific and Technological Development (CNPq/MS/SCTIE/DECIT/DAB/CGAN), grant number 440809/2017-7. In part by the Coordination of Improvement of Higher Education Personnel—Brazil (CAPES)—Finance Code 001. And by *Unidad Científica de Excelencia Ejercicio y Salud (UCEES)*, University of Granada, Spain.

Conflicts of Interest: The authors declare no conflict of interest.

References

1. Mortensen, C.; Mølgaard, C.; Hauger, H.; Kristensen, M.; Damsgaard, C.T. Sun behaviour and physical activity associated with autumn vitamin D status in 4–8-year-old Danish children. *Public Health Nutr.* **2018**, *21*, 3158–3167. [CrossRef] [PubMed]
2. Wang, S.; Shen, G.; Jiang, S.; Xu, H.; Li, M.; Wang, Z.; Zhang, S.; Yu, Y. Nutrient status of vitamin D among chinese children. *Nutrients* **2017**, *9*, 319. [CrossRef] [PubMed]
3. Kamen, D.L.; Tangpricha, V. Vitamin D and molecular actions on the immune system: Modulation of innate and autoimmunity. *J. Mol. Med.* **2010**, *88*, 441–450. [CrossRef] [PubMed]
4. Institute of Medicine. *Dietary Reference Intakes for Calcium and Vitamin D*; Ross, A.C., Taylor, C.L., Yaktine, A.L., Del, H.B., Eds.; National Academy of Sciences: Washington, DC, USA, 2011; ISBN 978-0-309-16394-1.
5. Forrest, K.Y.Z.; Stuhldreher, W.L. Prevalence and correlates of vitamin D deficiency in US adults. *Nutr. Res.* **2011**, *31*, 48–54. [CrossRef] [PubMed]
6. Mithal, A.; Wahl, D.A.; Bonjour, J.P.; Burckhardt, P.; Dawson-Hughes, B.; Eisman, J.A.; El-Hajj Fuleihan, G.; Josse, R.G.; Lips, P.; Morales-Torres, J. Global vitamin D status and determinants of hypovitaminosis D. *Osteoporos. Int.* **2009**, *20*, 1807–1820. [CrossRef] [PubMed]
7. Wacker, M.; Holick, M.F. Sunlight and Vitamin D: A global perspective for health. *Derm. Endocrinol.* **2013**, *5*, 51–108. [CrossRef]
8. Hossein-nezhad, A.; Holick, M.F.; Holick, M.F.; Heaney, R.; Singh, R.J.; Pettifor, J.M. Vitamin D for Health: A Global Perspective. *Mayo Clin. Proc.* **2013**, *88*, 720–755. [CrossRef]
9. Holick, M.F. The vitamin D deficiency pandemic: Approaches for diagnosis, treatment and prevention. *Rev. Endocr. Metab. Disord.* **2017**, *18*, 153–165. [CrossRef]
10. Eloi, M.; Horvath, D.V.; Szejnfeld, V.L.; Ortega, J.C.; Rocha, D.A.C.; Szejnfeld, J.; Castro, C.H.M. Vitamin D deficiency and seasonal variation over the years in São Paulo, Brazil. *Osteoporos. Int.* **2016**, *27*, 3449–3456. [CrossRef]
11. Binkley, N.; Novotny, R.; Krueger, D.; Kawahara, T.; Daida, Y.G.; Lensmeyer, G.; Hollis, B.W.; Drezner, M.K. Low Vitamin D Status despite Abundant Sun Exposure. *J. Clin. Endocrinol. Metab.* **2007**, *92*, 2130–2135. [CrossRef]
12. Lopes, V.M.; Lopes, J.R.; Brasileiro, J.P.; Oliveira, I.D.; Lacerda, R.P.; Andrade, M.R.; Tierno, N.I.; Souza, R.C.; Motta, L.A. Highly prevalence of vitamin D deficiency among Brazilian women of reproductive age. *Arch. Endocrinol. Metab.* **2017**, *61*, 21–27. [CrossRef] [PubMed]
13. Harinarayan, C.V.; Holick, M.F.; Prasad, U.V.; Vani, P.S.; Himabindu, G. Vitamin D status and sun exposure in India. *Derm. Endocrinol.* **2013**, *5*, 130–141. [CrossRef]
14. Hower, J.; Knoll, A.; Ritzenthaler, K.L.; Steiner, C.; Berwind, R. Vitamin D fortification of growing up milk prevents decrease of serum 25-hydroxyvitamin D concentrations during winter: A clinical intervention study in Germany. *Eur. J. Pediatr.* **2013**, *172*, 1597–1605. [CrossRef] [PubMed]
15. Black, L.J.; Seamans, K.M.; Cashman, K.D.; Kiely, M. An Updated Systematic Review and Meta-Analysis of the Efficacy of Vitamin D Food Fortification. *J. Nutr.* **2012**, *142*, 1102–1108. [CrossRef] [PubMed]
16. Brett, N.R.; Lavery, P.; Agellon, S.; Vanstone, C.A.; Maguire, J.L.; Rauch, F.; Weiler, H.A. Dietary vitamin D dose-response in healthy children 2 to 8 y of age: A 12-wk randomized controlled trial using fortified foods. *Am. J. Clin. Nutr.* **2016**, *103*, 144–152. [CrossRef] [PubMed]

17. Brett, N.R.; Parks, C.A.; Lavery, P.; Agellon, S.; Vanstone, C.A.; Kaufmann, M.; Jones, G.; Maguire, J.L.; Rauch, F.; Weiler, H.A. Vitamin D status and functional health outcomes in children aged 2–8 y: A 6-mo Vitamin D randomized controlled trial. *Am. J. Clin. Nutr.* **2018**, *107*, 355–364. [CrossRef]
18. Rich-Edwards, J.W.; Ganmaa, D.; Kleinman, K.; Sumberzul, N.; Holick, M.F.; Lkhagvasuren, T.; Dulguun, B.; Burke, A.; Frazier, A.L. Randomized trial of fortified milk and supplements to raise 25-hydroxyvitamin D concentrations in schoolchildren in Mongolia. *Am. J. Clin. Nutr.* **2011**, *94*, 578–584. [CrossRef]
19. Öhlund, I.; Lind, T.; Hernell, O.; Silfverdal, S.A.; Åkeson, P.K. Increased Vitamin D intake differentiated according to skin color is needed to meet requirements in young Swedish children during winter: A double-blind randomized clinical trial. *Am. J. Clin. Nutr.* **2017**, *106*, 105–112. [CrossRef]
20. Brett, N.R.; Gharibeh, N.; Weiler, H.A. Effect of Vitamin D Supplementation, Food Fortification, or Bolus Injection on Vitamin D Status in Children Aged 2–18 Years: A Meta-Analysis. *Adv. Nutr.* **2018**, *9*, 454–464. [CrossRef]
21. Matsuyama, M.; Harb, T.; David, M.; Davies, P.S.; Hill, R.J. Effect of fortified milk on growth and nutritional status in young children: A systematic review and meta-analysis. *Public Health Nutr.* **2016**, *20*, 1214–1225. [CrossRef]
22. Ritu, G.; Ajay, G. Fortification of Foods With Vitamin D in India: Strategies Targeted at Children. *J. Am. Coll. Nutr.* **2015**, *34*, 265–272.
23. Moher, D.; Liberati, A.; Tetzlaff, J.; Altman, D.G.; Altman, D.; Antes, G.; Atkins, D.; Barbour, V.; Barrowman, N.; Berlin, J.A.; et al. Preferred reporting items for systematic reviews and meta-analyses: The PRISMA statement. *J. Chin. Integr. Med.* **2009**, *7*, 889–896. [CrossRef]
24. Higgins, J.P.; Green, S. *Cochrane Handbook for Systematic Reviews of Interventions Version 5.1.0 [Updated March 2011]*; The Cochrane Collaboration: London, UK, 2016; pp. 297–303. Available online: https://training.cochrane.org/handbook/archive/v5.1/ (accessed on 29 January 2018).
25. Landis, J.R.; Koch, G.G. The measurement of observer agreement for categorical data. *Biometrics* **1977**, *33*, 159–174. [CrossRef] [PubMed]
26. World Health Organization. *WHO Child Growth Standards*; World Health Organization: Geneva, Switzerland, 2006; pp. 7–16.
27. Hozo, S.P.; Djulbegovic, B.; Hozo, I. Estimating the mean and variance from the median, range, and the size of a sample. *BMC Med. Res. Methodol.* **2005**, *5*, 13. [CrossRef] [PubMed]
28. Wan, X.; Wang, W.; Liu, J.; Tong, T. Estimating the sample mean and standard deviation from the sample size, median, range and/or interquartile range. *BMC Med. Res. Methodol.* **2014**, *14*, 135. [CrossRef]
29. Donnell, S.O.; Cranney, A.; Horsley, T.; Weiler, H.A.; Atkinson, S.A.; Hanley, D.A.; Ooi, D.S.; Ward, L.; Barrowman, N.; Fang, M.; et al. Efficacy of food fortification on serum 25-hydroxyvitamin D concentrations: Systematic review. *Am. J. Clin. Nutr.* **2008**, *88*, 1528–1534. [CrossRef]
30. Jakobsen, J.; Knuthsen, P. Stability of vitamin D in foodstuffs during cooking. *Food Chem.* **2014**, *148*, 170–175. [CrossRef]
31. Agency, C.F.I. Dairy Vitamin Addition. Available online: http://www.inspection.gc.ca/food/archived-food-guidance/dairy-products/manuals-inspection-procedures/dairy-vitamin-addition/eng/1378179097522/1378180040706 (accessed on 28 March 2019).
32. FAO/WHO. *Human Vitamin and Mineral Requirements*; FAO/WHO: Bangkok, Thailand, 2001.
33. Cashman, K.D.; van den Heuvel, E.G.; Schoemaker, R.J.; Préveraud, D.P.; Macdonald, H.M.; Arcot, J. 25-Hydroxyvitamin D as a Biomarker of Vitamin D Status and Its Modeling to Inform Strategies for Prevention of Vitamin D Deficiency within the Population. *Adv. Nutr.* **2017**, *8*, 947–957. [CrossRef]
34. Hayes, A.; Cashman, K.D. Irish Section Postgraduate Meeting Food-based solutions for Vitamin D deficiency: Putting policy into practice and the key role for research. *Proc. Nutr. Soc.* **2017**, *76*, 54–63. [CrossRef]
35. Corte-Real, J.; Bohn, T. Interaction of divalent minerals with liposoluble nutrients and phytochemicals during digestion and influences on their bioavailability—A review. *Food Chem.* **2018**, *252*, 285–293. [CrossRef]
36. Saggese, G.; Vierucci, F.; Boot, A.M.; Czech-kowalska, J.; Weber, G., Jr.; Camargo, A.C.; Mallet, E.; Fanos, M.; Shaw, N.J.; Holick, M.F.; et al. Vitamin D in childhood and adolescence: An expert position statement. *Am. Acad. Pediatr.* **2015**, *174*, 565–576. [CrossRef] [PubMed]
37. Livsmedelsverket (Swedish National Food Administration). *Föreskrifter om Berikning av Vissa Livsmedel*; Livsmedelsverket: Uppsala, Sweden, 2018; pp. 1–4.

38. Ministry of Health of Mongolia. *Nutrition Status of the Population of Mongolia*; Ministry of Health of Mongolia: Ulaanbaatar, Mongolia, 2017; ISBN 9789997859266.
39. Aloia, J.F.; Patel, M.; DiMaano, R.; Li-Ng, M.; Talwar, S.A.; Mikhail, M.; Pollack, S.; Yeh, J.K. Vitamin D intake to attain a desired serum 25-hydroxyvitamin D concentration. *Am. J. Clin. Nutr.* **2008**, *87*, 1952–1958. [CrossRef] [PubMed]
40. Haddad, J.G.; Rojanasathit, S. Acute Administration of 25-Hydroxycholecalciferol in Man. *J. Clin. Endocrinol. Metab.* **1976**, *42*, 284–290. [CrossRef] [PubMed]
41. Lo, C.W.; Paris, P.W.; Clemens, T.L.; Nolan, J.; Holick, M.F. Vitamin patients D absorption in healthy subjects with intestinal malabsorption and in. *Am. J. Clin. Nutr.* **1985**, *42*, 644–649. [CrossRef] [PubMed]
42. Hollis, B.W.; Wagner, C.L. The Role of the Parent Compound Vitamin D with Respect to Metabolism and Function: Why Clinical Dose Intervals Can Affect Clinical Outcomes. *J. Clin. Endocrinol. Metab.* **2013**, *98*, 4619–4628. [CrossRef] [PubMed]
43. Vieth, R.; Chan, P.R.; Macfarlane, G.D. Efficacy and safety of vitamin D3 intake exceeding the lowest observed adverse effect level. *Am. J. Clin. Nutr.* **2001**, *73*, 288–294. [CrossRef]
44. Heaney, R.P.; Recker, R.R.; Grote, J.; Horst, R.L.; Armas, L.A.G. Vitamin D3 Is More Potent Than Vitamin D 2 in Humans. *J. Clin. Endocrinol. Metab.* **2011**, *96*, 447–452. [CrossRef]
45. Ross, A.C.; Manson, J.E.; Abrams, S.A.; Aloia, J.F.; Brannon, P.M.; Clinton, S.K.; Durazo-arvizu, R.A.; Gallagher, J.C.; Gallo, R.L.; Jones, G.; et al. The 2011 Report on Dietary Reference Intakes for Calcium and Vitamin D from the Institute of Medicine: What Clinicians Need to Know. *J. Clin. Endocrinol. Metab.* **2011**, *96*, 53–58. [CrossRef]
46. Chung, M.; Balk, E.M.; Brendel, M.; Ip, S.; Lau, J.; Lee, J.; Lichtenstein, A.; Patel, K.; Raman, G.; Tatsioni, A.; et al. Vitamin D and Calcium: A Systematic Review of Health Outcomes. *Evid. Rep. Technol. Assess.* **2009**, *183*, 1–420.
47. Alonso, M.A.; Mantecón, L.; Santos, F. Vitamin D deficiency in children: A challenging diagnosis! *Pediatr. Res.* **2019**, *85*, 596–601. [CrossRef]
48. Holick, M.F.; Herman, R.H.; Award, M. Vitamin D: Importance in the prevention of cancers, type 1 diabetes, heart disease, and osteoporosis. *Am. J. Clin. Nutr.* **2004**, *79*, 362–371. [CrossRef] [PubMed]
49. EFSA Panel on Dietetic Products, Nutrition and Allergies (NDA). Scientific Opinion on nutrient requirements and dietary intakes of infants and young children in the European Union. *EFSA J.* **2013**, *11*, 3408.
50. Holick, M.F.; Binkley, N.C.; Bischoff-Ferrari, H.A.; Gordon, C.M.; Hanley, D.A.; Heaney, R.P.; Murad, M.H.; Weaver, C.M. Evaluation, treatment, and prevention of vitamin D deficiency: An endocrine society clinical practice guideline. *J. Clin. Endocrinol. Metab.* **2011**, *96*, 1911–1930. [CrossRef] [PubMed]
51. Ruiz-Ojeda, F.J.; Anguita-Ruiz, A.; Leis, R.; Aguilera, C.M. Genetic factors and molecular mechanisms of Vitamin D and obesity relationship. *Ann. Nutr. Metab.* **2018**, *73*, 89–99. [CrossRef] [PubMed]
52. Bonilla, C.; Ness, A.R.; Wills, A.K.; Lawlor, D.A.; Lewis, S.J.; Davey Smith, G. Skin pigmentation, sun exposure and vitamin D levels in children of the avon longitudinal study of parents and children. *BMC Public Health* **2014**, *14*, 597. [CrossRef] [PubMed]
53. Ebanks, J.P.; Koshoffer, A.; Wickett, R.R.; Schwemberger, S.; Babcock, G.; Hakozaki, T.; Boissy, R.E. Epidermal keratinocytes from light vs. Dark skin exhibit differential degradation of melanosomes. *J. Investig. Dermatol.* **2011**, *131*, 1226–1233. [CrossRef]
54. Card, D.J.; Carter, G. *Methods for Assessment of Vitamin D*; Elsevier Inc.: Amsterdam, The Netherlands, 2018; ISBN 9780128130506.

 © 2019 by the authors. Licensee MDPI, Basel, Switzerland. This article is an open access article distributed under the terms and conditions of the Creative Commons Attribution (CC BY) license (http://creativecommons.org/licenses/by/4.0/).

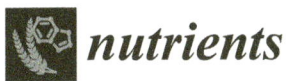

Review

Extra-Skeletal Effects of Vitamin D

Rose Marino and Madhusmita Misra *

Pediatric Endocrine Unit, Massachusetts General Hospital and Harvard Medical School, Boston, MA 02114, USA
* Correspondence: mmisra@mgh.harvard.edu; Tel.: +1-617-726-5790

Received: 30 May 2019; Accepted: 25 June 2019; Published: 27 June 2019

Abstract: The vitamin D receptor is expressed in multiple cells of the body (other than osteoblasts), including beta cells and cells involved in immune modulation (such as mononuclear cells, and activated T and B lymphocytes), and most organs in the body including the brain, heart, skin, gonads, prostate, breast, and gut. Consequently, the extra-skeletal impact of vitamin D deficiency has been an active area of research. While epidemiological and case-control studies have often suggested a link between vitamin D deficiency and conditions such as type 1 and type 2 diabetes, connective tissue disorders, inflammatory bowel disorders, chronic hepatitis, food allergies, asthma and respiratory infections, and cancer, interventional studies for the most part have failed to confirm a causative link. This review examines available evidence to date for the extra-skeletal effects of vitamin D deficiency, with a focus on randomized controlled trials and meta-analyses.

Keywords: vitamin D; type 1 diabetes; type 2 diabetes; metabolic syndrome; autoimmune; children; cancer

1. Introduction

While the skeletal effects of vitamin D are well recognized and described extensively in the literature [1–3], its extra-skeletal effects have been subject to some controversy with conflicting data reported, particularly for case-control or epidemiologic vs. prospective and interventional studies. This review aims to summarize and synthesize data regarding many extra-skeletal effects of vitamin D. Given the extensive literature reported in this area over the last two decades, we have discussed key papers that illustrate variations in data reported from the various kinds of studies, with a focus on randomized controlled trials (RCTs) and meta-analyses of existing studies.

Vitamin D_3 (cholecalciferol) is synthesized primarily in the skin on exposure to ultraviolet radiation, while vitamin D_2 (ergocalciferol) is derived from plant sources. 7-dehydrocholesterol (provitamin D; present in the stratum basale and stratum spinosum of the epidermis), is converted to previtamin D on exposure to ultraviolet radiation-B (UV-B), which is then isomerized to vitamin D. Vitamin D passes into dermal capillaries and is carried by vitamin D binding protein (DBP) to the liver, where microsomal vitamin D 25-hydroxylase catalyzes its conversion to 25-hydroxy vitamin D [25(OH)D], the storage form of vitamin D. 25(OH)D is what is reported when we ask for levels of vitamin D, and most assays report both 25(OH)D_2 and 25(OH)D_3. While controversy persists around the normative range for 25(OH)D levels, the Institute of Medicine has indicated that a 25(OH)D level at or above 20 ng/mL (50 nmol/L) is likely sufficient to optimize its skeletal effects [4]. Normative ranges for its possible extra-skeletal effects remain to be determined. Vitamin D supplements may contain either vitamin D_2 or D_3, or alfacalcidiol (1-hydroxycholecalciferol). Overall, data suggest that vitamin D_3 may be more effective in raising 25(OH)D levels than vitamin D_2 (reviewed in [5]).

25(OH)D is transported to the kidney by DBP, where cytochromal 25-hydroxyvitamin D 1-α hydroxylase catalyzes its conversion to 1,25 dihydroxy vitamin D [1,25(OH)$_2$D], the active form of vitamin D. The vitamin D receptor (VDR) is expressed in multiple cells including the osteoblasts, mononuclear cells, activated T and B lymphocytes and beta cells, and most organs in the body including the brain, heart, skin, gonads, prostate, breast, and gut. How vitamin D deficiency affects disease states in these multiple organ systems has been an active area of research. Repletion of vitamin D stores to mitigate and improve disease processes has been attempted in certain conditions, although there is a paucity of data to direct clear treatment protocols, especially in the pediatric population.

2. Immune and Anti-Inflammatory Effects

There is evidence that vitamin D modulates B and T lymphocyte function [6–9], and vitamin D deficiency has been associated with conditions such as multiple sclerosis, type 1 diabetes (T1D), rheumatoid arthritis, systemic lupus erythematosus, dermatomyositis, inflammatory bowel disease, hepatitis, asthma and respiratory infections.

2.1. Type 1 Diabetes

Data regarding associations of 25(OH)D levels or vitamin D sufficiency/insufficiency/deficiency status are conflicting with some [10,11], but not all [12–14], studies reporting an association between low vitamin D status and occurrence of T1D. Pancreatic beta cells have VDRs and express 1-α hydroxylase (encoded by *CYP27B1*) [15], and the human insulin gene promoter has a vitamin D response element [16]. Further, vitamin D plays a role in T-cell regulatory responses and may protect beta cells from immune attack [17]. In addition, T1D patients are reported to have lower 25(OH)D levels compared to age matched controls [11,18,19]. Cooper et al. [20] linked the genetic determinants of circulating 25(OH)D (*DHCR7* and *CYP2R1*, which encode 7-dehydrocholesterol reductase and 25-hydroxylase) and vitamin D signaling in T cells (*CYP27B1*) with risk of T1D, while others (including a meta-analysis of nine studies with 1053 patients and 1017 controls) have linked specific polymorphisms of the VDR gene with risk for T1D [21]. Another study linked T-cell proliferation with DBP, and reported higher levels and frequencies of serum anti-DBP antibodies in patients with T1D vs. controls. This study postulated that DBP (expressed in α-cells of pancreatic islets) may be an autoantigen in T1D [22]. Further, lower maternal third trimester DBP levels and cord blood DBP levels have been associated with risk of T1D in offspring [23,24]. Further investigation into the role of CYP27B1 in immune cells such as monocytes, macrophages and T-cells is needed to better understand the role of vitamin D in the pathogenesis and perhaps prevention of T1D. Under this umbrella of research, prospective studies of vitamin D supplementation have attempted to elucidate causality of T1D and use of vitamin D as a potential therapy.

Interventional studies: Table 1 describes details of some representative studies of vitamin D supplementation in T1D. a beneficial effect of cholecalciferol supplementation on regulatory T-cells (T-regs) has been reported, with an increase in T-reg percentage [25] and suppressive capacity [26], and reduced progression to undetectable C-peptide. Consistent with these findings, a meta-analysis of five observational studies reported a protective effect of vitamin D supplementation in early childhood against development of T1D with a dose response effect [27], while another reported that such supplementation may have prevented 27% of the predicted T1D cases in England and Wales in 2012 [28]. Similarly, a beneficial impact has been reported with respect to fasting C-peptide with lower daily insulin doses [29], peripheral vascular resistance and inflammatory renal markers [30]. However, many other studies have not demonstrated a beneficial effect of vitamin D supplementation in preventing or improving the course of T1D. Importantly, the prospective Environmental Determinants of Diabetes in the Young (TEDDY) Study demonstrated no benefit of maternal vitamin D supplementation during pregnancy on the risk of islet autoimmunity in the offspring [31]. Other studies have failed to demonstrate a beneficial impact on beta cell function [32], HbA1C levels [25,33,34] or insulin requirement [25,34]. While the reason for these conflicting results is unclear, one may speculate that differences in study design, sample size and vitamin D dosing may contribute. Overall, randomized controlled studies investigating vitamin D replacement in preventing T1D or treating at diagnosis to prolong endogenous insulin secretion are few. Vitamin D replacement is necessary in those deficient for optimal bone health. However, current data do not provide definitive evidence that supplementation will improve the inflammatory state in a clinically significant manner.

Table 1. Summary of studies of vitamin D administration in type 1 and type 2 diabetes.

Reference	Type of Study	Intervention	Participants	Results (Intervention)
Type 1 Diabetes				
Studies examining effects on immune modulation				
[25]	18-month randomized controlled trial (RCT)	2000 IUs vitamin D_3 daily or placebo	38 participants; 35 completers; 7–30 years old	Increase in regulatory T-cell (T-reg) percentage; lower cumulative incidence of progression to undetectable C-peptide; no difference in HbA1C, insulin requirement or BMI
[26]	12-month RCT	70 IUs/kg/day vitamin D_3 vs. placebo	29 Participants; >6 years old; <3 months duration of T1D	Increase in suppressive capacity of T-regs
Studies of prevention of islet autoimmunity or T1D				
[27]	Meta-analysis of four case-control and one cohort study	Vitamin D supplementation (variable doses)	Infants	Four case control studies: risk of T1D decreased; similar findings in cohort study; some evidence of a dose-response effect
[28]	Population impact number of eliminating a risk factor (PIN-ER-t) Statistical method	Vitamin D supplementation (variable doses)	Babies born in 2012	For a population of 729,674 babies born in England and Wales in 2012, 374 cases of T1D (out of 1357 total predicted cases) could be prevented over 18 years if all were supplemented with vitamin D
[31]	Cohort study; assessment every 3 months between 3–48 months, and then every 6 months	Maternal vitamin D supplementation during pregnancy (based on recall); cumulative intake of vitamin D supplements and n-3 FAs analyzed	8676 children with increased genetic risk for T1D in Finland, Germany, Sweden and the US	Vitamin D supplementation during pregnancy was not associated with risk for development of islet autoantibodies (any/none and cumulative intake)
Studies examining course or complications of T1D				
[29]	6-month RCT	0.25 mcg twice daily of alfacalcidol vs. placebo	61 participants; 54 completers; 8–15 years old; <8 weeks duration of T1D	Higher fasting C-peptide; lower daily insulin dose
[30]	12–24 weeks single arm intervention study	1000–2000 IUs of vitamin D_3 daily	271 adolescents with T1D with 25(OH)D <15 ng/mL	Improved endothelial function; decreased urinary inflammatory cytokines/chemokines; no change in systolic or diastolic blood pressure, lipids, HbA1C and albumin/creatinine ratio
[32]	2-year RCT	0.25 mcg daily of calcitriol or placebo	34 participants 11–35 years old with recent onset T1D and high basal C-peptide	No effect on beta cell function
[33]	Single dose single arm intervention study	Vitamin D_3: 100,000 IUs for those 2–10 years old; 160,000 IUs for those >10 years	40 children <19 years with T1D and vitamin D deficiency (<20 ng/mL) included in ITT analysis	No difference in HbA1C levels at 3 months or at 1 year
[34]	6-month RCT	Vitamin D_3 60,000 IUs once a month for 6 months	52 children with T1D 1–18 years old	Higher mean C-peptide level; no difference in HbA1C or insulin requirement

Table 1. Cont.

Reference	Type of Study	Intervention	Participants	Results (Intervention)
		Obesity, Prediabetes or Type 2 Diabetes		
			Adults	
[35]	Single arm intervention study	Vitamin D_3 two doses of 100,000 IUs at 2-week intervals	33 adults with vitamin D deficiency (25(OH)D < 20 ng/mL) and without T2D	No change in mean blood glucose or insulin, or insulin sensitivity (assessed using an OGTT)
[36]	6-month RCT	Vitamin D_3 4000 IUs daily or placebo	82 insulin resistant, vitamin D deficient (25(OH)D < 20 ng/mL) South Asian women in New Zealand without T2D	HOMA-IR improved when 25(OH)D level rose to >32 ng/mL; no differences in insulin secretion, CRP, BMI or lipid levels
[37]	6-month intervention study	Vitamin D_3 20,000 IUs or placebo given twice weekly over 6 months	104 adults with vitamin D deficiency; 94 completers	No difference in insulin secretion, insulin sensitivity (using a hyperglycemic clamp) or lipids
[38]	4-month RCT	Vitamin D_3 2500 IUs or placebo daily	114 post-menopausal women with 25(OH)D between 10–60 ng/mL	No improvement in blood pressure, endothelial function, arterial stiffness, inflammation and CRP
[39]	16-week RCT	Vitamin D_3 supplementation 200 IUs or placebo daily	165 healthy women 18–35 years	No change in lipids; modest change in systolic and diastolic blood pressure
[40]	5-year RCT	Vitamin D_3 20,000 IUs/week or placebo; followed every 6 months	556 adults 25–80 years old with prediabetes; 503 completers	25(OH)D increased from ~24 ng/mL to 48 ng/mL with supplementation; no effect on progression to T2D, measures of glucose metabolism, serum lipids or blood pressure in the group as a whole, or in those with vitamin D deficiency
[41]	Pooled meta-analysis of 28 RCTs	Vitamin D_3 supplementation, variable doses	Adults at risk for T2D (no T2D)	No effect on controlling fasting plasma glucose levels, improving insulin resistance, or preventing T2D; stratified analysis suggested a possible beneficial effect in those without obesity, those with prediabetes, when 25(OH)D levels were ≥20 ng/mL, and when the supplemental dose was >2000 IUs per day and given without calcium supplementation
[42]	RCT	Vitamin D_3 4000 IUs or placebo regardless of vitamin D status	2423 adult participants meeting criteria for prediabetes (2382 randomized)	No differences in baseline 25(OH)D; supplemented group had 25(OH)D levels about twice that in the placebo group; no difference in progression to T2D (9.4 vs. 10.7 events per 100 person-years respectively at a median follow-up of 2.5 years)
			Children	
[43]	6-month RCT	Vitamin D_3 4000 IUs daily or placebo	35 adolescents with obesity 9–19 years old	Improved HOMA-IR and QUICKI (but not fasting glucose, HbA1C, CRP, IL-6 or TNF-alpha) in those who received vitamin D
[44]	1-year open label parallel arm prospective study	Vitamin D_3 5000 IUs weekly for 8 weeks vs. no intervention	70 indigenous Argentinean children vs. 20 non-supplemented children	Improved HDL

Table 1. *Cont.*

Reference	Type of Study	Intervention	Participants	Results (Intervention)
[45]	12-week RCT	Vitamin D$_3$ 300,000 IUs weekly or placebo	50 children with obesity 10–16 years old	Improved serum insulin and HOMA-IR with no effect on lipids, fasting blood sugar or blood pressure
[46]	Retrospective study	Vitamin D supplementation	43 children 3–18 years old with T2D for >12 months and a diagnosis of vitamin D deficiency (25(OH)D < 20 ng/mL)	Decrease in BMI-SDS, HbA1C and ALT in supplemented group
[47]	12-week RCT	Vitamin D$_3$ 2000 IUs daily or placebo	58 adolescents with obesity 12–18 years old	No change in fasting glucose, insulin, HOMA-IR, lipids or CRP
[48]	12-week RCT	Vitamin D$_3$ two doses (400 IU/day and 2000 IU/day) for 12 weeks	51 Caucasian adolescents with obesity 12–18 years old; 46 completers	No change in 25(OH)D levels in the in 400 IU/day group and a modest increase in the 2000 IU/day group. No change in fasting HOMA-IR, insulin, glucose or lipid levels post-supplementation
[49]	2-year prospective study	Vitamin D$_3$ 100,00 IUs/year to both groups	104 children in Group a (treated in 2014) and 86 in Group B (treated in 2013)	Changes in 25(OH)D levels were significantly associated with lower LDL-C and Apo-B levels.
[50]	3-month open label, prospective study	Vitamin D$_3$ 100,000 IUs monthly for 3 months	19 children with obesity and vitamin D deficiency 13–18 years old 323 early pubertal children	No change in endothelial function, fasting lipids, glucose, insulin and CRP values
[51]	12-week RCT	Vitamin D$_3$ at either 0, 400, 1000, 2000 or 4000 IU/day for 12 weeks	At baseline, 15% had 25(OH)D levels that were insufficient <25 ng/mL, 6% had levels <16 ng/mL and 1% had levels lower than 12 ng/mL	At baseline, 25(OH)D levels were inversely associated with insulin and HOMA-IR. However, glucose, insulin and insulin resistance increased over 12 weeks in all dosage groups
[52]	12-week RCT	Vitamin D$_3$ 50,000 IUs per week vs. placebo	29 African American children with obesity 13–17 years old	No impact on insulin secretion or sensitivity

2.2. Multiple Sclerosis

The risk for multiple sclerosis (MS) is higher in people living above 35° latitudes than those who live below this latitude [53] (although effects were attenuated over time in this study), and studies have reported an association between risk for MS and lower sunlight exposure [54–59], vitamin D intake [60] and serum 25(OH)D levels [61–64]. Increased sun exposure in children has been linked to a lower risk of MS in studies out of Tasmania [57], twin studies where only one monozygotic twin developed MS [55], a study from Cuba, Martinique and Sicily [54], as well as studies in adults from Iran [58] and Sweden [59]. Other studies have linked the reduced risk of MS following sun exposure to the melanocortin 1 receptor genotype [56]. Further, polymorphisms in genes that impact 25(OH)D levels have been linked to risk of relapse in children with MS [65].

Munger et al. reported an inverse relationship between serum 25(OH)D and the risk of MS [61], and that before onset, MS risk decreases by 40% for every 20 ng/mL increase in 25(OH)D levels. In another study, women (but not men) with MS had lower 25(OH)D levels than controls 11 years after disease onset [62], with a 19% reduction in the odds for MS for every 4 ng/mL increase in winter 25(OH)D concentrations. Similar lower 25(OH)D in patients with MS versus controls has been reported in other studies for winter [63] or summer levels [64].

Data suggest that vitamin D sufficient states in the mother and infant may protect against MS [66]. Increased first trimester exposure to UVR reduced MS risk in the child in a dose dependent fashion [67]. Higher MS rates in children born in the summer or spring, and lower rates in those born in the fall may be related to maternal vitamin D insufficiency [68,69]. In the Nurses Health Study, women born to mothers with high vitamin D intake during pregnancy had a reduced risk of MS [70].

Interventional Studies: protective effects of vitamin D supplementation have been demonstrated against MS in a few studies [60]. The Nurses Health Study reported that women taking at least 400 IU of vitamin D supplements daily were at lower risk compared to those not on supplements [60,71]. a meta-analysis of 12 RCTs that included 950 adult patients with MS reported non-significant trends in improvement in annualized relapse rate Expanded Disability Status Scale scores and MRI findings in those who received vitamin D supplementation, although higher vitamin D doses (2850–10,400 IUs) performed significantly worse compared to lower doses (800–1000 IUs) [72]. One RCT did report an improvement in MRI lesions when vitamin D_3 was employed as add-on treatment to interferon beta-1b in patients with MS [73]. Data are lacking for effects of vitamin D supplementation in children with MS.

Overall, although case-control and epidemiological studies suggest that people with lower 25(OH)D levels may be at higher risk for MS, confounding factors, such as the association of higher latitudes (also a risk factor for MS) with lower 25(OH)D levels need to be considered. Interventional studies examining the preventive effect of vitamin D supplementation on the risk for developing MS are lacking. Existing RCTs in adult patients with established MS are not convincing for a significant role for vitamin D supplementation in reducing MS outcomes, although trends for a positive effect have been reported, particularly with low dose supplementation. Data to date indicate deleterious effects of high dose vitamin D supplementation on MS outcomes. RCTs assessing the impact of vitamin D supplementation on MS outcomes in children are lacking.

2.3. Rheumatoid Arthritis

One meta-analysis of 15 studies (including 1143 rheumatoid arthritis (RA) patients and 963 controls) confirmed lower 25(OH)D levels and a higher prevalence of vitamin D deficiency in patients compared with controls (55% vs. 33%) [74]. Similarly, a meta-analysis of three cohort studies that included 215,757 participants and 874 incident cases of RA reported that individuals in the highest quartile for vitamin D intake had a 24% lower risk of developing RA compared to those in the lowest quartile [75]. In addition, inverse associations of 25(OH)D levels with disease activity scores in RA patients have been reported [74,76–79]. Further, specific VDR polymorphisms have been demonstrated to contribute significantly to RA risk [80,81].

Interventional Studies: consistent with the findings from epidemiologic studies, protective effects of vitamin D supplementation have been demonstrated against RA in some studies [82]. Chandrashekara and Patted reported a reduction in disease severity scores following vitamin D replacement (60,000 IU of vitamin D weekly for six weeks followed by 60,000 IU monthly) over three months in RA patients who were vitamin D deficient (25(OH)D levels <20 ng/mL) and had persistent disease activity [83]. However, a meta-analysis that included five RCTs in patients with RA reported borderline significance for reduction in disease recurrence, but not for disease activity [84]. Calcitriol enhances inhibition of T cell activation by abatacept (CTLA-4-Ig), a CD28-ligand blocker to which patients with RA respond with variable efficacy [85], suggesting that vitamin D or calcitriol may be used as an adjunct therapy to improve efficacy of abatacept in RA patients. Overall, these data suggest that lower 25(OH)D levels may predict susceptibility to RA and its severity, but it is not clear that vitamin D supplementation reduces the risk of developing RA or its disease activity/severity. Further, data in children with RA are currently lacking.

2.4. Systemic Lupus Erythematosus (SLE) and Juvenile Dermatomyositis

Many studies have reported inverse associations of 25(OH)D levels with the occurrence and severity of SLE and dermatomyosits in adults and children [86–92]. In children, greater disease severity of SLE is reported in those with 25(OH)D levels <20 ng/mL [88].

Interventional Studies: in contrast to other autoimmune conditions, several interventional studies have reported an improvement in markers of severity of disease following vitamin D supplementation in patients with SLE. One study in adolescents and adults with juvenile onset SLE reported an improvement in disease severity scores and fatigue in those randomized to 50,000 IU per week of vitamin D supplementation compared to placebo over 6 months [93]. Similar findings are reported in studies of adults with SLE. a reduction in inflammatory and hemostatic markers, and disease activity was reported in those randomized to 2000 IU of vitamin D daily compared to placebo for 12 months [94]. Further, a meta-analysis of three RCTs of vitamin D supplementation in patients with SLE reported a significant reduction in anti-dsDNA positivity with supplementation [84]. Another study reported an increase of T-regs and a decrease of effector Th1 and Th17 cells, memory B cells and anti-DNA antibodies in adults with SLE given 100,000 IU of vitamin D weekly for 4 weeks followed by 100,000 IU monthly for 6 months [95]. No flares were observed over the study duration [95].

Overall, these data suggest that low 25(OH)D levels are concerning for greater risk of developing SLE and increased severity of the condition, and a possible beneficial effect of vitamin D supplementation on disease severity, particularly when levels are low. However, more RCTs, including in children, are necessary to confirm these data. Of note, symptoms of SLE can worsen after UV radiation exposure which will otherwise increase the vitamin D status of the individual [96]. Thus, excessive sun exposure to improve 25(OH)D levels in patients with SLE may worsen symptoms of the disease.

2.5. Psoriasis

Keratinocytes express the vitamin D receptor (VDR), and vitamin D inhibits the growth of keratinocytes, stimulates them to differentiate, and helps maintain the cutaneous barrier integrity [97]. This has led to the use of topical vitamin D analogs to treat psoriasis [98]. However, no VDR genotype (other than the TaqI polymorphsm in Caucasians) has been linked to an increased risk for psoriasis [99,100]. In addition, there is no correlation between the change in 25(OH)D post phototherapy and change in severity of symptoms of psoriasis [101,102].

Interventional Studies: a 6-month RCT of 60,000 IUs of vitamin D vs. placebo given every 2 weeks to 45 patients with psoriasis showed an increase in 25(OH)D levels in the active group associated with a reduction in the Psoriasis Area and Severity Index (PASI) [103]. Topical vitamin D analogs (calcipotriene/calcipotriol/maxacalcitol) given with topical betamethasone have also been shown to be effective in improving plaque psoriasis [104–106] by disrupting the IL-36 and IL-23/IL-17 positive feedback loop, key factors in the pathogenesis of psoriasis.

Overall, while studies suggest an association between 25(OH)D levels and psoriasis, causation is yet to be established. Additionally, RCTs to date are promising for an impact of vitamin D on psoriasis severity, but studies are small, and more and larger RCTs are necessary to confirm these preliminary findings. Data in children are lacking.

2.6. Inflammatory Bowel Disease (IBD)

Protective effects of vitamin D supplementation have been demonstrated against IBD [107]. Vitamin D deficient and vitamin D receptor (*Vdr*) null mice are at high risk of IBD [108], with more severe disease and more spontaneous recurrences. Further, polymorphisms in the *Vdr* gene (TaqI) may confer susceptibility to IBD [109]. a meta-analysis of VDR genotyping in relation to IBD reported that ApaI polymorphism may increase the risk of Crohn's disease, whereas the TaqI polymorphism may decrease the risk of ulcerative colitis, especially in Caucasians [110]. a connection has been proposed between seasonal vitamin D status and risk for both Crohn's disease and ulcerative colitis [111,112], with an association between vitamin D deficiency and more complicated disease course. a recent meta-analysis reported lower 25(OH)D levels in patients with both Crohn's disease and ulcerative colitis than controls, a two-fold risk of vitamin D deficiency in those with IBD, and greater severity of Crohn's disease in those with vitamin D deficiency [113,114]. However, these studies are associative and confounded by the fact that malabsorption (particularly in Crohn's disease) may contribute to lower 25(OH)D levels, with more severe disease being associated with more malabsorption.

Interventional studies: there are few randomized controlled trials that have examined the impact of vitamin D supplementation on disease occurrence or severity. One randomized controlled trial of 400 vs. 2000 IU of vitamin D supplementation in children and adolescents with IBD did report that the higher dose of vitamin D led to lower levels of pro-inflammatory markers [115]. Vitamin D has also been shown to exert marked anti-inflammatory effects on peripheral and intestinal CD4+ and CD8+ T cells of patients with inflammatory bowel disorders in vitro, and inhibit production of TH1 and TH17 cytokines in patients with Crohn's disease in vivo [116].

Overall, while data to date suggest that vitamin D deficiency may impact disease course in patients with inflammatory bowel disorders, we are in need of robust RCTs that will help determine whether vitamin D supplementation is indeed efficacious in reducing disease severity in these patients, including in children.

2.7. Food Allergies

Although associations of low 25(OH)D levels with a risk of atopy, asthma and food allergies have been reported [117], recent birth cohort studies demonstrate no association of 25(OH)D levels (including antenatal vitamin D exposure) with the incidence of food allergy [118,119]. One meta-analysis of more than 5000 children did not find a significant association between vitamin D status and food allergy [120].

Interventional Studies: data for the role of vitamin D supplementation in preventing food allergies is inconsistent, and large trials are necessary to determine the role if any of vitamin D in reducing the risk for food allergies [121]. One RCT of 400 vs. 1200 IUs of vitamin D supplementation in 975 infants from the age of 2 weeks found no impact of higher-dose vitamin D supplementation on allergic sensitization or allergic diseases (food or aeroallergen) at 12-months of age [122]. Overall, current data do not support a role of vitamin D status in impacting the risk for food allergies in children, and non-interventional studies may be confounded by variables such as associated malabsorption.

2.8. Chronic Hepatitis B and C

Certain vitamin D receptor gene (*VDR* a/a) polymorphisms have been linked to greater severity of hepatitis B infection and a higher viral load [123]. In addition, polymorphisms in the T/T allele of exon 9 of the *VDR* gene (but not intron 8 polymorphisms) are associated with occult hepatitis B infection [124]. Further, a meta-analysis of seven studies involving 814 patients with chronic hepatitis B and 696 controls showed lower 25(OH)D levels in patients with chronic hepatitis B associated with higher viral loads [125]. Petta et al. [126] reported that lower 25(OH)D levels in chronic hepatitis C infection were related to decreased CYP27A1 expression, female gender, necrosis and inflammation, severe fibrosis and poor viral response to interferon based therapy. Of note, polymorphisms in the VDR gene have been associated with development of hepatocellular carcinoma in patients with hepatitis C [127].

Interventional Studies: in in vitro studies, 25(OH)D has been shown to inhibit hepatitis C virus production by suppressing apolipoprotein expression [128]. In 42 patients with recurrent hepatitis C infections treated with INF-α and ribavirin for 48 weeks, vitamin D deficiency was associated with an unfavorable response to antiviral medication, and 15 patients given oral vitamin D supplements had a better and more sustained response to antiviral treatment [129]. One short 6-week RCT of vitamin D supplementation vs. placebo in 54 patients with chronic hepatitis C with vitamin D deficiency demonstrated improved serum markers of hepatic fibrogenesis upon correction of 25(OH)D levels [130].

Overall, data suggest deleterious effects of vitamin D deficiency on the course of chronic hepatitis B and C infections, with some studies suggesting a possible role (and mechanism) for vitamin D supplementation in improving outcomes in these patients. However, we are in need of larger RCTs and of longer duration to effectively confirm these findings, and data in children are lacking.

2.9. Asthma and Respiratory Infections

Several studies have reported an association between vitamin D deficiency (25(OH)D < 20 ng/mL) and increased airway inflammation, decreased lung function, increased exacerbations, and poor prognosis in patients with asthma (reviewed in [131]).

Interventional Studies: a literature review of RCTs of vitamin D supplementation in children older than 2 years found a possible effect of vitamin D supplementation in improving bronchial asthma exacerbation [132,133], but no effect on the severity of asthma [132]. a subsequent meta-analysis that included 435 children (seven trials) and 658 adults (two trials) similarly reported a reduction in asthma exacerbations requiring systemic corticosteroids and the risk for an exacerbation requiring an emergency department visit or hospitalization in those who received vitamin D supplementation, but not on measures of severity (% predicted forced expiratory volume in one second or Asthma Control test Scores [134]. The improvement in asthma exacerbation has been attributed to a decrease in respiratory infections [12].

RCTs of vitamin D supplementation (300–1200 IUs per day) vs. placebo report a potential effect of vitamin D in reducing the risk for influenza infections during the winter months [135], although a subsequent analysis reported that benefits observed in the first month of supplementation were lost in the second month, and overall there was no difference among groups for influenza prevalence over the entire season [136]. a meta-analysis of 25 RCTs using vitamin D supplementation of any duration in individuals 0–95 years old demonstrated that vitamin D reduced the risk for acute respiratory infections overall, with the greatest benefit in those with low 25(OH)D levels (<10 ng/mL), and those receiving daily or weekly vitamin D supplementation vs. bolus doses [137,138]. Effects may be less robust in those 1–5 years old [139], and a dose effect has not been demonstrated [140].

Overall, these data suggest that vitamin D may have an effect in reducing the risk for respiratory infections in children, with more pronounced effects after 5 years of age, and in those that are vitamin D deficient. This effect may explain the reduced risk of asthma exacerbations in children with vitamin D supplementation (although asthma severity does not appear to improve with vitamin D). The mechanism underlying the effect on respiratory infections needs to be determined, but may involve the impact of vitamin D on inflammatory pathways.

3. Metabolic Syndrome and Type 2 Diabetes Mellitus

Although, VDR polymorphisms are unlikely to play a major role in obesity-related phenotypes, as reported in a population of Caucasian adults [141], vitamin D deficiency has been associated with obesity in both pediatric and adult populations. The prevalence of vitamin D deficiency is about 50% in children with obesity [142,143], and attributable to decreased sun exposure secondary to low activity level, poor nutrition with decreased consumption of vitamin D containing foods such as milk, as well as storage in adipose tissue [142]. With the increased prevalence of obesity in children there has also been concern of increased prevalence of type 2 DM (T2D), dyslipidemia and hypertension, the metabolic syndrome [1]. The role vitamin D plays in contributing to these disorders has been of interest given the above association and implications for potential treatment. Exactly which aspects of the metabolic syndrome are associated with vitamin D deficiency have not been definitively delineated as studies show varied results. Olson et al. found a negative correlation between 25(OH)D levels and HOMA-IR (homeostasis model assessment of insulin resistance) and weaker but significant inverse correlations with 2-h glucose levels in an oral glucose tolerance test (OGTT). There was no correlation with HbA1C, systolic blood pressure (SBP) or diastolic blood pressure (DBP) [142]. In another study vitamin D deficiency in children with obesity was associated with higher BMI and SBP, and decreased HDL-C [143]. After adjusting for BMI in Native American children, 25(OH)D levels were inversely associated with log transformed fasting 2-h glucose, fasting insulin, HOMA-IR, triglyceride and CRP levels, and SBP and DBP. There was a positive correlation with HDL but no correlation with total or LDL cholesterol [144]. Studies have postulated that adipokines such as adiponectin and resistin may be involved in the pathogenesis of insulin resistance and vitamin D deficiency. a study of 125 children and adolescents with obesity showed a trend toward lower 25(OH)D levels being associated with low adiponectin levels and higher insulin resistance even after adjusting for body mass, though there was no correlation between 25(OH)D levels and resistin [145].

Conversely, Poomthavorn et al. [146] found no correlation between vitamin D deficiency and abnormal glucose homeostasis in 150 children and adolescents with obesity living in Thailand. In fact, the five children identified with T2D in this study were all vitamin D sufficient. They also found the same degree of vitamin D deficiency in 29 healthy children without obesity [146]. Similarly, Bril et al. found no relationship between lower 25(OH)D levels and insulin resistance (using an euglycemic insulin clamp), liver fat accumulation or steatohepatitis when adult patients with the latter were matched for BMI and total adiposity with controls [147]. More recently, in a study of 215 children with T1D and 326 children with T2D vs. youth of similar age without diabetes from the 2005–2006 NHANES Survey, the prevalence of vitamin D deficiency or insufficiency did not differ in children with vs. those without diabetes [14]. Additionally, although latitude and the winter months have been associated with a higher risk of hypertension, recent studies suggest that the effect of ultraviolet light on blood pressure is likely mediated via nitric oxide synthesis and not through vitamin D production [148]. Limitations of pediatric studies include the fact that these associative studies often do not include controls matched for measures of adiposity, or use euglycemic clamps to assess insulin resistance. In addition, sample sizes are small and length of studies short. Associations of vitamin D deficiency with worsening insulin resistance or other aspects of the metabolic syndrome are yet to be proven.

Interventional studies in adults and adolescents are described in detail in Table 1 and are summarized here.

Interventional Studies in Adults with Obesity, Prediabetes and T2D: the contribution of vitamin D to the metabolic phenotype of obesity is of interest given implications for treatment. If these associations have a biological basis, repleting vitamin D should improve the phenotype. How this should be done, to what level of replacement, and the actual efficacy have been the basis of several studies. Vitamin D administration in adults has had mixed results for progression to T2D and cardio-metabolic outcomes. Among short-term studies with small numbers of participants, most have reported no changes in insulin sensitivity [35], insulin secretion [36,37], CRP [36,38], BMI [36], lipids [36,37,39], blood pressure, endothelial function, and arterial stiffness [38] following vitamin D administration, while a few have reported an improvement in insulin sensitivity [36] and blood pressure [39]. Among larger and longer-term studies, a five-year interventional study in 556 adults 25–80 years old at risk for developing T2D, reported no impact of vitamin D administration on progression to T2D, measures of glucose metabolism, serum lipids or blood pressure [40]. a subsequent pooled meta-analysis of 23 RCTs similarly found no effect of vitamin D supplementation in controlling fasting plasma glucose levels, improving insulin resistance, or preventing T2D; however, stratified analysis suggested a possible beneficial effect in those without obesity, those with prediabetes, when 25(OH)D levels were at least 20 ng/mL, and when the supplemental dose was >2000 IUs per day and given without calcium supplementation [41]. Yet, an RCT in adult participants meeting criteria for prediabetes (but not diabetes) reported no difference between groups for onset of diabetes over the study duration [42].

Interventional Studies in Children with Obesity, Prediabetes and T2D: similar to the adult literature, the pediatric literature includes conflicting data regarding effects of vitamin D supplementation [43–52] (Table 1). a retrospective study of vitamin D supplementation in 43 children 3–18 years old with T2D reported a decrease in BMI-SDS and HbA1C in those supplemented with vitamin D [46]. A few prospective studies in adolescents with obesity have similarly reported improved HOMA-IR and QUICKI (but not in fasting glucose, HbA1C, CRP, inflammatory markers, blood pressure) [43,45] following vitamin D administration, and an association of reductions in Apo-B and LDL-C, and increases in HDL with increases in 25(OH)D levels after supplementation [44,49]. However, most prospective interventional studies in children with obesity have failed to demonstrate a beneficial effect of vitamin D administration on fasting lipids, glucose, insulin and CRP values [47,48,50,51], and insulin secretion or sensitivity [52], and dose response studies have similarly not been able to demonstrate an effect of increasing vitamin D doses on fasting glucose, insulin and insulin resistance [48,51] or lipid levels [48].

Overall data indicate that there is an association between obesity and vitamin D deficiency (likely related to sequestration of vitamin D in adipose depots). However, the biological effect of vitamin D deficiency on insulin resistance, hypertension, hyperlipidemia and progression to T2D is likely small. Data are conflicting regarding associations of vitamin D deficiency with components of the metabolic syndrome, as well as a treatment effect. Some differences may be attributable to the type of study, sample size, and dose of vitamin D used (Table 1). Larger and longer-term prospective studies are needed to definitively determine causality.

4. Cancer

In cell culture studies, 25(OH)D concentrations of >30 ng/mL prevent unregulated cell growth [149–151]. There are very little data for the role of vitamin D in preventing or ameliorating the course of cancer in children, although low 25(OH)vitamin D levels may contribute to poor bone health in children with hematological and other malignancies [152–154]. Much of the data for the impact of vitamin D in preventing or reducing the morbidity of cancer comes from studies in adults, particularly in the context of breast, colorectal and prostate cancer. This section briefly reviews existing literature for these three kinds of cancer.

In breast cancer cell lines, vitamin D signaling inhibits expression of a tumor progression gene (Id1), and ablation of VDR expression causes increased tumor growth and development of metastases [155]. This pathway is inhibited in murine models of breast cancer associated with vitamin D deficiency, and epidemiological studies in humans suggest associations of vitamin D deficiency and the risk of breast, prostate and colon cancer [156–158]. However, data are conflicting regarding the impact of vitamin D receptor genotype and cancer risk at this time [159]. One study reported that *VDR* single nucleotide polymorphisms and haplotypes may determine how inflammatory markers change in breast cancer survivors with vitamin D deficiency, following vitamin D supplementation [160].

In general, vitamin D deficiency is associated with increased risk of progression and mortality in breast cancers [161–163]. Of note, these data have been questioned in that meta-analyses indicate that while case control studies suggest a reduction in breast cancer risk in those with higher 25(OH)D levels, this is not evident in prospective studies [163,164]. Data suggest that weight and alcohol intake may modify associations between vitamin D intake and breast cancer risk [165]. Of note, the Women's Health Initiative demonstrated no reduction in risk for breast cancer in women receiving 400 IU vitamin D_3 and 1000 mg of calcium vs. placebo [166]. However, a decreased risk was noted in postmenopausal women on hormone replacement therapy from daily vitamin D and calcium supplements [167], and another study reported improved breast cancer survival in patients after surgery of invasive breast cancer in de novo vitamin D users [168]. One recent 12-month RCT of 20,000 IUs of vitamin D vs. placebo in 208 premenopausal women at high risk for breast cancer found no effect of vitamin D supplementation in reducing breast cancer risk (assessed using mammographic density) [169]. Similarly, an RCT of 2000 IUs of vitamin D and omega-3 fatty acids (1 g daily) (2 × 2 factorial design) in women 55 and older and men 50 and older found no effect of vitamin D supplementation in lowering the incidence of invasive cancer compared to placebo [170].

Meta-analyses have reported inverse associations of 25(OH)D levels and vitamin D intake with the incidence and recurrence of colorectal adenoma [171–174]. One meta-analysis suggested a 10%–20% reduction in risk of incidence or recurrence of colorectal adenomas with every 20 ng/mL increase in 25(OH)D levels [171]. Another meta-analysis suggested a 26% reduction in risk with every 10 ng/mL increase in 25(OH)D levels [175,176]. However, a large Mendelian randomization study that included 10,725 colorectal cancer cases and 30,794 controls found no evidence for a causal relationship between circulating 25(OH)D and colorectal cancer risk. These authors suggested that circulating vitamin D may be a biomarker of colorectal cancer, rather than a causative factor [177]. Thus far, data for a role of VDR polymorphisms in mediating the risk of colorectal adenomas are conflicting, with no associations reported in more recent studies [176,178].

Some studies have suggested that vitamin D with or without calcium supplementation promotes colorectal epithelial cell differentiation, reduces proliferation, and promotes apoptosis, and is thus chemopreventive against colorectal neoplasms [179]. Further, a higher expression of CYP24A1, which reduces local 1,25-D (3) availability and thus its antiproliferative effect, has been demonstrated in colorectal adenocarcinomas, associated with increased expression of the proliferation marker Ki-67 [180]. Despite these data and consistent with the Mendelian randomization study, randomized controlled trials and meta-analyses do not support a role of vitamin D supplementation in preventing these cancers [161,181,182] or relapses [183–185]. Baron et al. disappointingly reported that daily supplementation with vitamin D_3 (1000 IU), calcium (1200 mg), or both after removal of colorectal adenomas did not reduce the risk of recurrence over a 3–5 year period [184]. Similarly, Urashima et al. reported no improvement in relapse free survival in patients with digestive tract cancers (48% were colorectal cancers) randomized to 2000 IUs of vitamin D vs. placebo (AMATERASU RCT) [185]. However, in the SUNSHINE trial (a phase 2 RCT in which 139 patients with advanced or metastatic colorectal cancer were randomized to chemotherapy plus high-dose vitamin D_3 supplementation (8000 IUs daily for one month followed by 4000 IUs daily vs. chemotherapy plus standard-dose vitamin D_3 (400 IUs daily)) the higher vitamin D dose was associated with a multivariable hazard ratio of 0.64 for progression-free survival or death that was statistically significant [186].

Sun exposure may delay the onset of prostate cancer [157] while serum 25(OH)D levels of at least 20 ng/mL appear to reduce the risk for prostate cancer by 50% [187]. However, data for associations of vitamin D deficiency with incidence of prostate cancer are weaker than those for colon cancer, and data for associations with progression are inconsistent [161,188].

Overall, at this time, data do not support a significant role of vitamin D supplementation in preventing or changing the course of breast, colorectal or prostate cancer.

5. Conclusions

In conclusion, vitamin D may have biological effects well beyond the skeleton. While it is important to maintain adequate 25(OH)D levels for optimal bone health, this may have benefits in a variety of different organ systems. However, interventional studies to prevent or ameliorate disease processes attributable to vitamin D deficiency in large populations have been disappointing thus far for the most part. More investigation is needed to determine optimal dosing and serum levels to effect positive biological outcomes.

Author Contributions: R.M. and M.M. contributed equally to the concept of this manuscript, the required literature review, and the writing of this manuscript. Both authors approved the submitted version of the manuscript.

Funding: This research was funded in part by K24 HD071843 (Misra).

Conflicts of Interest: The authors have no conflict of interest to disclose relevant to this manuscript.

References

1. Misra, M.; Pacaud, D.; Petryk, A.; Collett-Solberg, P.F.; Kappy, M. Vitamin D deficiency in children and its management: Review of current knowledge and recommendations. *Pediatrics* **2008**, *122*, 398–417. [CrossRef] [PubMed]
2. Holick, M.F.; Binkley, N.C.; Bischoff-Ferrari, H.A.; Gordon, C.M.; Hanley, D.A.; Heaney, R.P.; Murad, M.H.; Weaver, C.M. Guidelines for preventing and treating vitamin D deficiency and insufficiency revisited. *J. Clin. Endocrinol. Metab.* **2012**, *97*, 1153–1158. [CrossRef] [PubMed]
3. Holick, M.F.; Binkley, N.C.; Bischoff-Ferrari, H.A.; Gordon, C.M.; Hanley, D.A.; Heaney, R.P.; Murad, M.H.; Weaver, C.M. Evaluation, treatment, and prevention of vitamin D deficiency: An Endocrine Society clinical practice guideline. *J. Clin. Endocrinol. Metab.* **2011**, *96*, 1911–1930. [CrossRef] [PubMed]
4. Ross, A.C.; Manson, J.E.; Abrams, S.A.; Aloia, J.F.; Brannon, P.M.; Clinton, S.K.; Durazo-Arvizu, R.A.; Gallagher, J.C.; Gallo, R.L.; Jones, G.; et al. The 2011 report on dietary reference intakes for calcium and vitamin D from the Institute of Medicine: What clinicians need to know. *J. Clin. Endocrinol. Metab.* **2011**, *96*, 53–58. [CrossRef] [PubMed]
5. Guo, J.; Lovegrove, J.A.; Givens, D.I. 25(OH)D_3-enriched or fortified foods are more efficient at tackling inadequate vitamin D status than vitamin D_3. *Proc. Nutr. Soc.* **2018**, *77*, 282–291. [CrossRef] [PubMed]
6. Tsoukas, C.D.; Provvedini, D.M.; Manolagas, S.C. 1,25-dihydroxyvitamin D_3: A novel immunoregulatory hormone. *Science* **1984**, *224*, 1438–1440. [CrossRef] [PubMed]
7. Bhalla, A.K.; Amento, E.P.; Clemens, T.L.; Holick, M.F.; Krane, S.M. Specific high-affinity receptors for 1,25-dihydroxyvitamin D_3 in human peripheral blood mononuclear cells: Presence in monocytes and induction in T lymphocytes following activation. *J. Clin. Endocrinol. Metab.* **1983**, *57*, 1308–1310. [CrossRef] [PubMed]
8. Drozdenko, G.; Scheel, T.; Heine, G.; Baumgrass, R.; Worm, M. Impaired T cell activation and cytokine production by calcitriol-primed human B cells. *Clin. Exp. Immunol.* **2014**, *178*, 364–372. [CrossRef] [PubMed]
9. Milliken, S.V.; Wassall, H.; Lewis, B.J.; Logie, J.; Barker, R.N.; Macdonald, H.; Vickers, M.A.; Ormerod, A.D. Effects of ultraviolet light on human serum 25-hydroxyvitamin D and systemic immune function. *J. Allergy Clin. Immunol.* **2012**, *129*, 1554–1561. [CrossRef]
10. Al-Zubeidi, H.; Leon-Chi, L.; Newfield, R.S. Low vitamin D level in pediatric patients with new onset type 1 diabetes is common, especially if in ketoacidosis. *Pediatr. Diabetes* **2016**, *17*, 592–598. [CrossRef]
11. Savastio, S.; Cadario, F.; Genoni, G.; Bellomo, G.; Bagnati, M.; Secco, G.; Picchi, R.; Giglione, E.; Bona, G. Vitamin D Deficiency and Glycemic Status in Children and Adolescents with Type 1 Diabetes Mellitus. *PLoS ONE* **2016**, *11*, e0162554. [CrossRef] [PubMed]
12. Makinen, M.; Mykkanen, J.; Koskinen, M.; Simell, V.; Veijola, R.; Hyoty, H.; Ilonen, J.; Knip, M.; Simell, O.; Toppari, J. Serum 25-Hydroxyvitamin D Concentrations in Children Progressing to Autoimmunity and Clinical Type 1 Diabetes. *J. Clin. Endocrinol. Metab.* **2016**, *101*, 723–729. [CrossRef] [PubMed]
13. Granfors, M.; Augustin, H.; Ludvigsson, J.; Brekke, H.K. No association between use of multivitamin supplement containing vitamin D during pregnancy and risk of Type 1 Diabetes in the child. *Pediatr. Diabetes* **2016**, *17*, 525–530. [CrossRef] [PubMed]
14. Wood, J.R.; Connor, C.G.; Cheng, P.; Ruedy, K.J.; Tamborlane, W.V.; Klingensmith, G.; Schatz, D.; Gregg, B.; Cengiz, E.; Willi, S.; et al. Vitamin D status in youth with type 1 and type 2 diabetes enrolled in the Pediatric Diabetes Consortium (PDC) is not worse than in youth without diabetes. *Pediatr. Diabetes* **2016**, *17*, 584–591. [CrossRef] [PubMed]
15. Bland, R.; Markovic, D.; Hills, C.E.; Hughes, S.V.; Chan, S.L.; Squires, P.E.; Hewison, M. Expression of 25-hydroxyvitamin D_3-1alpha-hydroxylase in pancreatic islets. *J. Steroid Biochem. Mol. Biol.* **2004**, *89*, 121–125. [CrossRef] [PubMed]
16. Maestro, B.; Davila, N.; Carranza, M.C.; Calle, C. Identification of a Vitamin D response element in the human insulin receptor gene promoter. *J. Steroid Biochem. Mol. Biol.* **2003**, *84*, 223–230. [CrossRef]
17. El-Fakhri, N.; McDevitt, H.; Shaikh, M.G.; Halsey, C.; Ahmed, S.F. Vitamin D and its effects on glucose homeostasis, cardiovascular function and immune function. *Horm. Res. Paediatr.* **2014**, *81*, 363–378. [CrossRef]
18. Bae, K.N.; Nam, H.K.; Rhie, Y.J.; Song, D.J.; Lee, K.H. Low levels of 25-hydroxyvitamin D in children and adolescents with type 1 diabetes mellitus: A single center experience. *Ann. Pediatr. Endocrinol. Metab.* **2018**, *23*, 21–27. [CrossRef]

19. Federico, G.; Genoni, A.; Puggioni, A.; Saba, A.; Gallo, D.; Randazzo, E.; Salvatoni, A.; Toniolo, A. Vitamin D status, enterovirus infection, and type 1 diabetes in Italian children/adolescents. *Pediatr. Diabetes* **2018**, *19*, 923–929. [CrossRef]
20. Cooper, J.D.; Smyth, D.J.; Walker, N.M.; Stevens, H.; Burren, O.S.; Wallace, C.; Greissl, C.; Ramos-Lopez, E.; Hypponen, E.; Dunger, D.B.; et al. Inherited variation in vitamin D genes is associated with predisposition to autoimmune disease type 1 diabetes. *Diabetes* **2011**, *60*, 1624–1631. [CrossRef]
21. Sahin, O.A.; Goksen, D.; Ozpinar, A.; Serdar, M.; Onay, H. Association of vitamin D receptor polymorphisms and type 1 diabetes susceptibility in children: A meta-analysis. *Endocr. Connect.* **2017**, *6*, 159–171. [CrossRef] [PubMed]
22. Kodama, K.; Zhao, Z.; Toda, K.; Yip, L.; Fuhlbrigge, R.; Miao, D.; Fathman, C.G.; Yamada, S.; Butte, A.J.; Yu, L. Expression-Based Genome-Wide Association Study Links Vitamin D-Binding Protein with Autoantigenicity in Type 1 Diabetes. *Diabetes* **2016**, *65*, 1341–1349. [CrossRef] [PubMed]
23. Sorensen, I.M.; Joner, G.; Jenum, P.A.; Eskild, A.; Brunborg, C.; Torjesen, P.A.; Stene, L.C. Vitamin D-binding protein and 25-hydroxyvitamin D during pregnancy in mothers whose children later developed type 1 diabetes. *Diabetes Metab. Res. Rev.* **2016**, *32*, 883–890. [CrossRef] [PubMed]
24. Tapia, G.; Marild, K.; Dahl, S.R.; Lund-Blix, N.A.; Viken, M.K.; Lie, B.A.; Njolstad, P.R.; Joner, G.; Skrivarhaug, T.; Cohen, A.S.; et al. Maternal and Newborn Vitamin D-Binding Protein, Vitamin D Levels, Vitamin D Receptor Genotype, and Childhood Type 1 Diabetes. *Diabetes Care* **2019**, *42*, 553–559. [CrossRef] [PubMed]
25. Gabbay, M.A.; Sato, M.N.; Finazzo, C.; Duarte, A.J.; Dib, S.A. Effect of cholecalciferol as adjunctive therapy with insulin on protective immunologic profile and decline of residual beta-cell function in new-onset type 1 diabetes mellitus. *Arch. Pediatr. Adolesc. Med.* **2012**, *166*, 601–607. [CrossRef]
26. Treiber, G.; Prietl, B.; Frohlich-Reiterer, E.; Lechner, E.; Ribitsch, A.; Fritsch, M.; Rami-Merhar, B.; Steigleder-Schweiger, C.; Graninger, W.; Borkenstein, M.; et al. Cholecalciferol supplementation improves suppressive capacity of regulatory T-cells in young patients with new-onset type 1 diabetes mellitus—A randomized clinical trial. *Clin. Immunol.* **2015**, *161*, 217–224. [CrossRef] [PubMed]
27. Zipitis, C.S.; Akobeng, A.K. Vitamin D supplementation in early childhood and risk of type 1 diabetes: A systematic review and meta-analysis. *Arch. Dis. Child.* **2008**, *93*, 512–517. [CrossRef] [PubMed]
28. Zipitis, C.S.; Mughal, Z.M.; Clayton, P.E. Assessing the population impact of low rates of vitamin D supplementation on type 1 diabetes using a new statistical method. *JRSM Open* **2016**, *7*. [CrossRef] [PubMed]
29. Ataie-Jafari, A.; Loke, S.C.; Rahmat, A.B.; Larijani, B.; Abbasi, F.; Leow, M.K.; Yassin, Z. a randomized placebo-controlled trial of alphacalcidol on the preservation of beta cell function in children with recent onset type 1 diabetes. *Clin. Nutr.* **2013**, *32*, 911–917. [CrossRef]
30. Deda, L.; Yeshayahu, Y.; Sud, S.; Cuerden, M.; Cherney, D.Z.; Sochett, E.B.; Mahmud, F.H. Improvements in peripheral vascular function with vitamin D treatment in deficient adolescents with type 1 diabetes. *Pediatr. Diabetes* **2018**, *19*, 457–463. [CrossRef] [PubMed]
31. Silvis, K.; Aronsson, C.A.; Liu, X.; Uusitalo, U.; Yang, J.; Tamura, R.; Lernmark, A.; Rewers, M.; Hagopian, W.; She, J.X.; et al. Maternal dietary supplement use and development of islet autoimmunity in the offspring: TEDDY study. *Pediatr. Diabetes* **2019**, *20*, 86–92. [CrossRef] [PubMed]
32. Bizzarri, C.; Pitocco, D.; Napoli, N.; Di Stasio, E.; Maggi, D.; Manfrini, S.; Suraci, C.; Cavallo, M.G.; Cappa, M.; Ghirlanda, G.; et al. No protective effect of calcitriol on beta-cell function in recent-onset type 1 diabetes: The IMDIAB XIII trial. *Diabetes Care* **2010**, *33*, 1962–1963. [CrossRef] [PubMed]
33. Perchard, R.; Magee, L.; Whatmore, A.; Ivison, F.; Murray, P.; Stevens, A.; Mughal, M.Z.; Ehtisham, S.; Campbell, J.; Ainsworth, S.; et al. a pilot interventional study to evaluate the impact of cholecalciferol treatment on HbA1c in type 1 diabetes (T1D). *Endocr. Connect.* **2017**, *6*, 225–231. [CrossRef] [PubMed]
34. Sharma, S.; Biswal, N.; Bethou, A.; Rajappa, M.; Kumar, S.; Vinayagam, V. Does Vitamin D Supplementation Improve Glycaemic Control in Children with Type 1 Diabetes Mellitus?—A Randomized Controlled Trial. *J. Clin. Diagn. Res.* **2017**, *11*, SC15. [CrossRef] [PubMed]
35. Tai, K.; Need, A.G.; Horowitz, M.; Chapman, I.M. Glucose tolerance and vitamin D: Effects of treating vitamin D deficiency. *Nutrition* **2008**, *24*, 950–956. [CrossRef] [PubMed]
36. Von Hurst, P.R.; Stonehouse, W.; Coad, J. Vitamin D supplementation reduces insulin resistance in South Asian women living in New Zealand who are insulin resistant and vitamin D deficient—A randomised, placebo-controlled trial. *Br. J. Nutr.* **2010**, *103*, 549–555. [CrossRef] [PubMed]

37. Grimnes, G.; Figenschau, Y.; Almas, B.; Jorde, R. Vitamin D insulin secretion, sensitivity, and lipids: Results from a case-control study and a randomized controlled trial using hyperglycemic clamp technique. *Diabetes* **2011**, *60*, 2748–2757. [CrossRef]
38. Gepner, A.D.; Ramamurthy, R.; Krueger, D.C.; Korcarz, C.E.; Binkley, N.; Stein, J.H. a prospective randomized controlled trial of the effects of vitamin D supplementation on cardiovascular disease risk. *PLoS ONE* **2012**, *7*, e36617. [CrossRef]
39. Toxqui, L.; Blanco-Rojo, R.; Wright, I.; Perez-Granados, A.M.; Vaquero, M.P. Changes in blood pressure and lipid levels in young women consuming a vitamin D-fortified skimmed milk: A randomised controlled trial. *Nutrients* **2013**, *5*, 4966–4977. [CrossRef]
40. Jorde, R.; Sollid, S.T.; Svartberg, J.; Schirmer, H.; Joakimsen, R.M.; Njolstad, I.; Fuskevag, O.M.; Figenschau, Y.; Hutchinson, M.Y. Vitamin D 20,000 IU per Week for Five Years Does Not Prevent Progression from Prediabetes to Diabetes. *J. Clin. Endocrinol. Metab.* **2016**, *101*, 1647–1655. [CrossRef]
41. He, S.; Yu, S.; Zhou, Z.; Wang, C.; Wu, Y.; Li, W. Effect of vitamin D supplementation on fasting plasma glucose, insulin resistance and prevention of type 2 diabetes mellitus in non-diabetics: A systematic review and meta-analysis. *Biomed. Rep.* **2018**, *8*, 475–484. [CrossRef] [PubMed]
42. Pittas, A.G.; Dawson-Hughes, B.; Sheehan, P.; Ware, J.H.; Knowler, W.C.; Aroda, V.R.; Brodsky, I.; Ceglia, L.; Chadha, C.; Chatterjee, R.; et al. Vitamin D Supplementation and Prevention of Type 2 Diabetes. *N. Engl. J. Med.* **2019**. [CrossRef] [PubMed]
43. Belenchia, A.M.; Tosh, A.K.; Hillman, L.S.; Peterson, C.A. Correcting vitamin D insufficiency improves insulin sensitivity in obese adolescents: A randomized controlled trial. *Am. J. Clin. Nutr.* **2013**, *97*, 774–781. [CrossRef] [PubMed]
44. Hirschler, V.; Maccallini, G.; Sanchez, M.; Claudio, G.; Molinari, C.; Figueroa, M.; Arnada, C.; Hidalgo, M. Improvement of Apolipoprotein B in Argentine Indigenous School Children after Vitamin D Supplementation. *Cardiovasc. Hematol. Agents Med. Chem.* **2015**, *13*, 137–145. [CrossRef] [PubMed]
45. Kelishadi, R.; Salek, S.; Salek, M.; Hashemipour, M.; Movahedian, M. Effects of vitamin D supplementation on insulin resistance and cardiometabolic risk factors in children with metabolic syndrome: A triple-masked controlled trial. *J. Pediatr.* **2014**, *90*, 28–34. [CrossRef] [PubMed]
46. Nwosu, B.U.; Maranda, L. The effects of vitamin D supplementation on hepatic dysfunction, vitamin D status, and glycemic control in children and adolescents with vitamin D deficiency and either type 1 or type 2 diabetes mellitus. *PLoS ONE* **2014**, *9*, e99646. [CrossRef] [PubMed]
47. Nader, N.S.; Aguirre Castaneda, R.; Wallace, J.; Singh, R.; Weaver, A.; Kumar, S. Effect of vitamin D_3 supplementation on serum 25(OH)D, lipids and markers of insulin resistance in obese adolescents: A prospective, randomized, placebo-controlled pilot trial. *Horm. Res. Paediatr.* **2014**, *82*, 107–112. [CrossRef] [PubMed]
48. Javed, A.; Vella, A.; Balagopal, P.B.; Fischer, P.R.; Weaver, A.L.; Piccinini, F.; Dalla Man, C.; Cobelli, C.; Giesler, P.D.; Laugen, J.M.; et al. Cholecalciferol supplementation does not influence beta-cell function and insulin action in obese adolescents: A prospective double-blind randomized trial. *J. Nutr.* **2015**, *145*, 284–290. [CrossRef] [PubMed]
49. Hirschler, V.; Maccallini, G.; Sanchez, M.S.; Castano, L.; Molinari, C. Improvement in high-density lipoprotein cholesterol levels in argentine Indian school children after vitamin D supplementation. *Horm. Res. Paediatr.* **2013**, *80*, 335–342. [CrossRef] [PubMed]
50. Javed, A.; Kullo, I.J.; Balagopal, P.B.; Kumar, S. Effect of vitamin D_3 treatment on endothelial function in obese adolescents. *Pediatr. Obes.* **2016**, *11*, 279–284. [CrossRef] [PubMed]
51. Ferira, A.J.; Laing, E.M.; Hausman, D.B.; Hall, D.B.; McCabe, G.P.; Martin, B.R.; Hill Gallant, K.M.; Warden, S.J.; Weaver, C.M.; Peacock, M.; et al. Vitamin D Supplementation Does Not Impact Insulin Resistance in Black and White Children. *J. Clin. Endocrinol. Metab.* **2016**, *101*, 1710–1718. [CrossRef] [PubMed]
52. Sethuraman, U.; Zidan, M.A.; Hanks, L.; Bagheri, M.; Ashraf, A. Impact of vitamin D treatment on 25 hydroxy vitamin D levels and insulin homeostasis in obese African American adolescents in a randomized trial. *J. Clin. Transl. Endocrinol.* **2018**, *12*, 13–19. [CrossRef] [PubMed]
53. Hernan, M.A.; Olek, M.J.; Ascherio, A. Geographic variation of MS incidence in two prospective studies of US women. *Neurology* **1999**, *53*, 1711–1718. [CrossRef] [PubMed]

54. Dalmay, F.; Bhalla, D.; Nicoletti, A.; Cabrera-Gomez, J.A.; Cabre, P.; Ruiz, F.; Druet-Cabanac, M.; Dumas, M.; Preux, P.M. Multiple sclerosis and solar exposure before the age of 15 years: Case-control study in Cuba, Martinique and Sicily. *Mult. Scler.* **2010**, *16*, 899–908. [CrossRef] [PubMed]
55. Islam, T.; Gauderman, W.J.; Cozen, W.; Mack, T.M. Childhood sun exposure influences risk of multiple sclerosis in monozygotic twins. *Neurology* **2007**, *69*, 381–388. [CrossRef] [PubMed]
56. Dwyer, T.; van der Mei, I.; Ponsonby, A.L.; Taylor, B.V.; Stankovich, J.; McKay, J.D.; Thomson, R.J.; Polanowski, A.M.; Dickinson, J.L. Melanocortin 1 receptor genotype, past environmental sun exposure, and risk of multiple sclerosis. *Neurology* **2008**, *71*, 583–589. [CrossRef] [PubMed]
57. van der Mei, I.A.; Ponsonby, A.L.; Dwyer, T.; Blizzard, L.; Simmons, R.; Taylor, B.V.; Butzkueven, H.; Kilpatrick, T. Past exposure to sun, skin phenotype, and risk of multiple sclerosis: Case-control study. *BMJ* **2003**, *327*, 316. [CrossRef]
58. Alonso, A.; Cook, S.D.; Maghzi, A.H.; Divani, A.A. a case-control study of risk factors for multiple sclerosis in Iran. *Mult. Scler.* **2011**, *17*, 550–555. [CrossRef]
59. Baarnhielm, M.; Hedstrom, A.K.; Kockum, I.; Sundqvist, E.; Gustafsson, S.A.; Hillert, J.; Olsson, T.; Alfredsson, L. Sunlight is associated with decreased multiple sclerosis risk: No interaction with human leukocyte antigen-DRB1*15. *Eur. J. Neurol.* **2012**, *19*, 955–962. [CrossRef]
60. Munger, K.L.; Zhang, S.M.; O'Reilly, E.; Hernan, M.A.; Olek, M.J.; Willett, W.C.; Ascherio, A. Vitamin D intake and incidence of multiple sclerosis. *Neurology* **2004**, *62*, 60–65. [CrossRef]
61. Munger, K.L.; Levin, L.I.; Hollis, B.W.; Howard, N.S.; Ascherio, A. Serum 25-hydroxyvitamin D levels and risk of multiple sclerosis. *JAMA* **2006**, *296*, 2832–2838. [CrossRef]
62. Kragt, J.; van Amerongen, B.; Killestein, J.; Dijkstra, C.; Uitdehaag, B.; Polman, C.; Lips, P. Higher levels of 25-hydroxyvitamin D are associated with a lower incidence of multiple sclerosis only in women. *Mult. Scler.* **2009**, *15*, 9–15. [CrossRef]
63. Shaygannejad, V.; Golabchi, K.; Haghighi, S.; Dehghan, H.; Moshayedi, A. a Comparative Study of 25 (OH) Vitamin D Serum Levels in Patients with Multiple Sclerosis and Control Group in Isfahan, Iran. *Int. J. Prev. Med.* **2010**, *1*, 195–201.
64. Soilu-Hanninen, M.; Airas, L.; Mononen, I.; Heikkila, A.; Viljanen, M.; Hanninen, A. 25-Hydroxyvitamin D levels in serum at the onset of multiple sclerosis. *Mult. Scler.* **2005**, *11*, 266–271. [CrossRef]
65. Graves, J.S.; Barcellos, L.F.; Krupp, L.; Belman, A.; Shao, X.; Quach, H.; Hart, J.; Chitnis, T.; Weinstock-Guttman, B.; Aaen, G.; et al. Vitamin D genes influence MS relapses in children. *Mult. Scler.* **2019**. [CrossRef]
66. Willer, C.J.; Dyment, D.A.; Sadovnick, A.D.; Rothwell, P.M.; Murray, T.J.; Ebers, G.C. Timing of birth and risk of multiple sclerosis: Population based study. *BMJ* **2005**, *330*, 120. [CrossRef]
67. Staples, J.; Ponsonby, A.L.; Lim, L. Low maternal exposure to ultraviolet radiation in pregnancy, month of birth, and risk of multiple sclerosis in offspring: Longitudinal analysis. *BMJ* **2010**, *340*, c1640.
68. Torkildsen, O.; Grytten, N.; Aarseth, J.; Myhr, K.M.; Kampman, M.T. Month of birth as a risk factor for multiple sclerosis: An update. *Acta Neurol. Scand. Suppl.* **2012**, *126*, 58–62. [CrossRef]
69. Disanto, G.; Morahan, J.M.; Ramagopalan, S.V. Multiple sclerosis: Risk factors and their interactions. *CNS Neurol. Disord. Drug Targets* **2012**, *11*, 545–555. [CrossRef]
70. Mirzaei, F.; Michels, K.B.; Munger, K.; O'Reilly, E.; Chitnis, T.; Forman, M.R.; Giovannucci, E.; Rosner, B.; Ascherio, A. Gestational vitamin D and the risk of multiple sclerosis in offspring. *Ann. Neurol.* **2011**, *70*, 30–40. [CrossRef]
71. McKay, K.A.; Jahanfar, S.; Duggan, T.; Tkachuk, S.; Tremlett, H. Factors associated with onset, relapses or progression in multiple sclerosis: A systematic review. *Neurotoxicology* **2016**, *61*, 189–212. [CrossRef]
72. McLaughlin, L.; Clarke, L.; Khalilidehkordi, E.; Butzkueven, H.; Taylor, B.; Broadley, S.A. Vitamin D for the treatment of multiple sclerosis: A meta-analysis. *J. Neurol.* **2018**, *265*, 2893–2905. [CrossRef]
73. Soilu-Hanninen, M.; Aivo, J.; Lindstrom, B.M.; Elovaara, I.; Sumelahti, M.L.; Farkkila, M.; Tienari, P.; Atula, S.; Sarasoja, T.; Herrala, L.; et al. a randomised, double blind, placebo controlled trial with vitamin D_3 as an add on treatment to interferon beta-1b in patients with multiple sclerosis. *J. Neurol. Neurosurg. Psychiatry* **2012**, *83*, 565–571. [CrossRef]
74. Lee, Y.H.; Bae, S.C. Vitamin D level in rheumatoid arthritis and its correlation with the disease activity: A meta-analysis. *Clin. Exp. Rheumatol.* **2016**, *34*, 827–833.
75. Son, K.M.; Song, S.H.; Lim, S.K.; Seo, Y.I.; Kim, H.A. Characteristics of patients with rheumatoid arthritis in clinical remission: The many aspects of DAS28 remission. *Clin. Exp. Rheumatol.* **2012**, *30*, 947–950.

76. Song, G.G.; Bae, S.C.; Lee, Y.H. Association between vitamin D intake and the risk of rheumatoid arthritis: A meta-analysis. *Clin. Rheumatol.* **2012**, *31*, 1733–1739. [CrossRef]
77. Lin, J.; Liu, J.; Davies, M.L.; Chen, W. Serum Vitamin D Level and Rheumatoid Arthritis Disease Activity: Review and Meta-Analysis. *PLoS ONE* **2016**, *11*, e0146351. [CrossRef]
78. Wang, Y.; Zhang, F.; Wang, S.; Shang, X.; Luo, S.; Zhou, H.; Shi, H.; Cai, L. Serum Vitamin D Level is Inversely Associated with Anti-Cyclic Citrullinated Peptide Antibody Level and Disease Activity in Rheumatoid Arthritis Patients. *Arch. Rheumatol.* **2016**, *31*, 64–70. [CrossRef]
79. Zakeri, Z.; Sandoughi, M.; Mashhadi, M.A.; Raeesi, V.; Shahbakhsh, S. Serum vitamin D level and disease activity in patients with recent onset rheumatoid arthritis. *Int. J. Rheum. Dis.* **2016**, *19*, 343–347. [CrossRef]
80. Tizaoui, K.; Hamzaoui, K. Association between VDR polymorphisms and rheumatoid arthritis disease: Systematic review and updated meta-analysis of case-control studies. *Immunobiology* **2015**, *220*, 807–816. [CrossRef]
81. Song, G.G.; Bae, S.C.; Lee, Y.H. Vitamin D receptor FokI, BsmI, and TaqI polymorphisms and susceptibility to rheumatoid arthritis: A meta-analysis. *Z. Rheumatol.* **2016**, *75*, 322–329. [CrossRef]
82. Merlino, L.A.; Curtis, J.; Mikuls, T.R.; Cerhan, J.R.; Criswell, L.A.; Saag, K.G. Vitamin D intake is inversely associated with rheumatoid arthritis: Results from the Iowa Women's Health Study. *Arthritis Rheum.* **2004**, *50*, 72–77. [CrossRef]
83. Chandrashekara, S.; Patted, A. Role of vitamin D supplementation in improving disease activity in rheumatoid arthritis: An exploratory study. *Int. J. Rheum. Dis.* **2015**, *20*, 825–831. [CrossRef]
84. Franco, A.S.; Freitas, T.Q.; Bernardo, W.M.; Pereira, R.M.R. Vitamin D supplementation and disease activity in patients with immune-mediated rheumatic diseases: A systematic review and meta-analysis. *Medicine* **2017**, *96*, e7024. [CrossRef] [PubMed]
85. Gardner, D.H.; Jeffery, L.E.; Soskic, B.; Briggs, Z.; Hou, T.Z.; Raza, K.; Sansom, D.M. 1,25(OH)$_2$D$_3$ Promotes the Efficacy of CD28 Costimulation Blockade by Abatacept. *J. Immunol.* **2015**, *195*, 2657–2665. [CrossRef]
86. Amital, H.; Szekanecz, Z.; Szucs, G.; Danko, K.; Nagy, E.; Csepany, T.; Kiss, E.; Rovensky, J.; Tuchynova, A.; Kozakova, D.; et al. Serum concentrations of 25-OH vitamin D in patients with systemic lupus erythematosus (SLE) are inversely related to disease activity: Is it time to routinely supplement patients with SLE with vitamin D? *Ann. Rheum. Dis.* **2010**, *69*, 1155–1157. [CrossRef]
87. Robinson, A.B.; Thierry-Palmer, M.; Gibson, K.L.; Rabinovich, C.E. Disease activity, proteinuria, and vitamin D status in children with systemic lupus erythematosus and juvenile dermatomyositis. *J. Pediatr.* **2012**, *160*, 297–302. [CrossRef]
88. Wright, T.B.; Shults, J.; Leonard, M.B.; Zemel, B.S.; Burnham, J.M. Hypovitaminosis D is associated with greater body mass index and disease activity in pediatric systemic lupus erythematosus. *J. Pediatr.* **2009**, *155*, 260–265. [CrossRef]
89. Kamen, D.; Aranow, C. Vitamin D in systemic lupus erythematosus. *Curr. Opin. Rheumatol.* **2008**, *20*, 532–537. [CrossRef]
90. AlSaleem, A.; AlE'ed, A.; AlSaghier, A.; Al-Mayouf, S.M. Vitamin D status in children with systemic lupus erythematosus and its association with clinical and laboratory parameters. *Clin. Rheumatol.* **2015**, *34*, 81–84. [CrossRef]
91. Borba, V.Z.; Vieira, J.G.; Kasamatsu, T.; Radominski, S.C.; Sato, E.I.; Lazaretti-Castro, M. Vitamin D deficiency in patients with active systemic lupus erythematosus. *Osteoporos. Int.* **2009**, *20*, 427–433. [CrossRef] [PubMed]
92. Schneider, L.; Dos Santos, A.S.; Santos, M.; da Silva Chakr, R.M.; Monticielo, O.A. Vitamin D and systemic lupus erythematosus: State of the art. *Clin. Rheumatol.* **2014**, *33*, 1033–1038. [CrossRef] [PubMed]
93. Lima, G.L.; Paupitz, J.; Aikawa, N.E.; Takayama, L.; Bonfa, E.; Pereira, R.M. Vitamin D Supplementation in Adolescents and Young Adults with Juvenile Systemic Lupus Erythematosus for Improvement in Disease Activity and Fatigue Scores: A Randomized, Double-Blind, Placebo-Controlled Trial. *Arthritis Care Res.* **2016**, *68*, 91–98. [CrossRef] [PubMed]
94. Abou-Raya, A.; Abou-Raya, S.; Helmii, M. The effect of vitamin D supplementation on inflammatory and hemostatic markers and disease activity in patients with systemic lupus erythematosus: A randomized placebo-controlled trial. *J. Rheumatol.* **2013**, *40*, 265–272. [CrossRef] [PubMed]

95. Terrier, B.; Derian, N.; Schoindre, Y.; Chaara, W.; Geri, G.; Zahr, N.; Mariampillai, K.; Rosenzwajg, M.; Carpentier, W.; Musset, L.; et al. Restoration of regulatory and effector T cell balance and B cell homeostasis in systemic lupus erythematosus patients through vitamin D supplementation. *Arthritis Res. Ther.* **2012**, *14*, R221. [CrossRef] [PubMed]
96. Shoenfeld, Y.; Giacomelli, R.; Azrielant, S.; Berardicurti, O.; Reynolds, J.A.; Bruce, I.N. Vitamin D and systemic lupus erythematosus—The hype and the hope. *Autoimmun. Rev.* **2018**, *17*, 19–23. [CrossRef] [PubMed]
97. Smith, E.L.; Walworth, N.C.; Holick, M.F. Effect of 1 alpha,25-dihydroxyvitamin D_3 on the morphologic and biochemical differentiation of cultured human epidermal keratinocytes grown in serum-free conditions. *J. Investig. Dermatol.* **1986**, *86*, 709–714. [CrossRef] [PubMed]
98. Smith, E.L.; Pincus, S.H.; Donovan, L.; Holick, M.F. a novel approach for the evaluation and treatment of psoriasis. Oral or topical use of 1,25-dihydroxyvitamin D_3 can be a safe and effective therapy for psoriasis. *J. Am. Acad. Dermatol.* **1988**, *19*, 516–528. [CrossRef]
99. Stefanic, M.; Rucevic, I.; Barisic-Drusko, V. Meta-analysis of vitamin D receptor polymorphisms and psoriasis risk. *Int. J. Dermatol.* **2013**, *52*, 705–710. [CrossRef]
100. Lee, Y.H. Vitamin D receptor ApaI, TaqI, BsmI, and FokI polymorphisms and psoriasis susceptibility: An updated meta-analysis. *Clin. Exp. Dermatol.* **2019**, *44*, 498–505. [CrossRef]
101. Saleky, S.; Bulur, I.; Saracoglu, Z.N. Narrowband UVB treatment increases serum 25-hydroxyvitamin D levels in patients with chronic plaque psoriasis. *Cutis* **2017**, *99*, 431–435. [PubMed]
102. Gupta, A.; Arora, T.C.; Jindal, A.; Bhadoria, A.S. Efficacy of narrowband ultraviolet B phototherapy and levels of serum vitamin D_3 in psoriasis: A prospective study. *Indian Dermatol. Online J.* **2016**, *7*, 87–92. [CrossRef] [PubMed]
103. Disphanurat, W.; Viarasilpa, W.; Chakkavittumrong, P.; Pongcharoen, P. The Clinical Effect of Oral Vitamin D_2 Supplementation on Psoriasis: A Double-Blind, Randomized, Placebo-Controlled Study. *Dermatol. Res. Pract.* **2019**, *2019*. [CrossRef] [PubMed]
104. Del Rosso, J.Q.; Kircik, L.H. The Effect of Calcipotriene-Betamethasone Dipropionate Aerosol Foam versus Vehicle on Target Lesions in Moderate Severity Plaque Psoriasis: Focus on Elbows and Knees. *J. Drugs Dermatol.* **2019**, *18*, 358–361. [PubMed]
105. German, B.; Wei, R.; Hener, P.; Martins, C.; Ye, T.; Gottwick, C.; Yang, J.; Seneschal, J.; Boniface, K.; Li, M. Disrupting the IL-36 and IL-23/IL-17 loop underlies the efficacy of calcipotriol and corticosteroid therapy for psoriasis. *JCI Insight.* **2019**, *4*. [CrossRef] [PubMed]
106. Hau, C.S.; Shimizu, T.; Tada, Y.; Kamata, M.; Takeoka, S.; Shibata, S.; Mitsui, A.; Asano, Y.; Sugaya, M.; Kadono, T.; et al. The vitamin D_3 analog, maxacalcitol, reduces psoriasiform skin inflammation by inducing regulatory T cells and downregulating IL-23 and IL-17 production. *J. Dermatol. Sci.* **2018**, *92*, 117–126. [CrossRef] [PubMed]
107. Cantorna, M.T.; Munsick, C.; Bemiss, C.; Mahon, B.D. 1,25-Dihydroxycholecalciferol prevents and ameliorates symptoms of experimental murine inflammatory bowel disease. *J. Nutr.* **2000**, *130*, 2648–2652. [CrossRef]
108. Bouillon, R.; Carmeliet, G.; Verlinden, L.; van Etten, E.; Verstuyf, A.; Luderer, H.F.; Lieben, L.; Mathieu, C.; Demay, M. Vitamin D and human health: Lessons from vitamin D receptor null mice. *Endocr. Rev.* **2008**, *29*, 726–776. [CrossRef]
109. Simmons, J.D.; Mullighan, C.; Welsh, K.I.; Jewell, D.P. Vitamin D receptor gene polymorphism: Association with Crohn's disease susceptibility. *Gut* **2000**, *47*, 211–214. [CrossRef]
110. Wang, L.; Wang, Z.T.; Hu, J.J.; Fan, R.; Zhou, J.; Zhong, J. Polymorphisms of the vitamin D receptor gene and the risk of inflammatory bowel disease: A meta-analysis. *Genet. Mol. Res.* **2014**, *13*, 2598–2610. [CrossRef]
111. Peyrin-Biroulet, L.; Oussalah, A.; Boucekkine, T.; Bigard, M.A. TNF antagonists in the treatment of inflammatory bowel disease: Results of a survey of gastroenterologists in the French region of Lorraine. *Gastroenterol. Clin. Biol.* **2009**, *33*, 23–30. [CrossRef] [PubMed]
112. Janssen, C.E.; Globig, A.M.; Busse Grawitz, A.; Bettinger, D.; Hasselblatt, P. Seasonal variability of vitamin D status in patients with inflammatory bowel disease—A retrospective cohort study. *PLoS ONE* **2019**, *14*, e0217238. [CrossRef] [PubMed]
113. Lu, C.; Yang, J.; Yu, W.; Li, D.; Xiang, Z.; Lin, Y.; Yu, C. Association between 25(OH)D Level, Ultraviolet Exposure, Geographical Location, and Inflammatory Bowel Disease Activity: A Systematic Review and Meta-Analysis. *PLoS ONE* **2015**, *10*, e0132036. [CrossRef] [PubMed]

114. Del Pinto, R.; Pietropaoli, D.; Chandar, A.K.; Ferri, C.; Cominelli, F. Association between Inflammatory Bowel Disease and Vitamin D Deficiency: A Systematic Review and Meta-analysis. *Inflamm. Bowel Dis.* **2015**, *21*, 2708–2717. [CrossRef] [PubMed]
115. Pappa, H.M.; Mitchell, P.D.; Jiang, H.; Kassiff, S.; Filip-Dhima, R.; DiFabio, D.; Quinn, N.; Lawton, R.C.; Bronzwaer, M.E.; Koenen, M.; et al. Maintenance of optimal vitamin D status in children and adolescents with inflammatory bowel disease: A randomized clinical trial comparing two regimens. *J. Clin. Endocrinol. Metab.* **2014**, *99*, 3408–3417. [CrossRef]
116. Schardey, J.; Globig, A.M.; Janssen, C.; Hofmann, M.; Manegold, P.; Thimme, R.; Hasselblatt, P. Vitamin D inhibits pro-inflammatory T cell function in patients with inflammatory bowel disease. *J. Crohn's Colitis* **2019**. [CrossRef] [PubMed]
117. Guo, H.; Zheng, Y.; Cai, X.; Yang, H.; Zhang, Y.; Hao, L.; Jin, Y.; Yang, G. Correlation between serum vitamin D status and immunological changes in children affected by gastrointestinal food allergy. *Allergol. Immunopathol.* **2018**, *46*, 39–44. [CrossRef]
118. Hennessy, A.; Hourihane, J.O.; Malvisi, L.; Irvine, A.D.; Kenny, L.C.; Murray, D.M.; Kiely, M.E. Antenatal vitamin D exposure and childhood eczema, food allergy, asthma and allergic rhinitis at 2 and 5 years of age in the atopic disease-specific Cork BASELINE Birth Cohort Study. *Allergy* **2018**, *73*, 2182–2191. [CrossRef]
119. Molloy, J.; Koplin, J.J.; Allen, K.J.; Tang, M.L.K.; Collier, F.; Carlin, J.B.; Saffery, R.; Burgner, D.; Ranganathan, S.; Dwyer, T.; et al. Vitamin D insufficiency in the first 6 months of infancy and challenge-proven IgE-mediated food allergy at 1 year of age: A case-cohort study. *Allergy* **2017**, *72*, 1222–1231. [CrossRef]
120. Willits, E.K.; Wang, Z.; Jin, J.; Patel, B.; Motosue, M.; Bhagia, A.; Almasri, J.; Erwin, P.J.; Kumar, S.; Joshi, A.Y. Vitamin D and food allergies in children: A systematic review and meta-analysis. *Allergy Asthma Proc.* **2017**, *38*, 21–28. [CrossRef]
121. Peroni, D.G.; Boner, A.L. Food allergy: The perspectives of prevention using vitamin, D. *Curr. Opin. Allergy Clin. Immunol.* **2013**, *13*, 287–292. [CrossRef] [PubMed]
122. Rosendahl, J.; Pelkonen, A.S.; Helve, O.; Hauta-Alus, H.; Holmlund-Suila, E.; Valkama, S.; Enlund-Cerullo, M.; Viljakainen, H.; Hytinantti, T.; Makitie, O.; et al. High-Dose Vitamin D Supplementation Does Not Prevent Allergic Sensitization of Infants. *J. Pediatr.* **2019**, *209*, 139–145.e1. [CrossRef] [PubMed]
123. Suneetha, P.V.; Sarin, S.K.; Goyal, A.; Kumar, G.T.; Shukla, D.K.; Hissar, S. Association between vitamin D receptor, CCR5, TNF-alpha and TNF-beta gene polymorphisms and HBV infection and severity of liver disease. *J. Hepatol.* **2006**, *44*, 856–863. [CrossRef] [PubMed]
124. Nosratabadi, R.; Arababadi, M.K.; Salehabad, V.A.; Shamsizadeh, A.; Mahmoodi, M.; Sayadi, A.R.; Kennedy, D. Polymorphisms within exon 9 but not intron 8 of the vitamin D receptor are associated with the nephropathic complication of type-2 diabetes. *Int. J. Immunogenet.* **2010**, *37*, 493–497. [CrossRef] [PubMed]
125. Hu, Y.C.; Wang, W.W.; Jiang, W.Y.; Li, C.Q.; Guo, J.C.; Xun, Y.H. Low vitamin D levels are associated with high viral loads in patients with chronic hepatitis B: A systematic review and meta-analysis. *BMC Gastroenterol.* **2019**, *19*, 84. [CrossRef] [PubMed]
126. Petta, S.; Camma, C.; Scazzone, C.; Tripodo, C.; Di Marco, V.; Bono, A.; Cabibi, D.; Licata, G.; Porcasi, R.; Marchesini, G.; et al. Low vitamin D serum level is related to severe fibrosis and low responsiveness to interferon-based therapy in genotype 1 chronic hepatitis, C. *Hepatology* **2010**, *51*, 1158–1167. [CrossRef]
127. Barooah, P.; Saikia, S.; Bharadwaj, R.; Sarmah, P.; Bhattacharyya, M.; Goswami, B.; Medhi, S. Role of VDR, GC, and CYP2R1 Polymorphisms in the Development of Hepatocellular Carcinoma in Hepatitis C Virus-Infected Patients. *Genet. Test. Mol. Biomark.* **2019**, *23*, 325–331. [CrossRef]
128. Murayama, A.; Saitoh, H.; Takeuchi, A.; Yamada, N.; Matsumura, T.; Shiina, M.; Muramatsu, M.; Wakita, T.; Imawari, M.; Kato, T. Vitamin D derivatives inhibit hepatitis C virus production through the suppression of apolipoprotein. *Antivir. Res.* **2018**, *160*, 55–63. [CrossRef]
129. Bitetto, D.; Fabris, C.; Fornasiere, E.; Pipan, C.; Fumolo, E.; Cussigh, A.; Bignulin, S.; Cmet, S.; Fontanini, E.; Falleti, E.; et al. Vitamin D supplementation improves response to antiviral treatment for recurrent hepatitis C. *Transpl. Int.* **2011**, *24*, 43–50. [CrossRef]
130. Komolmit, P.; Kimtrakool, S.; Suksawatamnuay, S.; Thanapirom, K.; Chattrasophon, K.; Thaimai, P.; Chirathaworn, C.; Poovorawan, Y. Vitamin D supplementation improves serum markers associated with hepatic fibrogenesis in chronic hepatitis C patients: A randomized, double-blind, placebo-controlled study. *Sci. Rep.* **2017**, *7*, 8905. [CrossRef]

131. Hall, S.C.; Agrawal, D.K. Vitamin D and Bronchial Asthma: An Overview of Data from the Past 5 Years. *Clin. Ther.* **2017**, *39*, 917–929. [CrossRef]
132. Reinehr, T.; Schnabel, D.; Wabitsch, M.; Bechtold-Dalla Pozza, S.; Buhrer, C.; Heidtmann, B.; Jochum, F.; Kauth, T.; Korner, A.; Mihatsch, W.; et al. Vitamin D supplementation after the second year of life: Joint position of the Committee on Nutrition, German Society for Pediatric and Adolescent Medicine (DGKJ e.V.), and the German Society for Pediatric Endocrinology and Diabetology (DGKED e.V.). *Mol. Cell. Pediatr.* **2019**, *6*, 3. [CrossRef] [PubMed]
133. Jolliffe, D.A.; Greenberg, L.; Hooper, R.L.; Griffiths, C.J.; Camargo, C.A., Jr.; Kerley, C.P.; Jensen, M.E.; Mauger, D.; Stelmach, I.; Urashima, M.; et al. Vitamin D supplementation to prevent asthma exacerbations: A systematic review and meta-analysis of individual participant data. *Lancet Respir. Med.* **2017**, *5*, 881–890. [CrossRef]
134. Martineau, A.R.; Cates, C.J.; Urashima, M.; Jensen, M.; Griffiths, A.P.; Nurmatov, U.; Sheikh, A.; Griffiths, C.J. Vitamin D for the management of asthma. *Cochrane Database Syst. Rev.* **2016**, *9*, CD011511. [CrossRef] [PubMed]
135. Urashima, M.; Segawa, T.; Okazaki, M.; Kurihara, M.; Wada, Y.; Ida, H. Randomized trial of vitamin D supplementation to prevent seasonal influenza a in schoolchildren. *Am. J. Clin. Nutr.* **2010**, *91*, 1255–1260. [CrossRef] [PubMed]
136. Urashima, M.; Mezawa, H.; Noya, M.; Camargo, C.A., Jr. Effects of vitamin D supplements on influenza a illness during the 2009 H1N1 pandemic: A randomized controlled trial. *Food Funct.* **2014**, *5*, 2365–2370. [CrossRef] [PubMed]
137. Martineau, A.R.; Jolliffe, D.A.; Hooper, R.L.; Greenberg, L.; Aloia, J.F.; Bergman, P.; Dubnov-Raz, G.; Esposito, S.; Ganmaa, D.; Ginde, A.A.; et al. Vitamin D supplementation to prevent acute respiratory tract infections: Systematic review and meta-analysis of individual participant data. *BMJ* **2017**, *356*, i6583. [CrossRef] [PubMed]
138. Martineau, A.R.; Jolliffe, D.A.; Greenberg, L.; Aloia, J.F.; Bergman, P.; Dubnov-Raz, G.; Esposito, S.; Ganmaa, D.; Ginde, A.A.; Goodall, E.C.; et al. Vitamin D supplementation to prevent acute respiratory infections: Individual participant data meta-analysis. *Health Technol. Assess.* **2019**, *23*, 1–44. [CrossRef] [PubMed]
139. Yakoob, M.Y.; Salam, R.A.; Khan, F.R.; Bhutta, Z.A. Vitamin D supplementation for preventing infections in children under five years of age. *Cochrane Database Syst. Rev.* **2016**, *11*, CD008824. [CrossRef]
140. Aglipay, M.; Birken, C.S.; Parkin, P.C.; Loeb, M.B.; Thorpe, K.; Chen, Y.; Laupacis, A.; Mamdani, M.; Macarthur, C.; Hoch, J.S.; et al. Effect of High-Dose vs Standard-Dose Wintertime Vitamin D Supplementation on Viral Upper Respiratory Tract Infections in Young Healthy Children. *JAMA* **2017**, *318*, 245–254. [CrossRef]
141. Correa-Rodriguez, M.; Carrillo-Avila, J.A.; Schmidt-RioValle, J.; Gonzalez-Jimenez, E.; Vargas, S.; Martin, J.; Rueda-Medina, B. Genetic association analysis of vitamin D receptor gene polymorphisms and obesity-related phenotypes. *Gene* **2018**, *640*, 51–56. [CrossRef]
142. Olson, M.L.; Maalouf, N.M.; Oden, J.D.; White, P.C.; Hutchison, M.R. Vitamin D deficiency in obese children and its relationship to glucose homeostasis. *J. Clin. Endocrinol. Metab.* **2012**, *97*, 279–285. [CrossRef]
143. Smotkin-Tangorra, M.; Purushothaman, R.; Gupta, A.; Nejati, G.; Anhalt, H.; Ten, S. Prevalence of vitamin D insufficiency in obese children and adolescents. *J. Pediatr. Endocrinol. Metab.* **2007**, *20*, 817–823. [CrossRef] [PubMed]
144. Nsiah-Kumi, P.A.; Erickson, J.M.; Beals, J.L.; Ogle, E.A.; Whiting, M.; Brushbreaker, C.; Borgeson, C.D.; Qiu, F.; Yu, F.; Larsen, J.L. Vitamin D insufficiency is associated with diabetes risk in Native American children. *Clin. Pediatr.* **2012**, *51*, 146–153. [CrossRef] [PubMed]
145. Roth, C.L.; Elfers, C.; Kratz, M.; Hoofnagle, A.N. Vitamin d deficiency in obese children and its relationship to insulin resistance and adipokines. *J. Obes.* **2011**, *2011*, 495101. [CrossRef] [PubMed]
146. Poomthavorn, P.; Saowan, S.; Mahachoklertwattana, P.; Chailurkit, L.; Khlairit, P. Vitamin D status and glucose homeostasis in obese children and adolescents living in the tropics. *Int. J. Obes.* **2012**, *36*, 491–495. [CrossRef] [PubMed]
147. Bril, F.; Maximos, M.; Portillo-Sanchez, P.; Biernacki, D.; Lomonaco, R.; Subbarayan, S.; Correa, M.; Lo, M.; Suman, A.; Cusi, K. Relationship of vitamin D with insulin resistance and disease severity in non-alcoholic steatohepatitis. *J. Hepatol.* **2015**, *62*, 405–411. [CrossRef]

148. Liu, D.; Fernandez, B.O.; Hamilton, A.; Lang, N.N.; Gallagher, J.M.C.; Newby, D.E.; Feelisch, M.; Weller, R.B. UVA irradiation of human skin vasodilates arterial vasculature and lowers blood pressure independently of nitric oxide synthase. *J. Investig. Dermatol.* **2014**, *134*, 1839–1846. [CrossRef]
149. Tangpricha, V.; Flanagan, J.N.; Whitlatch, L.W.; Tseng, C.C.; Chen, T.C.; Holt, P.R.; Lipkin, M.S.; Holick, M.F. 25-hydroxyvitamin D-1alpha-hydroxylase in normal and malignant colon tissue. *Lancet* **2001**, *357*, 1673–1674. [CrossRef]
150. Mawer, E.B.; Hayes, M.E.; Heys, S.E.; Davies, M.; White, A.; Stewart, M.F.; Smith, G.N. Constitutive synthesis of 1,25-dihydroxyvitamin D_3 by a human small cell lung cancer cell line. *J. Clin. Endocrinol. Metab.* **1994**, *79*, 554–560. [PubMed]
151. Cross, H.S.; Bareis, P.; Hofer, H.; Bischof, M.G.; Bajna, E.; Kriwanek, S.; Bonner, E.; Peterlik, M. 25-Hydroxyvitamin D(3)-1alpha-hydroxylase and vitamin D receptor gene expression in human colonic mucosa is elevated during early cancerogenesis. *Steroids* **2001**, *66*, 287–292. [CrossRef]
152. Fouda, A.; Kandil, S.; Boujettif, K.; Fayea, N. Hypovitamininosis D in Childhood Cancer Survivors: Importance of Vitamin D Supplementation and Measurement Over Different Points of Time. *J. Pediatr. Hematol. Oncol.* **2018**, *40*, e83–e90. [CrossRef] [PubMed]
153. Demirsoy, U.; Sarper, N.; Aylan Gelen, S.; Zengin, E.; Kum, T.; Demir, H. The Association of Oral Vitamin D and Calcium Supplementation with Bone Mineral Density in Pediatric Acute Lymphoblastic Leukemia Patients. *J. Pediatr. Hematol. Oncol.* **2017**, *39*, 287–292. [CrossRef] [PubMed]
154. Genc, D.B.; Vural, S.; Yagar, G. The Incidence of and Factors Associated with Vitamin D Deficiency in Newly Diagnosed Children with Cancer. *Nutr. Cancer* **2016**, *68*, 756–761. [CrossRef] [PubMed]
155. Williams, J.D.; Aggarwal, A.; Swami, S.; Krishnan, A.V.; Ji, L.; Albertelli, M.A.; Feldman, B.J. Tumor Autonomous Effects of Vitamin D Deficiency Promote Breast Cancer Metastasis. *Endocrinology* **2016**, *157*, 1341–1347. [CrossRef] [PubMed]
156. Grant, W.B. An ecologic study of dietary and solar ultraviolet-B links to breast carcinoma mortality rates. *Cancer* **2002**, *94*, 272–281. [CrossRef] [PubMed]
157. Bodiwala, D.; Luscombe, C.J.; French, M.E.; Liu, S.; Saxby, M.F.; Jones, P.W.; Ramachandran, S.; Fryer, A.A.; Strange, R.C. Susceptibility to prostate cancer: Studies on interactions between UVR exposure and skin type. *Carcinogenesis* **2003**, *24*, 711–717. [CrossRef] [PubMed]
158. Pritchard, R.S.; Baron, J.A.; de Verdier, M.G. Dietary calcium, vitamin, D.; and the risk of colorectal cancer in Stockholm, Sweden. *Cancer Epidemiol. Biomark. Prev.* **1996**, *5*, 897–900.
159. Gandini, S.; Gnagnarella, P.; Serrano, D.; Pasquali, E.; Raimondi, S. Vitamin D receptor polymorphisms and cancer. *Adv. Exp. Med. Biol.* **2014**, *810*, 69–105.
160. Kazemian, E.; Akbari, M.E.; Moradi, N.; Gharibzadeh, S.; Mondul, A.M.; Jamshidi-Naeini, Y.; Khademolmele, M.; Zarins, K.R.; Ghodoosi, N.; Amouzegar, A.; et al. Vitamin D Receptor Genetic Variation and Cancer Biomarkers among Breast Cancer Patients Supplemented with Vitamin D_3: A Single-Arm Non-Randomized Before and After Trial. *Nutrients* **2019**, *11*, 1264. [CrossRef]
161. Jacobs, E.T.; Kohler, L.N.; Kunihiro, A.G.; Jurutka, P.W. Vitamin D and Colorectal, Breast, and Prostate Cancers: A Review of the Epidemiological Evidence. *J. Cancer* **2016**, *7*, 232–240. [CrossRef] [PubMed]
162. Yin, L.; Grandi, N.; Raum, E.; Haug, U.; Arndt, V.; Brenner, H. Meta-analysis: Serum vitamin D and breast cancer risk. *Eur. J. Cancer* **2010**, *46*, 2196–2205. [CrossRef] [PubMed]
163. Kim, Y.; Je, Y. Vitamin D intake, blood 25(OH)D levels, and breast cancer risk or mortality: A meta-analysis. *Br. J. Cancer* **2014**, *110*, 2772–2784. [CrossRef] [PubMed]
164. Gandini, S.; Boniol, M.; Haukka, J.; Byrnes, G.; Cox, B.; Sneyd, M.J.; Mullie, P.; Autier, P. Meta-analysis of observational studies of serum 25-hydroxyvitamin D levels and colorectal, breast and prostate cancer and colorectal adenoma. *Int. J. Cancer* **2011**, *128*, 1414–1424. [CrossRef] [PubMed]
165. Deschasaux, M.; Souberbielle, J.C.; Latino-Martel, P.; Sutton, A.; Charnaux, N.; Druesne-Pecollo, N.; Galan, P.; Hercberg, S.; Le Clerc, S.; Kesse-Guyot, E.; et al. Weight Status and Alcohol Intake Modify the Association between Vitamin D and Breast Cancer Risk. *J. Nutr.* **2016**, *146*, 576–585. [CrossRef]
166. Chlebowski, R.T.; Johnson, K.C.; Kooperberg, C.; Pettinger, M.; Wactawski-Wende, J.; Rohan, T.; Rossouw, J.; Lane, D.; O'Sullivan, M.J.; Yasmeen, S.; et al. Calcium plus vitamin D supplementation and the risk of breast cancer. *J. Natl. Cancer Inst.* **2008**, *100*, 1581–1591. [CrossRef]

167. Cadeau, C.; Fournier, A.; Mesrine, S.; Clavel-Chapelon, F.; Fagherazzi, G.; Boutron-Ruault, M.C. Interaction between current vitamin D supplementation and menopausal hormone therapy use on breast cancer risk: Evidence from the E3N cohort. *Am. J. Clin. Nutr.* **2015**, *102*, 966–973. [CrossRef]
168. Madden, J.M.; Murphy, L.; Zgaga, L.; Bennett, K. De novo vitamin D supplement use post-diagnosis is associated with breast cancer survival. *Breast Cancer Res. Treat.* **2018**, *172*, 179–190. [CrossRef]
169. Crew, K.D.; Anderson, G.L.; Hershman, D.L.; Terry, M.B.; Tehranifar, P.; Lew, D.L.; Yee, M.; Brown, E.A.; Kairouz, S.S.; Kuwajerwala, N.; et al. Randomized Double-Blind Placebo-Controlled Biomarker Modulation Study of Vitamin D in Premenopausal Women at High Risk for Breast Cancer (SWOG S0812). *Cancer Prev. Res.* **2019**. [CrossRef]
170. Manson, J.E.; Cook, N.R.; Lee, I.M.; Christen, W.; Bassuk, S.S.; Mora, S.; Gibson, H.; Gordon, D.; Copeland, T.; D'Agostino, D.; et al. Vitamin D Supplements and Prevention of Cancer and Cardiovascular Disease. *N. Engl. J. Med.* **2019**, *380*, 33–44. [CrossRef]
171. Yin, L.; Grandi, N.; Raum, E.; Haug, U.; Arndt, V.; Brenner, H. Meta-analysis: Serum vitamin D and colorectal adenoma risk. *Prev. Med.* **2011**, *53*, 10–16. [CrossRef] [PubMed]
172. Wei, M.Y.; Garland, C.F.; Gorham, E.D.; Mohr, S.B.; Giovannucci, E. Vitamin D and prevention of colorectal adenoma: A meta-analysis. *Cancer Epidemiol. Biomark. Prev.* **2008**, *17*, 2958–2969. [CrossRef] [PubMed]
173. Jacobs, E.T.; Hibler, E.A.; Lance, P.; Sardo, C.L.; Jurutka, P.W. Association between circulating concentrations of 25(OH)D and colorectal adenoma: A pooled analysis. *Int. J. Cancer* **2013**, *133*, 2980–2988. [CrossRef] [PubMed]
174. Garland, C.F.; Gorham, E.D. Dose-response of serum 25-hydroxyvitamin D in association with risk of colorectal cancer: A meta-analysis. *J. Steroid Biochem. Mol. Biol.* **2017**, *168*, 1–8. [CrossRef] [PubMed]
175. Ma, Y.; Zhang, P.; Wang, F.; Yang, J.; Liu, Z.; Qin, H. Association between vitamin D and risk of colorectal cancer: A systematic review of prospective studies. *J. Clin. Oncol.* **2011**, *29*, 3775–3782. [CrossRef] [PubMed]
176. Sheng, S.; Chen, Y.; Shen, Z. Correlation between polymorphism of vitamin D receptor TaqI and susceptibility to colorectal cancer: A meta-analysis. *Medicine* **2017**, *96*, e7242. [CrossRef] [PubMed]
177. He, Y.; Timofeeva, M.; Farrington, S.M.; Vaughan-Shaw, P.; Svinti, V.; Walker, M.; Zgaga, L.; Meng, X.; Li, X.; Spiliopoulou, A.; et al. Exploring causality in the association between circulating 25-hydroxyvitamin D and colorectal cancer risk: A large Mendelian randomisation study. *BMC Med.* **2018**, *16*, 142. [CrossRef]
178. Grau, M.V.; Baron, J.A.; Sandler, R.S.; Haile, R.W.; Beach, M.L.; Church, T.R.; Heber, D. Vitamin D calcium supplementation, and colorectal adenomas: Results of a randomized trial. *J. Natl. Cancer Inst.* **2003**, *95*, 1765–1771. [CrossRef]
179. Gao, Y.; Um, C.Y.; Fedirko, V.; Rutherford, R.E.; Seabrook, M.E.; Barry, E.L.; Baron, J.A.; Bostick, R.M. Effects of supplemental vitamin D and calcium on markers of proliferation, differentiation, and apoptosis in the normal colorectal mucosa of colorectal adenoma patients. *PLoS ONE* **2018**, *13*, e0208762. [CrossRef]
180. Horvath, H.C.; Lakatos, P.; Kosa, J.P.; Bacsi, K.; Borka, K.; Bises, G.; Nittke, T.; Hershberger, P.A.; Speer, G.; Kallay, E. The candidate oncogene CYP24A1: A potential biomarker for colorectal tumorigenesis. *J. Histochem. Cytochem.* **2010**, *58*, 277–285. [CrossRef]
181. Wactawski-Wende, J.; Kotchen, J.M.; Anderson, G.L.; Assaf, A.R.; Brunner, R.L.; O'Sullivan, M.J.; Margolis, K.L.; Ockene, J.K.; Phillips, L.; Pottern, L.; et al. Calcium plus vitamin D supplementation and the risk of colorectal cancer. *N. Engl. J. Med.* **2006**, *354*, 684–696. [CrossRef] [PubMed]
182. Autier, P.; Mullie, P.; Macacu, A.; Dragomir, M.; Boniol, M.; Coppens, K.; Pizot, C. Effect of vitamin D supplementation on non-skeletal disorders: A systematic review of meta-analyses and randomised trials. *Lancet Diabetes Endocrinol.* **2017**, *5*, 986–1004. [CrossRef]
183. Calderwood, A.H.; Baron, J.A.; Mott, L.A.; Ahnen, D.J.; Bostick, R.M.; Figueiredo, J.C.; Passarelli, M.N.; Rees, J.R.; Robertson, D.J.; Barry, E.L. No Evidence for Posttreatment Effects of Vitamin D and Calcium Supplementation on Risk of Colorectal Adenomas in a Randomized Trial. *Cancer Prev. Res.* **2019**, *12*, 295–304. [CrossRef] [PubMed]
184. Baron, J.A.; Barry, E.L.; Ivanova, A. Calcium and Vitamin D for the Prevention of Colorectal Adenomas. *N. Engl. J. Med.* **2016**, *374*, 791–792. [CrossRef] [PubMed]
185. Urashima, M.; Ohdaira, H.; Akutsu, T.; Okada, S.; Yoshida, M.; Kitajima, M.; Suzuki, Y. Effect of Vitamin D Supplementation on Relapse-Free Survival among Patients with Digestive Tract Cancers: The AMATERASU Randomized Clinical Trial. *JAMA* **2019**, *321*, 1361–1369. [CrossRef] [PubMed]

186. Ng, K.; Nimeiri, H.S.; McCleary, N.J.; Abrams, T.A.; Yurgelun, M.B.; Cleary, J.M.; Rubinson, D.A.; Schrag, D.; Miksad, R.; Bullock, A.J.; et al. Effect of High-Dose vs Standard-Dose Vitamin D_3 Supplementation on Progression-Free Survival among Patients with Advanced or Metastatic Colorectal Cancer: The SUNSHINE Randomized Clinical Trial. *JAMA* **2019**, *321*, 1370–1379. [CrossRef] [PubMed]
187. Tuohimaa, P.; Tenkanen, L.; Ahonen, M.; Lumme, S.; Jellum, E.; Hallmans, G.; Stattin, P.; Harvei, S.; Hakulinen, T.; Luostarinen, T.; et al. Both high and low levels of blood vitamin D are associated with a higher prostate cancer risk: A longitudinal, nested case-control study in the Nordic countries. *Int. J. Cancer* **2004**, *108*, 104–108. [CrossRef] [PubMed]
188. Petrou, S.; Mamais, I.; Lavranos, G.; Tzanetakou, P.T.; Chrysostomou, S. Effect of Vitamin D Supplementation in Prostate Cancer: A Systematic Review of Randomized Control Trials. *Int. J. Vitam. Nutr. Res.* **2018**, *88*, 100–112. [CrossRef] [PubMed]

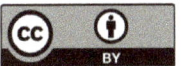

© 2019 by the authors. Licensee MDPI, Basel, Switzerland. This article is an open access article distributed under the terms and conditions of the Creative Commons Attribution (CC BY) license (http://creativecommons.org/licenses/by/4.0/).

MDPI
St. Alban-Anlage 66
4052 Basel
Switzerland
Tel. +41 61 683 77 34
Fax +41 61 302 89 18
www.mdpi.com

Nutrients Editorial Office
E-mail: nutrients@mdpi.com
www.mdpi.com/journal/nutrients